Textbook of
INDUSTRIAL
PHARMACOGNOSY

Textbook of INDUSTRIAL PHARMACOGNOSY

Prof. (Dr.) A.N. KALIA Ph.D.
Prof. & Head, Deptt. of Pharmacognosy,
I.S.F. College of Pharmacy, Moga (Punjab)
Former Prof. & Head, Deptt. of Pharmaceutical Sciences,
M.D. University, Rohtak (Haryana)

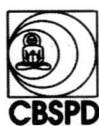

CBSPD

CBS Publishers & Distributors Pvt Ltd

New Delhi • Bengaluru • Chennai • Kochi • Kolkata • Lucknow • Mumbai
Gujarat • Hyderabad • Jharkhand • Nagpur • Patna • Pune • Uttarakhand

**Textbook of Industrial
Pharmacognosy**

ISBN: 81-239-1209-9 (PB)
ISBN: 81-239-1240-4 (HB)

Copyright © Publisher

First Edition: 2005
   Reprint: 2005, 2007, 2008, 2009, 2010, 2011, 2012, 2015, 2017, 2018, 2019, 2020, 2023, 2025, **2026**

Published by **Satish Kumar** Jain and Produced by **Varun Jain** for

CBS Publishers & Distributors Pvt Ltd
4819/XI Prahlad Street, 24 Ansari Road, Daryaganj, New Delhi 110 002, India.

Ph: 011-23289259, 23266361, 23266867   Fax: 011-23243014   Website: www.cbspd.com
                                                             e-mail: delhi@cbspd.com; cbspubs@airtelmail.in.
Corporate Office: 204 FIE, Industrial Area, Patparganj, Delhi 110 092, India
Ph: 011-4934 4934   Fax: 011-4934 4935   e-mail: publishing@cbspd.com; publicity@cbspd.com

Branches

* **Bengaluru:** Seema House 2975, 17th Cross, KR Road, Banasankari 2nd Stage, Bengaluru 560 070, Karnataka, India
  Ph: +91-80-26771678/79   Fax: +91-80-26771680   e-mail: bangalore@cbspd.com
* **Chennai:** 18/8B, Subbaraya Street, Shenoy Nagar, Chennai 600 030, Tamil Nadu, India
  Ph: +91-044-42032115, 044-2681266   e-mail: chennai@cbspd.com
* **Kochi:** 42/1325, 1326, Power House Road, Opp KSEB, Power House, Ernakulum Kochi 682 018, Kerala, India
  Ph: +91-484-4059061-65, 67   Fax: +91-484-4059065   e-mail: kochi@cbspd.com
* **Kolkata:** 147, Hind Ceramics Compound, 1st Floor, Nilgunj Road, Belghoria, Kolkata-700056, West Bengal, India
  Ph: +033-25633055, 033-25633056   e-mail: kolkata@cbspd.com
* **Lucknow:** Basement, Khushnuma Complex, 7 Meerabai Marg (Behind Jawahar Bhawan), Lucknow-226001, UP, India
  Ph: +0522-4000032   e-mail: tiwari.lucknow@cbspd.com
* **Mumbai:** PWD Shed, Gala no 25/26, Ramchandra Bhatt Marg, Next to JJ Hospital Gate no. 2, Opp. Union Bank of India, Noorbaug, Mumbai-400009, Maharashtra, India
  Ph: 022-66661880/89
                                      e-mail: mumbai@cbspd.com

Representatives

* Gujarat   0-9879558667   * Hyderabad   0-98851,   * Jharkhand   0-9811541605
* Nagpur   0-8692091830   * Patna   0-933415 ₃   * Pune   0-9664372571
* Uttarakhand   0-9716462459

Printed at   SRK Graphics, Delhi (India)

It is dedicated to the fond memory of my better half,
Mrs. Swaraj Kalia

Preface

The course content of Pharmacognosy VI (Semester VIII) prescribed by AICTE, for B. Pharmacy is of multidisciplinary characters. It is industry, health and commerce orientated; no single book can meet the needs of the prescribed syllabus. Often teachers of Pharmacognosy, experience difficulties in providing requisite material as the books available on the subject partially meet the requirement of the course contents, hence there was a great demand for a consolidated text book on the subject covering diverse nature of topics. It was therefore aimed to compile-up the information collected from different sources in one place in the form of text book in Applied & Industrial Pharmacognosy.

I hope this book will fulfill the demands of undergraduates and be equally informative & beneficial to post-graduate students of pharmacognosy and those who desire to establish herbal based drug industry.

The book comprises following twelve chapters: (i) Role of medicinal plants in national economy, (ii) Worldwide trade in medicinal plants and derived products with special reference to Liquorice, Ginseng, Diosgenin, Plant containing laxative, Rauwolfia, Digitalis, Podophyllum, Cinchona, Tropane alkaloids, Papain, Valerian and Ipecac, (iii) Indian trade in medicinal and aromatic plants, (iv) Plants based Industry & Institutions involved in work on medicinal plants with special reference to Cinchona, Opium (poppy), Ergot, Digitalis, Ispaghula, Dioscorea, Vinca, Aloe, Ipecac, Senna, Tropane alkaloids and Solanum Khasianum, (v) Utilization of aromatic plants and their derived products, (vi) Plant tissue culture & its application in Pharmacognosy. (vii) Chemotaxonomy of medicinal plants, (viii) Marine Pharmacognosy, (ix) Natural allergens & allergenic extracts, (x) Photosensitizing agents, (xi) Herbs used as food, (xiii) Herbs used as Cosmetics.

In order to limit the size of the book, the text has been kept brief, to the point (relevant to the topic) easily understood and lot of information has been incorporated in form of tables, schematic diagrams and important chemical structures. The information cited in this book are procured from scientific periodicals, Websites of Govt. agencies, WHO, Current Sciences, Economic Times, UNCTAD/WTO, Market News Services as well as from the books of various authors cited in the reference keeping in mind the academic interest of the students. Inspite of my best efforts the book is bound to have deficiencies, I will be grateful if readers kindly make reference for those and send their valuable suggestions to the author to improve the utility of the book.

A.N. Kalia

Acknowledgement

In the completion of this text book, I am highly grateful to Almighty for the spirit, inspiration & stamina to write this text.

In writing this book, I would like to acknowledge the valuable help received from Dr. Karan Vasisht, Reader, Institute of Pharmaceutical Sciences, Panjab University, Chandigarh for providing special information on Worldwide trade in medicinal plants. I also acknowledge the help of Dr. P.K. Jaiwal, Reader Biosciences Dept., Maharshi Dayanand University, Rohtak for graciously accepting to review the chapter of Tissue Culture and make extensive useful observations and suggestions.

I am obliged to Prof. A.K. Madan, Dean and Head, Faculty of Pharmaceutical Sciences, Maharshi Dayanand University, Rohtak for his nice cooperation, Dr. Arun Nanda, Reader, Pharmaceutics, Maharshi Dayanand University, for valuable suggestions and my other fellow colleagues for their support in the completion of this book.

While writing this book I had to consult number of books and journals. It is difficult to mention about all those authors and publishers. I acknowledge all of them with gratitude.

I am highly obliged to my daughter Dr. Vandana Kalia, Scientist, Ranbaxy Research Lab., Gurgaon, for her continuous support throughout the progress of this book by going through the text of each and every chapter.

In the last but not the least I would like to thank M/s CBS Publishers & Distributors, New Delhi for their keen interest and cooperation in publishing this Book of Applied and Industrial Pharmacognosy.

A.N. Kalia

Contents

CHAPTER 12   HERBS AND HERBAL PRODUCTS AS COSMETICS 240–271

Plate 1

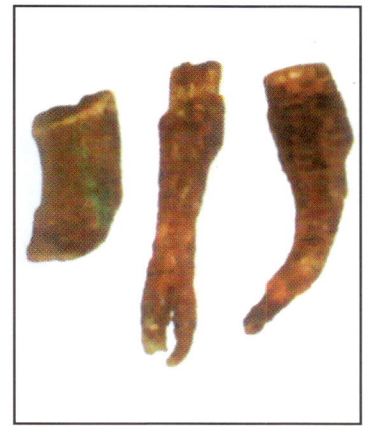

RHUBARB *(Rheum officinale)*

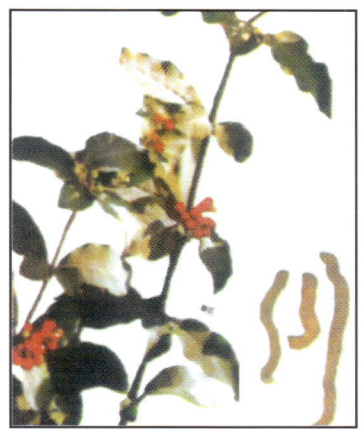

RAUWOLFIA *(R. serpentina)*

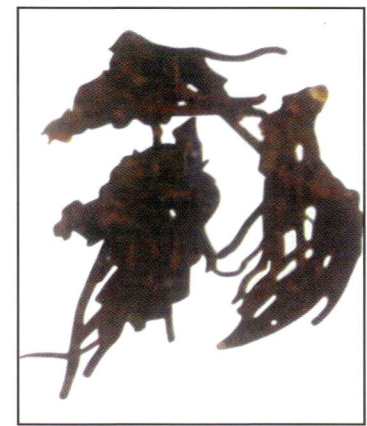

PODOPHYLLUM *(P. hexandrum)*

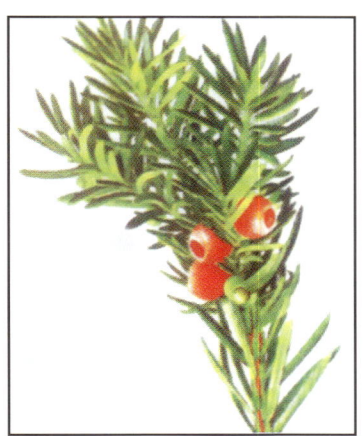

TAXUS *(Taxus wallichiana)*

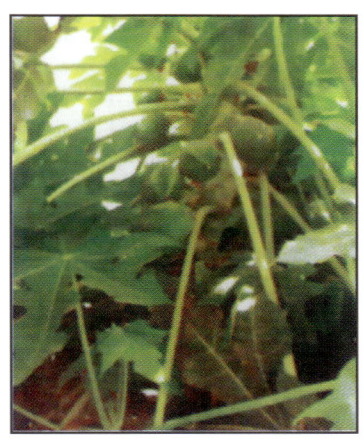

PAPAIN *(Carica papaya)*

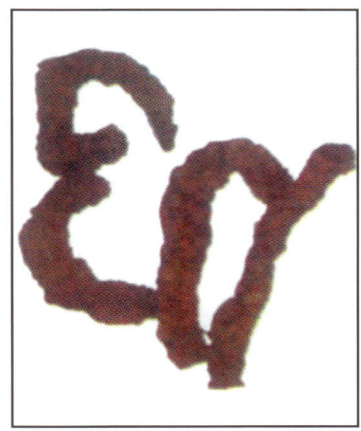

VALERIAN ROOTS
(Valeriana officinalis)

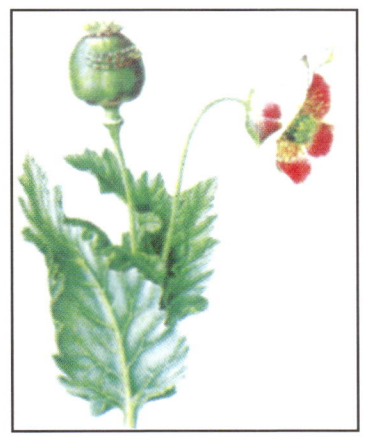

OPIUM POPPY
(Papaver somniferum)

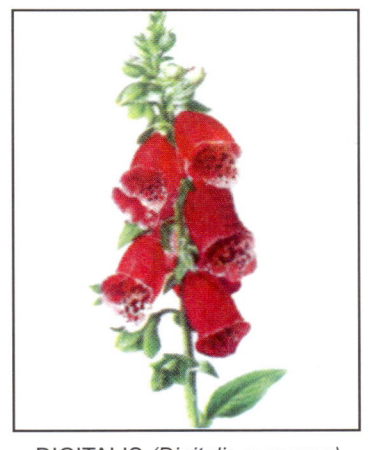

DIGITALIS *(Digitalis purpurea)*

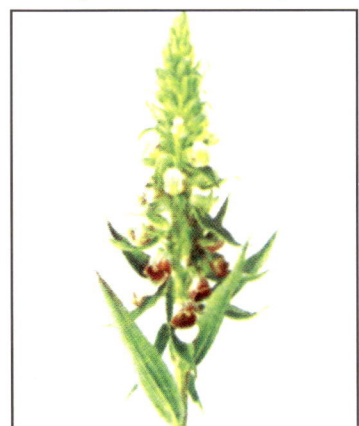

DIGITALIS *(Digitalis lanata)*

Plate 2

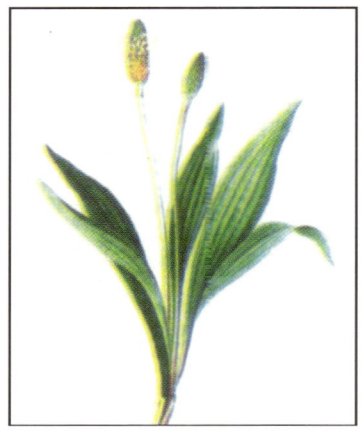
ISPAGHULA (ISAEGOL PLANT)
(Plantago ovata)

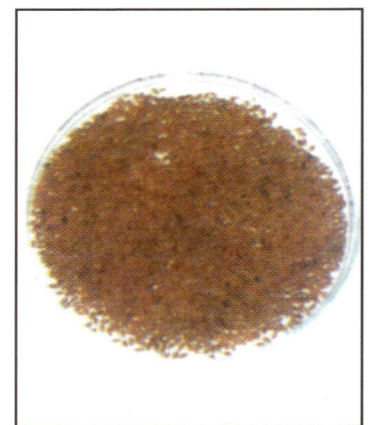
ISPAGHULA (ISABGOL SEEDS)
(Plantago ovata)

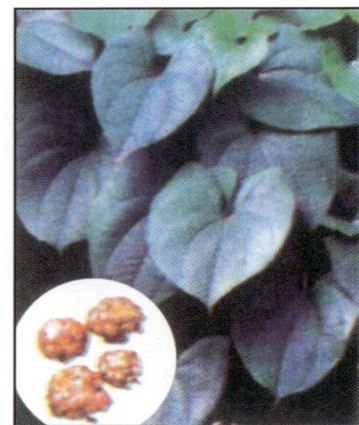
DIOSCOREA *(D. deltoidea)*

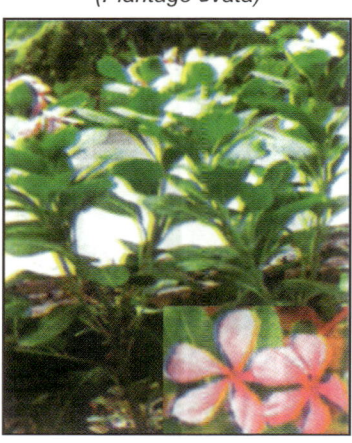
VINCA *(Catharanthus roseus)*

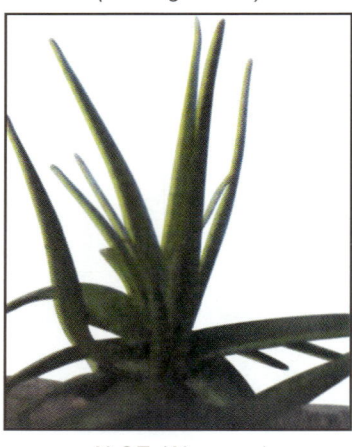
ALOE *(Aloe vera)*

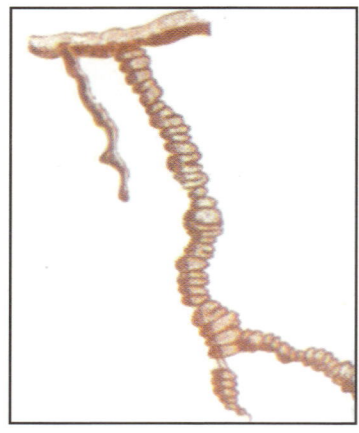
IPECAC ROOT
(Cephaelis ipecacuanha)

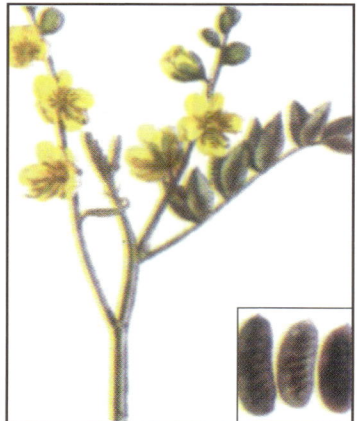
SENNA LEAVES & PODS BRANCH
(Cassia angustifolia)

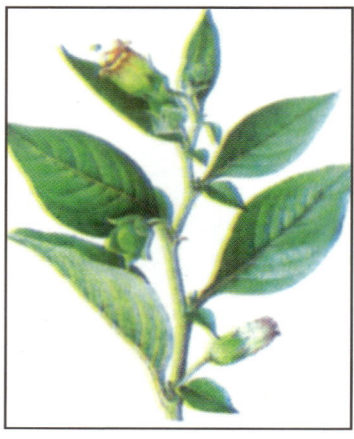
ATROPA *(A. belladonna)*

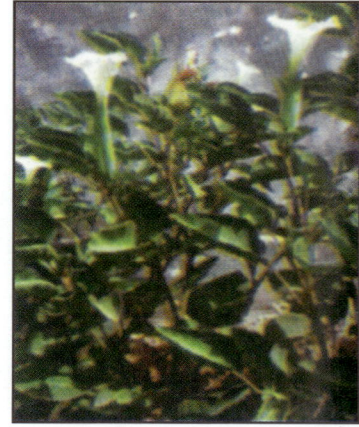
DATURA *(D. stramonium)*

Plate 3

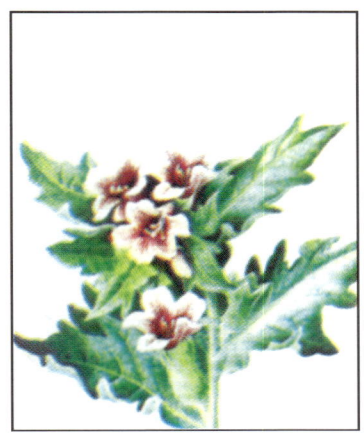

HENBANE *(Hyoscyamus niger)*

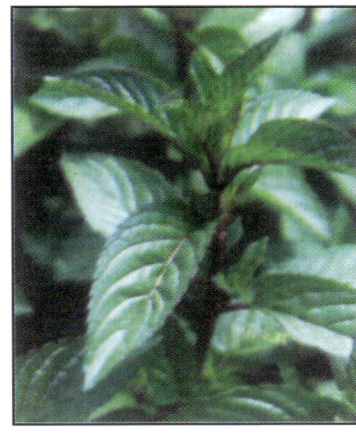

MENTHA (PEPPERMINT)
(M. piperita)

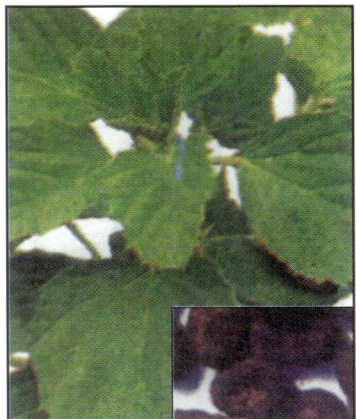

BABCHI (PSORALEA)
(P. corylifolia)

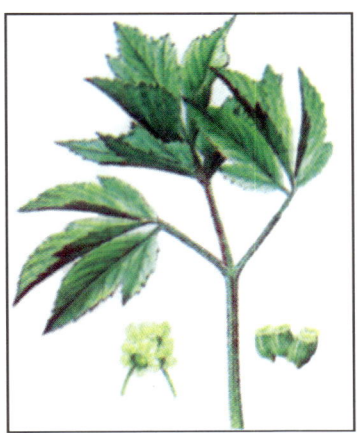

ANGELICA FRUIT & LEAF
(Angelica archangelica)

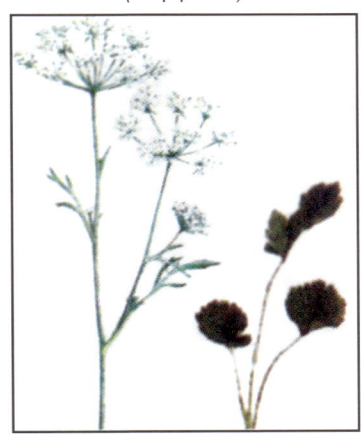

ANISEED PLANT
(Pimpinella anisum Linn.)

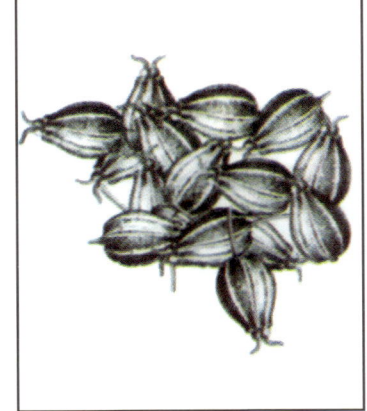

ANISEED SEED
(Pimpinella anisum Linn.)

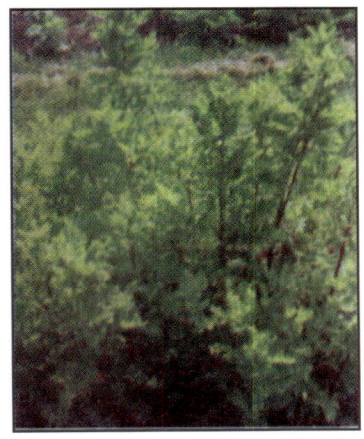

ASTRAGALUS *(A. membranaceus)*

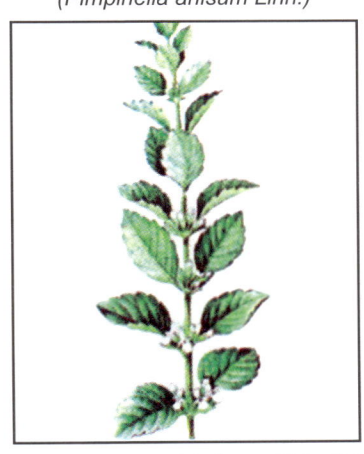

BALM LEMON *(Melissa officinalis)*

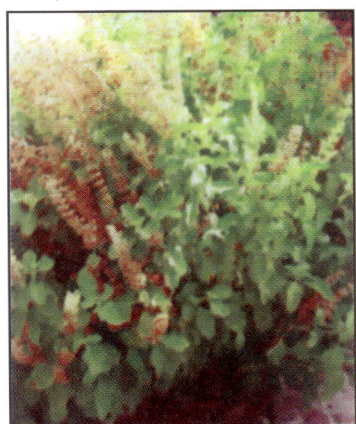

TULSI *(Ocimum basilicum)*

Plate 4

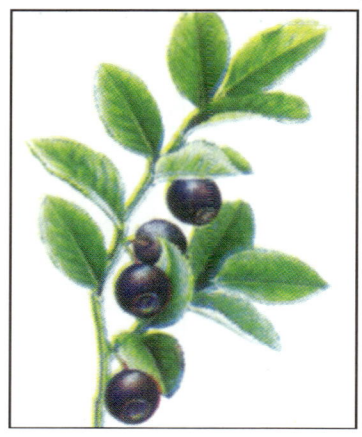

BILBERRY FRUITS BRANCH
(Vaccinum myrtillus)

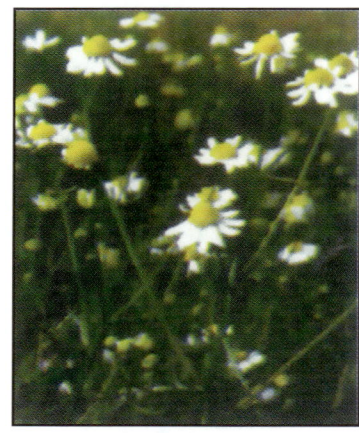

CHAMOMILE *(Matricaria recutita)*

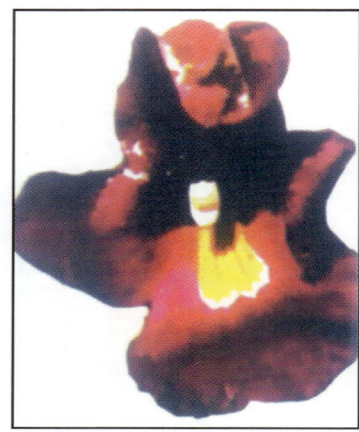

DEVIL'S CLAW
(Herpagophytum procumbens)

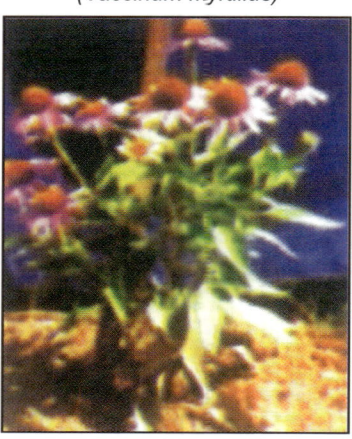

ECHINACEAE *(E. angustifolia)*

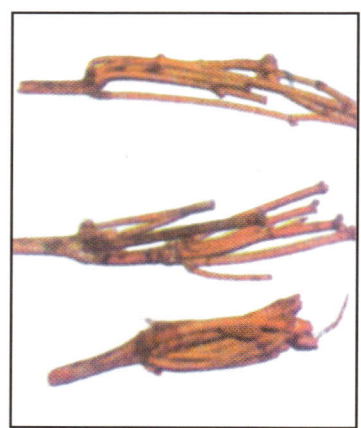

EPHEDRA *(E. sinica)*

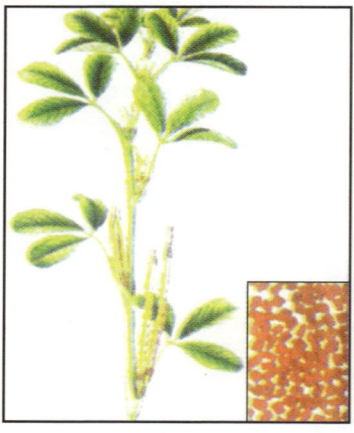

FENUGREEK PLANT AND SEEDS
(Trigonella foerum graecum)

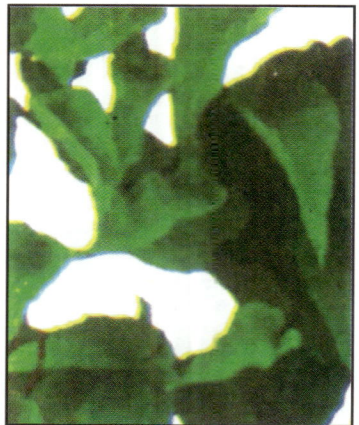

FO-TI *(Polygonum multiflorum)*

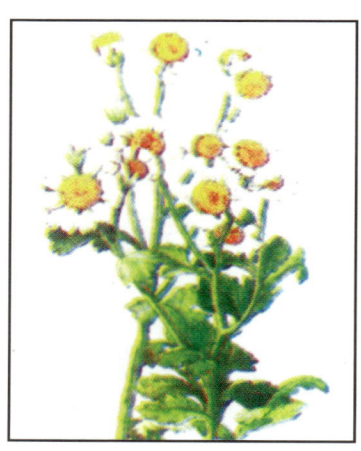

FEVERFEW *(Tanacetum parthenium
syn. chrysanthemum parthenium)*

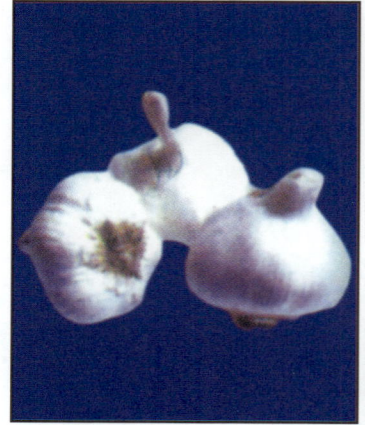

GARLIC *(Allium sativum)*

Plate 5

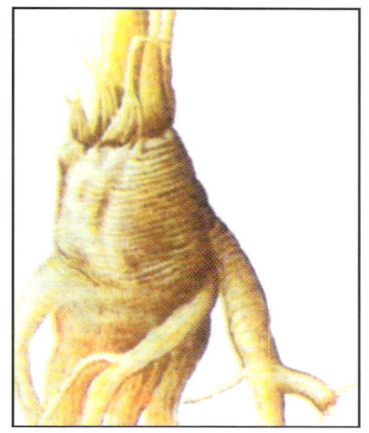

GENTIAN *(Gentiana lutea)*

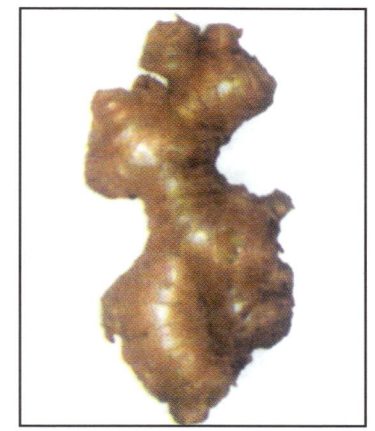

GINGER *(Zingiber officinale)*

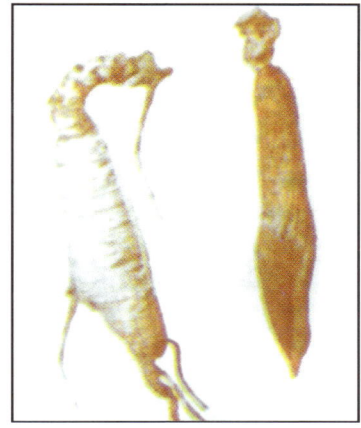

GINSENG ROOT *(Panax ginseng)*

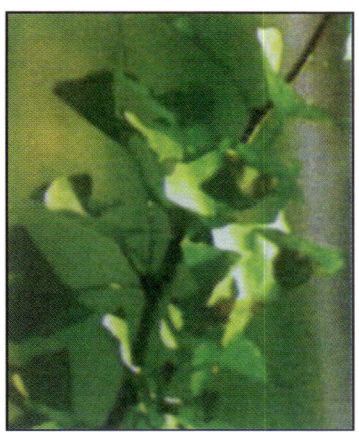

GINKGO *(G. biloba)*

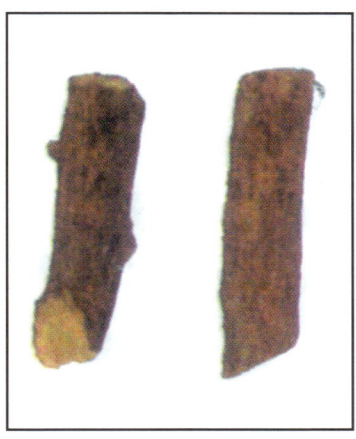

LIQUORICE ROOT
(Glycyrrhiza glabra)

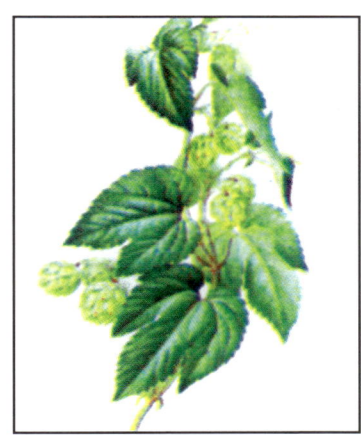

HOPS *(Humulus lupulus)*

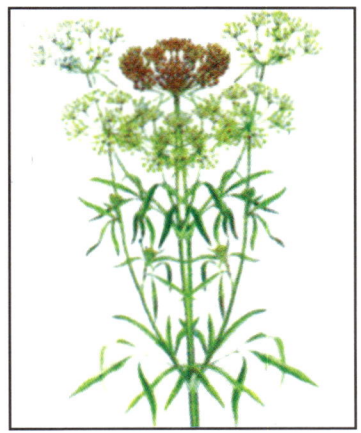

PARSLEY *(Petroselinum crispum)*

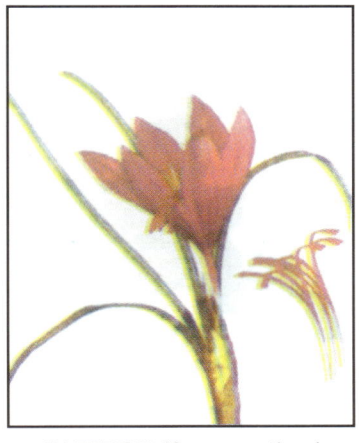

SAFFRON *(Crocus sativus)*

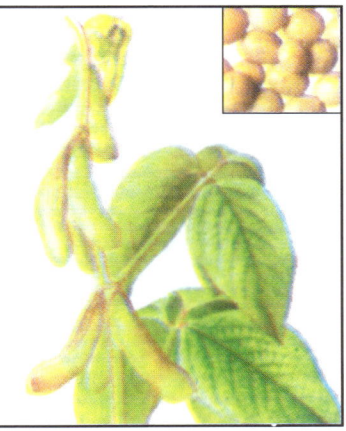

SOYBEAN BRANCH AND SEEDS
(Glycine soja)

Plate 6

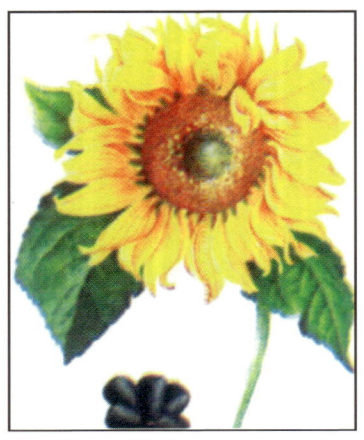

SUNFLOWER *(Helianthus annuus)*

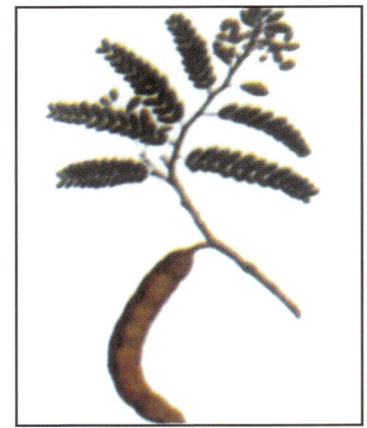

TAMARIND *(Tamarindus indica)*

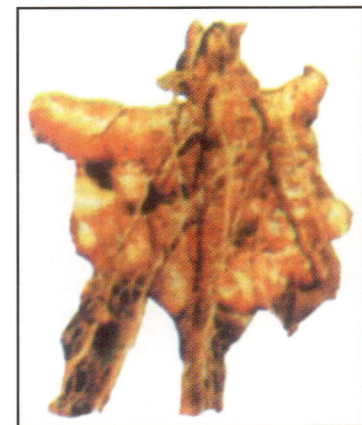

TURMERIC *(Curcuma longa)*

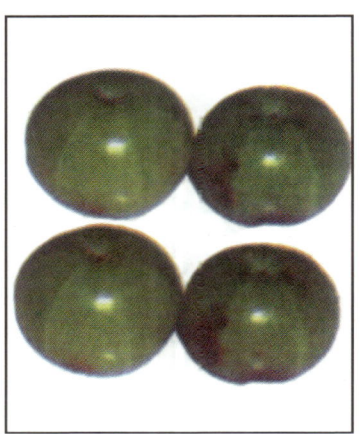

AMLA *(Emblica officinalis)*

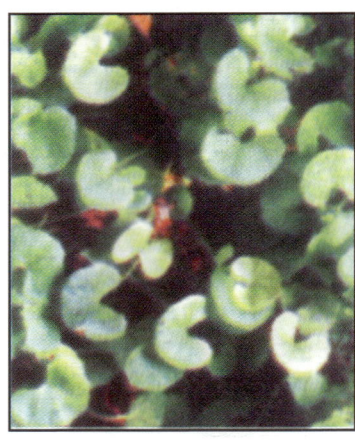

BRAHMI *(Centella asiatica)*

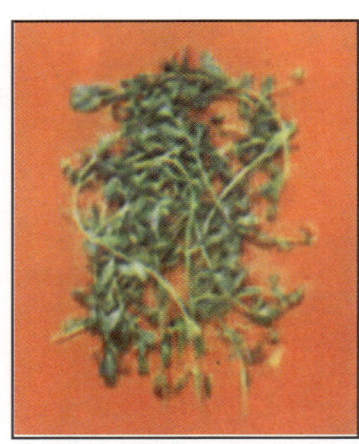

BRAHMI *(Bacopa monniera)*

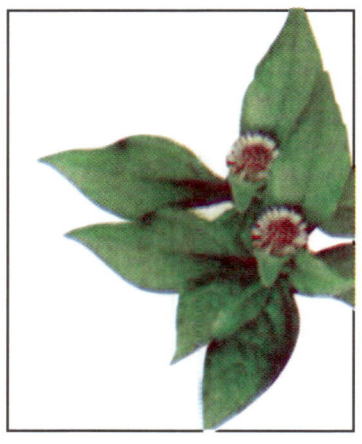

BHRINGRAJ *(Eclipta alba Hassk)*

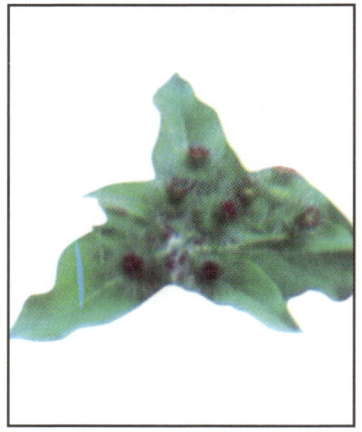

BURDOCK *(Arctium lappa Linn.)*

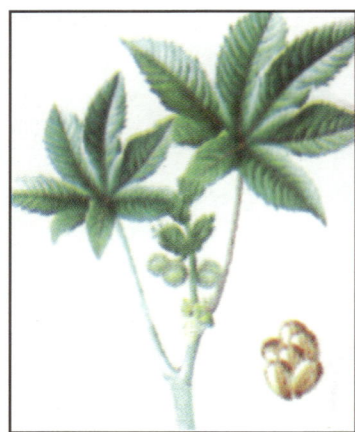

CASTOR OIL PLANT AND SEED
(Ricinus communis)

Plate 7

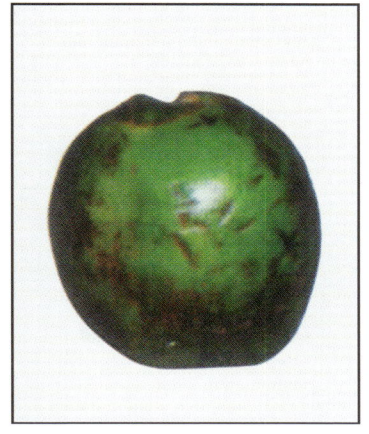

COCONUT FRUIT *(Cocos nucifera)*

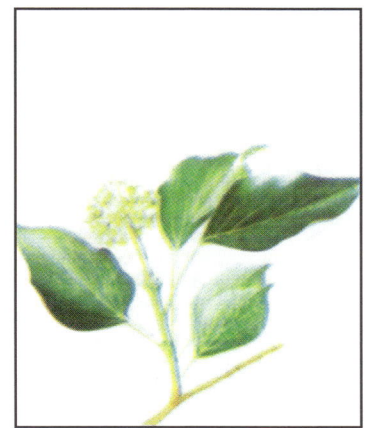

COMMON IVY *(Hedera helix)*

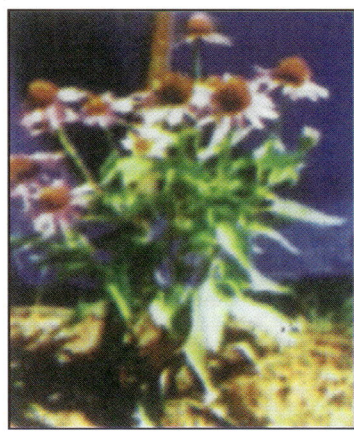

ECHINACEAE *(E. angustifolia)*

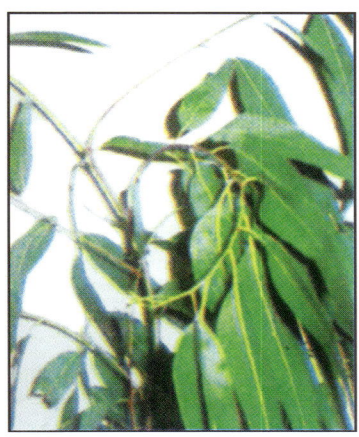

EUCALYPTUS LEAF BRANCH
(E. globulus)

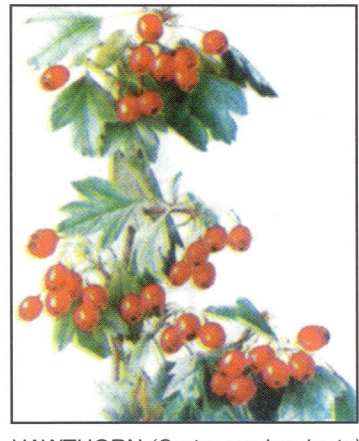

HAWTHORN *(Crataegus laevigata)*

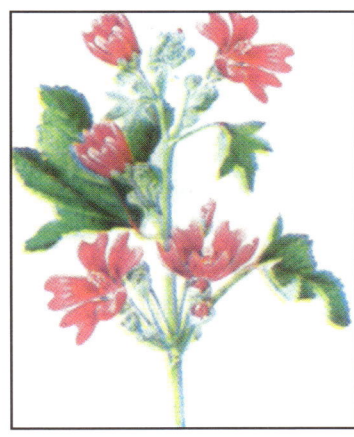

HIGH MALLOW *(Malva sylvestris)*

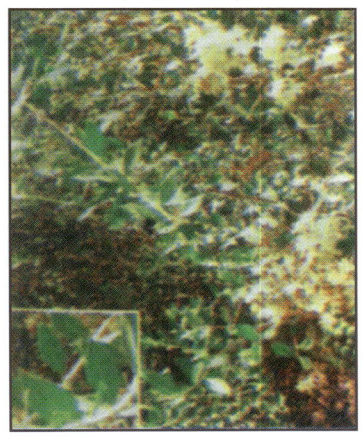

HENNA (MEHNDI)
(Lawsonia inermis)

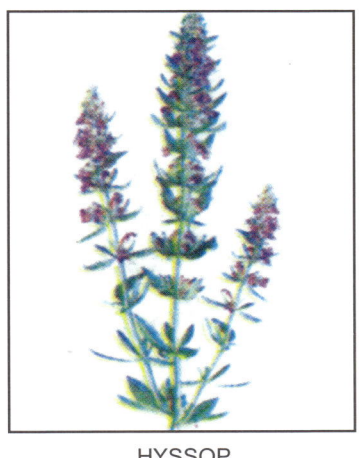

HYSSOP
(Hyssopus officinalis Linn.)

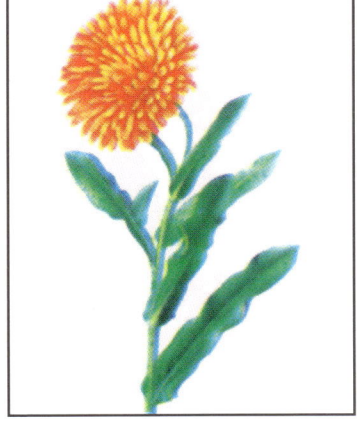

MARIGOLD
(Calendula officinalis)

Plate 8

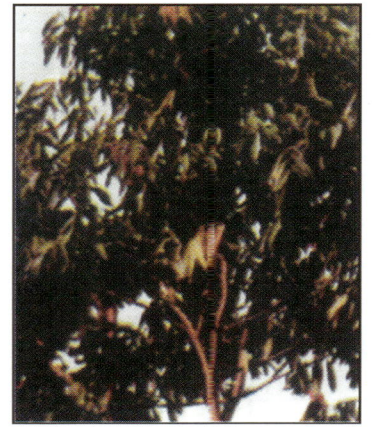

NAGKESAR *(Mesua ferrea)*

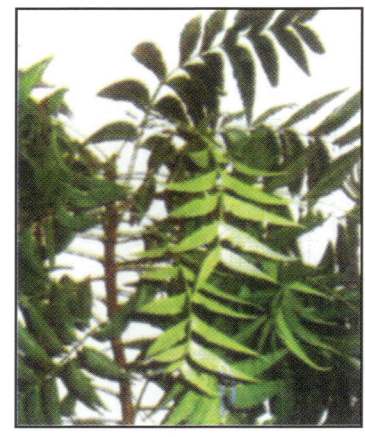

NEEM LEAVES *(Azadirachta indica)*

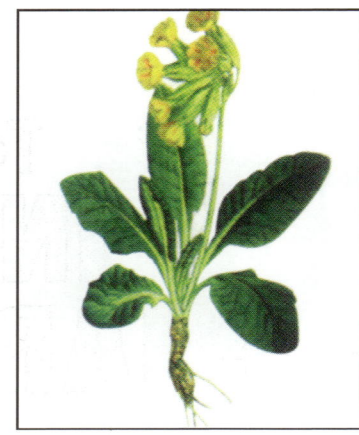

PRIMROSE *(Primula veris Linn.)*

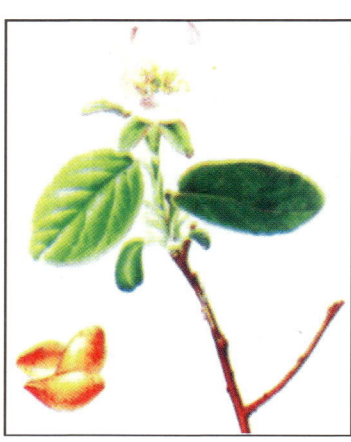

QUINCE PLANT AND SEEDS
(Cydonia oblonga)

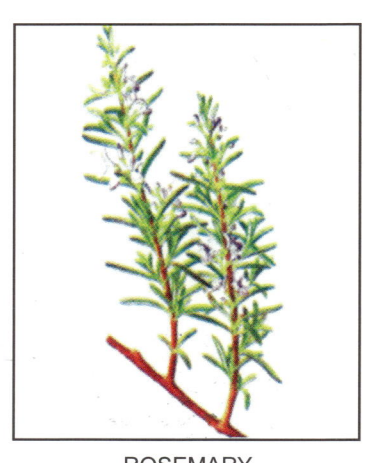

ROSEMARY
(Rosmarinus officinalis)

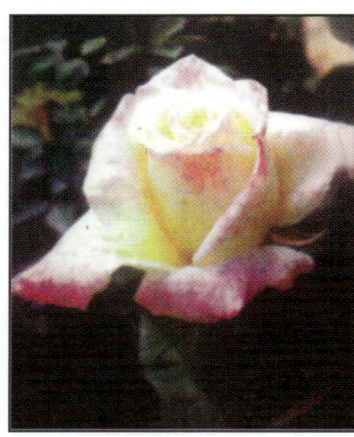

ROSE *(Rosa damascena)*

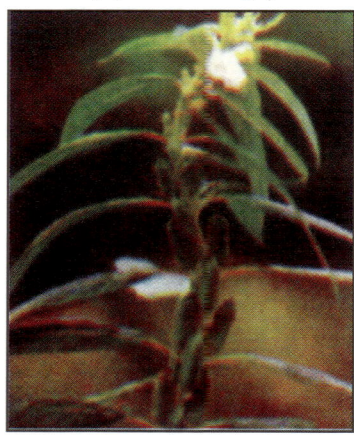

SESAME *(Sesamum indicum Linn.)*

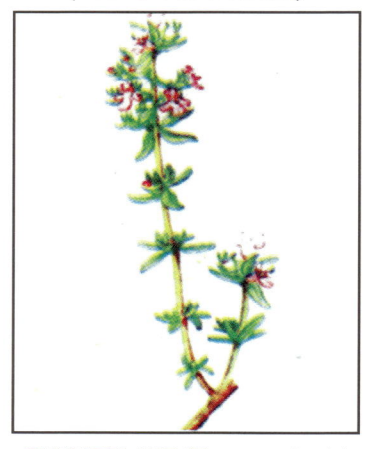

THYME PLANT *(Thymus vulgaris)*

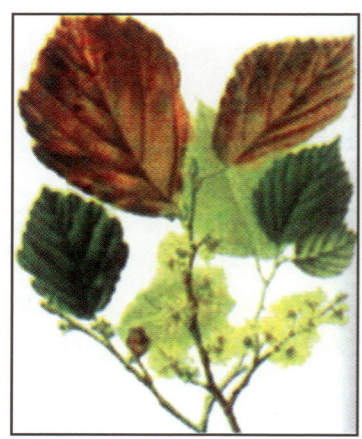

WITCH HAZEL
(Hamamelis virginiana Linn.)

Textbook of
INDUSTRIAL
PHARMACOGNOSY

Role of Medicinal Plants in National Economy

INTRODUCTION

Since ancient times, mankind all over the world mainly depended upon plant kingdom to meet their all needs of medicines, for alleviating ailments, search for eternal health, longevity and to seek remedy to relieve pain and discomfort, fragrance, flavours and foods. It had prompted the early man to explore his immediate natural surrounding and try many plant, animal products, mineral and develop a variety of therapeutic agents. Medicinal plants still play an important role in emerging and developing countries of Asia, both in preventive and curative treatments, despite advances in modern western medicine. They also generate income to the people of many Asian countries who earn their livelihood from selling collected materials from the forest or by cultivating on their farms. Thus, the medicinal plants constitute a very important national resources. People in India and China are known to have used plants in organized health care regime for over 5000 years. European herbal medicines blossomed in the Graeco-Roman era and remained in mainstream until six decades ago. The ancient civilization of India, China, Greece, Arab and other countries of the world developed their own systems of medicine independent of each other but all of them were predominantly plant-based. But the theoretical foundation and the in sights or in depth understanding on the practice of medicine was much superior in **Ayurveda** among organized system of medicine. It is perhaps the oldest (6000 BC) among the organized traditional medicine. People from other countries of the world as China, Cambodia, Indonesia and Baghdad used to come to the **ancient universities of India like Takshila (700 BC)** and **Nalanda (500 BC)** to learn health sciences of India particularly "Ayurveda". From history we learn that since ancient times, plants remained major natural resource in the world.

One of the oldest repositories of human knowledge, the **Righveda (4500-4600 BC)** mentioned the use of medicinal plants for the treatment of one or other disease. In the long struggle to overcome the powerful forces of nature, the human beings have always turned to plants. There are reports available about the local communities in the Asian, African & Latin American countries having a long history of dependence on traditional remedies, largely based on plants, for immediate access to relatively safe, cost effective, efficacious and culturally acceptable solutions to primary health care.

World Health Organization (WHO) estimated that 80% of the population of developing countries relies on traditional medicines, mostly plant drugs for their primary health care needs. Even the modern pharmacopoeia still contains at least 25% drugs derived from plants and many others which are semi-synthetic, built on prototype compounds isolated from plants. Medicinal plants are the major components of all **indigenous or alternative systems of medicine**. For example, they are common elements in Ayurveda, Homeopathy, Naturopathy, Oriental and Native American Indian medicine. Demand for herbal drugs is increasing throughout the world due to growing recognition of natural plant-based products, being non-toxic, having no-side effects, easily available at affordable prices and sometimes the only source of health care available to the poor. Hence, medicinal plant sector has traditionally occupied an important position in the sociocultural, spiritual, economic values of rural and tribal lives of both developing and developed countries. Millions of rural household are using medicinal plants in self-help mode.

About 90% of medicinal plants used by the industries are collected from the wild. While over 800 species are used by industries, not more than 20 species of plant are under the commercial cultivation. Hence, more than 70% plant collection involved destructive harvesting because of the use of parts like root, bark, stem, wood and whole plant (in the case of herbs). This process is a definite threat to the genetic stock and diversity of medicinal plant resources and ultimately economy of the country if the biodiversity is not sustainably used.

The other main source of medicinal plants is from cultivation. The cultivated material is definitely more appropriate for use in the production of drugs. Indeed standardisation whether for pure products, extracts or crude drugs is critical and becomes easier. Hence, higher cost for cultivated material and cultivation often done under contract.

More recently growers have set up cooperative or collaborative ventures in an attempt to improve their negotiating power and achieve higher prices and thus medicinal plants in a wider context generate income to the people of many Asian countries who earn their livelihood from selling collected materials from the wild forest, or by cultivating on their farms.

International trade in medicinal plants both within South asian countries and East Asia, Europe and North America is growing in economic importance, e.g. Nepal is earning an estimated US\$ 8.6 million annually from the export of medicinal plants, thus the medicinal plants and other forest products influence local, national and international economics.

There is wide spread belief that "green" drugs are healthier than synthetic product. Recent reports have witnessed an upsurge in the popularity of herbal medicines. In most industrialized countries, use of medicinal plants has increased dramatically in the last decade, there has been a rising trend in Ayurvedic (herbal) products, an area where India's expertise dates back centuries. But it is not only in the last decade that the country has truly seen the commercialisation on the herbal concept. Herbal has now become full-fledged wave composing of both in beauty-care and health-care products. As well as herbal Over The Counter (OTC) drugs have gained substantial ground. Currently, according to industry estimate, total **pharmaceutical market** is around Rs.5000 crores, the total herbal market share is Rs.1200 crores, of which the OTC market constitute around Rs.400 crores.

The importance and value of traditional and indigenous herbal medicine was the subject of campaign of the WHO. Its effort, in the 1970s, led an appeal to all member countries to do their utmost to preserve their national heritage in the form of ethno-medicine and ethno-pharmacology and to bring back the use of known and tested medicinal plants and derivatives into primary health care in rural areas as alternatives when modern medicines are not available.

In India, plants have been **traditionally** used for human and veterinary health care and also, in the food and textile industry. Ninety percent of the local food resources known to indigenous people were undocumented to nutritional literature, trade, cosmetics and perfumes; but India has a special position in area of herbal medicines, since it is one of the few countries which are capable of cultivating most of the important plants used both in modern and traditional systems of medicine. This is because India has vast area with wide variation in climate, soil, altitude/latitude and rich flora.

The **herbal drug market** itself is growing at a rate of between 20–30% annually, with individual company registering different growth rates. The healthy growth rate of this market can also be attributed to the Government policy of encouraging the manufacturers of purely herbal products. This coupled with absence of any pricing guidelines. Unlike 'Drug Price Control Order (DPCO)' pricing guidelines for ethical drugs has resulted in this segment being perceived as a highly lucrative alternative source of revenue. The new patent policy under 'GATT', which will come into effective by the year 2005 has encouraged the herbal market.

While the domestic market (about US$ one billion of Ayurvedic medicine) is opening up to the herbal phenomenon, the export market is also showing promise. Many pharmaceutical companies are targeting export as the prime source in the coming years. **World trade** in plant medicines is of billions dollar. In 1994 China exported US$ five billion of plant drugs. Germany imported about US$ 105 millions of plant drugs. The number of medicinal plants trade too is astonishing. Now

Germany export market is about Rs.600 crores and is expected to expand to Rs.20,000 crores in the next decade. The present export volume of crude drugs from India stands at 36,200 tonnes valued around US$ 24 millions. China and India are two great producers of medicinal plants having more than 40% of global diversity.

In developing countries, plants are the main source of **Alternative medicine**. According to the World Health Organization as many as 80% of the world's people rely on traditional medicines, for their primary health care, most types of which use remedies from plants. The use of traditional medicine in developing countries is increasing because population is increasing. Govt. wants to encourage indigenous forms of medicine rather than to rely on imported drugs and there are strong moves to revive traditional cultures; being easy access and cost effective and ultimately affect the national economy.

For example, traditional medicine is an important part of African culture. It varies with cultural group and region. The Western pharmaceuticals are inaccessible especially to rural based population. Therefore, more than 80% of Africans rely on plant-based medicine. About 70-90% of the population in South Africa, Zambia, Nigeria, Mozambique, Ethopia and Democratic Republic of Congo, among others, rely on traditional medicine for their health care. In South Africa, at national level, 20,000 tonnes of medicinal plant materials are traded, corresponding to a value of about US$ 60 millions. In Zambia, trade in traditional medicine is worth over US$ 43 millions per annum. Traditional systems of medicine are also predominant medical systems in practice in Malawian rural areas.

Medicinal plants based medicine also has significant role in most Latin American countries. About 70-80% of the Latin American population rely on traditional medicines for their health care needs. For example, about 80% of Ecuadorians, rely on medicinal plants or products derived from plants. There is lack of access to modern drugs in a significant part of Latin America. In India, annual turnover of **herbal industry** was estimated around US$ 250 million in 1995. According to Chemexcil report, export value of Ayurvedic and Unani medicine was about US$ 41.6 million during 1999-2000; the major OTC products contribute around US$ 30.5 million.

ECONOMIC GROWTH POTENTIAL IN NATURAL HEALTH AND COSMETIC PRODUCTS

Medicinal plants also play a great role in food supplements for health care as well as in personal care of the mankind alongside the therapeutically active substances, thus medicinal plant-based nutraceutical and cosmeceutical industry is a promising sector with enormous economic growth potential. The USA leads the market, following countries of Western Europe and Japan. In 1999 the global health food products market was US$ 6.8 billion, almost thrice the value in 1987. The global demand for **herbal extract** in food products grew to US$ 3.0 billion in 1999 from US$ 0.76 million in 1997, almost 4.5 fold rise in demand (Table 1.1). There are reports that Asia and Pacific Latin America, Africa and Middle East are

set to provide the fastest growth for food based (nutraceutical) industry. USA, Japan and major European countries are the largest global producers and consumers of nutraceuticals, owing to higher level of consumer income.

Globally, the market for plant-based cosmeceuticals has been estimated to US$ 22 billions and the fastest growing sector in this market is anti-aging products. The developed countries like USA, Japan, Australia and Europe are the most dominant market for cosmeceuticals and China, Malaysia, Russia and Latin America have a strong potential for long-term growth. In USA, the market for cosmeceuticals was estimated at US$ 2.5 billion where the market for medicinal plant ingredients used in cosmetics and toiletries stood at US$ 345 million in 1998, forecasted to increase 7.9% annually to reach US$ 503 million by 2005 and 760 million by 2008.

FUTURE ECONOMIC GROWTH

Throughout the world, about 35,000-70,000 species of plants have been used at one time or another for **medicinal, nutraceuticals and cosmeceuticals** purposes. **In India**, about 1000 plant species, **in Nepal** about **700 species**, about 700 species in Peninsular Malaysia and its neighbouring Islands and in Chinese medicine about 9905 plant materials are used but only a relatively very small number of them are used in any significant volume. According to the International Trade Centre (ITC) report, there is generally upward trend except for 1990, when it dipped slightly before rising again to US$ 1.08 billion in 1991. The world trade in medicinal plants and raw material from plants parts averaged US$ 1.28 billion during 1995–1999. **Thus there is lot of scope in future for new plant-based drugs which are still to be introduced and the economic significance of these plant-based pharmaceuticals is considerable which is based on the following two aspects:**

Table 1.1. Medicinal plant extracts demand in cosmetics from 1989 to 1998

Item	Demand value (million US$)		
	1989	1993	1998
Aloe extract	38	46	63
Botanical extract	180	230	345
Others	22	34	67
Plant acids/enzymes	19	37	65
Essential oils	101	113	150
Other natural products	85	115	180
Total	**445**	**575**	**870**

(1) The value of the current plant-based pharmaceuticals, and

(2) The value of potential plant-based pharmaceuticals, which are yet to be introduced.

The values of these drugs are described both in terms of their market value and their economic value.

Market value is a subset of economic value, which includes all benefits to society. Market value of the drugs is attributable to the plants raw materials, development and manufacturing costs as well as the incorporation of research cost for the failed efforts and above all the existence of consumer's surplus.

Economic value represents all the social benefits of particular type of product including market value. Economic value can be viewed as an expression of the total benefit of a product.

The relationship between the economic value of a medicinal plant species and market price of the drugs derived from it, is not a direct one. However, it is true that the market prices are minimum valuations assuming that:

- The demand for the drug is inelastic, and
- That it is appropriate to value an essential input as its own cost plants.
- The economic rent obtained from it plus the associated consumer's surplus.

For example, the market value of a stand of forest could be measured by translating the wood volume there in into an equivalent quantity of paper and then taking the market value of the paper. In contrast, economic value to society includes not only the value of the paper (or whatever the other commodity is selected), but also what may be referred to as the "in situ" benefit of trees as forest that is the contribution as:

- The forest checks the soil erosion, stabilizing the water table, converting carbon dioxide into oxygen (environmental effects);

- Providing protection to wild life, and;
- Providing recreational opportunities, hence, the economic value is much larger in magnitude but also much more difficult to quantify. For example:

An economic value for medicinal plant species would be examining the current cost to society of a disease whose impact might be diminished in the future by drug derived from plants e.g. in the case of cancer disease which is the major cause of about 5 lakhs deaths per year in United States and cost about US$ 14 billion annually in treatment, where as the value of each life estimated to be about US$ 8 million, then the total value will be about US$ 4 trillion annually. **Anti-cancer** drugs save about 75,000 lives annually in the United States (an estimated 15% of 500000 lives) and plant-based drugs comprises about 40% of total group of anticancer drugs. Combining those estimates approximately 30,000 lives are saved annually in United States as result of the use of plant-based drugs. Multiplying the lives saved by the value per life, the annual **economic value** of plant-based drugs in the United States alone is estimated to be about US$ 250 billion. Since this estimate reflect only a part of the total economic value of all plant-based pharmaceuticals, moreover these values include none of the non-pharmaceuticals benefits provided by the plants responsible for these drugs, the above mentioned data is on the basis of information by Violette and Chestnut 1986, in EPA-230-06-86016 Feb. 1986 and information available from the economic value of biological diversity among medicinal plants. OECD environment monograph. These values would be tripled to US$ 750 billion annually to account for anticancer application in all OECD countries (The countries which are members of organisation for economic cooperation and development).

This reflects that medicinal plants and their products have taken an increasing medical and economical importance with respect to product categories like health food, cosmetics and personal care products containing natural ingredients, the demand for medicinal plants is growing exponentially. The fastest growing **world market** in herbal products is opening up new opportunities for the developing countries to benefit from the rising green consumerism, trend to develop their export potential. However this requires a grand strategic plan, which takes a holistic view of the entire situation to boost the export. For example:

- Development of herbal medicine industry
- Contribution to economy of the people
- Novelties

DEVELOPMENT OF HERBAL MEDICINE INDUSTRY

To cope up with the increasing demand for quality herbal medicines in the domestic as well as export markets, the successful development of herbal medicines industry will contribute positive impact for the development of the National health care systems, improvement of people welfare, creation of competitive pharmaceutical products and encouragement of new drug discovery in the pharmaceutical industry, which will ultimately contribute to **economy** of the people.

CONTRIBUTION TO ECONOMY OF THE PEOPLE

A partnership scheme among institutions involved i.e. the farmers, general public, research and higher education, Government health care services providers and the industry, taking into consideration the interest of each constituent is to be directed to an integrated National Herbal Medicine Industry.

The industry is expected to have better access to the market and the customers of the commodities for further processing to produce added value. The industry and its technology will play its role in creating and enhancing the competitiveness of the products and the results in the form of revenue will be distributed to the farmers through the procurement of farmer's products in an agreed reasonable price. Research and higher education institution with the support from Govt. will provide the knowledge, technical assistance required by the farmers. The farmers will then have all the requirements to participate and contribute to activities that ultimately will positively impact the economy of the farmer. The scheme will result multiplier effects through creation of new jobs.

Herbal medicines will be the leading products in pharmaceutical business in the future

The abundant sources of many varieties and uniqueness of medicinal plants for herbal medicines open opportunity for the development of competitive pharmaceutical products to supply the domestic and export market.

NOVELTIES

Forest medicinal plant are sources and can become a good start for the discovery of new chemical compounds, which will lead to new drugs.

Current level of international trade in medicinal plants (including categories referred to as pharmaceutical plants and "botanical drugs") is reported to be US$ 800 million this has been the average annual value during 1992-1995, according to information from International Trade Centre, Geneva.

Thus Medicinal and Aromatic plants play great role in the National Economy and to maintain its existing supplies to keep up with demand, they will need adequate protection through development of appropriate institutions, policies and legislation. Local communities need support and encouragement to protect these resources. To complement cultivation of adaptable species, harvesting from the wild must be guided by accurate inventories and knowledge about the species concerned. Above all, over exploitation of rare and endanger species must be avoided.

The health care systems are going to become more and more expensive. Therefore, we will have to develop technologies to essentially introduce and integrate herbal medicine systems into our health care. There is an enormous scope for India also to emerge as a major player in the global herbal product based medicines. However this requires a grand strategic plan, which takes a hilistic view of the entire situation to boost the export of Rs. 10,000 crores by 2010 and minimising the import.

2

Worldwide Trade in Medicinal Plants and Derived Products

INTRODUCTION

The term **"Medicinal Plants"** for the purpose of worldwide trade specifies the plants having substance or substances of medicinal value, which have been biologically proved useful as drug or contain drug constituents, that can be used as therapeutic agents or as starting material for the synthesis of therapeutic agents, or as models for new synthetic drugs and as instruments in drug development and diagnostic purposes.

The main difficulty in analysing world trade in herbal drugs is the extremely limited statistical data available on production and trade. No country has published production data; only USA provides the detailed breakdown of herbs imports. Even wherever trade data whatsoever is available that only provide information to consumption levels. The production and trade levels relating to individual herb vary widely. Moreover, the pattern of usage of individual herb differs in different countries.

The major brokers and importers of herbs are established in the major trading centres of major importing countries namely New York (USA), Hamburg (West Germany), Marseilles & Paris (France), London (UK), Tokyo (Japan) and Amsterdam & Routerdam (Netherland). Hence,

whatsoever data the author has presented in this chapter, is being collected from the databases of national level agencies, which still needs to update by the later information from time to time.

DEMAND FOR MEDICINAL PLANTS

The wide spread popularity towards the traditional medicines in Asia, Europe and USA has induced high growth and development in the worldwide trade of medicinal plants, in terms of crude herbs, nutrapharmaceuticals, health food, food supplements, essential oils, fixed oils, massage, cosmetic and medicines. In China about 50% of the total medicinal consumption is based on traditional medicines. World demand for medicinal plants is steadily increasing not only from the developing countries but also from the developed countries. This demand for medicinal plants is increasing as the drug pharmaceutical products are falling under more strict Government regulations. Herbal medicines industry is one of the fast growing industries in the world. **Global market in the herbal medicines** was estimated US$ 12.4 billion in 1994 increasing up to US$ 19.6 billion in 1999. The demand in herbal medicines was expected to grow about US$ 24.2 billion in 2002 but it has gone to about US$ 62 billion in 2002.

In India approximately 1800 plant species are used in Ayurveda, 600 for Siddha, about 400 for Unani and more than 400 for Homoeopathic system of medicine, with substantial overlaps of common plants among these systems. Thus the total number of plant species used in traditional systems of medicine in India comes to near about 8000.

Plants are used in crude or semi-processed form, often in mixture of drugs along with some non-botanical ingredients.

The US market for medicinal plant extracts in 1999 was estimated approximately US$ 500 million, which was equivalent to about 25% of the global market. Further it is reported that newly developed products such as extract i.e. grape seed and valerian extract, various multi-functional plant derivatives, such as lycopene and anthocyanin will register growth exceeding 8% per annum in 2005.

A few species are the source of refined compounds used in pharmaceutical industry. Example: **terpenoids** contributed major part of the worldwide trade of plant derived refined compounds, valued about US$ 7.7 billion, followed by **glycosides** US$ 7.2 billion, **alkaloids** US$ 3.6 billion and other plant derived compound were about US$ 4 billion. Their sales value have been estimated to reach US$ 10.79 billion, 10.03 billion, 5.1 billion and 5.6 billion respectively in 2005.

Approximately one quarter of prescription dispensed from Community Pharmacy in USA contain one or more ingredients derived from higher plants. In the mid-90s, it was estimated that more than US$ 2.5 billions resulted from the sales of plant based drugs. In **Japan**, herbal medicinal preparations are more in demand than the pharmaceutical preparations. In many tropical and sub-tropical countries like Africa, South and East Asia, majority of people resort to herbal medicines for their primary health care needs. In South Africa more than 500 species are commercialized trade products.

Botswana, Kenya, Madagascar, Mozambique, Namibia, South Africa, Sudan, Tanzania and Uganda are the African countries, which in 1994 exported a significant volume (about 8000 metric tonnes) of medicinal plants material from Africa to Germany.

In 1995–96, about 20,000 metric tonnes of medicinal plants material with an approximate value of US$ 60 million and finished products of worth US$ 215.6 million were traded from South Africa.

The following is the list of medicinal plants from South Africa, which are having place in the International trade market. These are:

- Cape aloe (*Aloe ferox*)
- Buchu (*B. crenulata*)
- Devil's claw (*Harpagophytum procumbens*)
- Umkcaloabo (*Pelarogonium sidoides*)
- *Prunus africana*
- *Catharanthus roseus*

Latin America export the medicinal plants in the form of dried crude drug, mainly collected from wild sources. **Chile** exports about US$ 20 million of medicinal plants in 1994 major of which is *Quillaja saponaria* amounting to US$ 80,000 other important exported plants were *Peumus boldus*, *Origanum majorana*, *Rosa perruna* and *Smilax medica*. The major export was to Brazil and Argentina, while *Origanum* and *Quillaja* species to Germany. The total export during the year 1992 to 1994 reached to 10,000–11,000 metric tonnes per year.

The import of medicinal plant extracts of glycosides, alkaloids, essential oils and steroid hormones from Brazil was reported to be of US$ 40–45 million per year in 1990s while total export was of 50 millions.

DEMAND FOR HERBAL MEDICINE

Demand for herbal medicine sector is growing fast, increasing by 12–15% value per year.

World market for herbal medicines was estimated to be about US$ 12.4 billion in 1994, raised to US$ 19.5 billion in 1999, was expected to grow at the rate of 15% annually and reached to about US$ 22.4 billion in 2002. Europe leads the world market for herbal medicine with the sale figure of US$ 7 billion approximately.

Europe represents the huge reservoir of global herbal market constituting about 45% of the total market followed by North America (18.8%) and Asia (17.2%).

Latin America and Eastern Europe have retail sale of US$ 600 million and US$ 400 million respectively. In Asia, the demand for herbal medicines was estimated to almost double during the early 2000s because of the increasing population factor and economy factor. Among the European countries, Germany leads the herbal medicine market with the sale amounting to about US$ 3.5 billion in 1997–98 followed by France, Italy, UK, Scandinavia and Netherland. According to the World Health Organization (WHO) reports about 4 billion people of the world population presently use herbal medicines for their primary health care as alternative system of medicine i.e. Ayurvedic, Homeopathic, Naturopathic, Oriental and Native American Indian medicine.

As per survey report there are more than 2000 herbal medicinal companies in Europe alone.

According to an estimate, there are more than 27 million consumers of herbal medicines alone in South Africa. Herbal medicines in Phillipines are now considered to be a strong partner in the health care and body care delivery systems. In Vietnam, the traditional medicines are in the list of national essential drugs. In Pakistan more than 55,000 Traditional Medical Practitioners (TMPs) serve over 70–80% of the population using their own prescription. Crude plant based drugs worth about US$ 120 million are used annually in Pakistan. Unani system of medicine is the most prevalent alternative system of medicine and uses both raw and semi processed plant material. About 40% of Indonesians use herbal drugs for self–care health services for different purposes.

TRENDS IN WORLDWIDE TRADE IN MEDICINAL PLANTS

Trade in medicinal plants is growing in volume and ultimately in export value. As per the International Trade Centre (ITC) information as far back as 1967, the value of global import of the medicinal plants for pharmaceutical and cosmetic industry was about US$ 52.9 million, which was raised to US$ 72.1 million in 1971 and then showed a steady rise in growth rate of approximately 5–7% till mid 1980s. From 1987 to 1991 the average value of worldwide trade in medicinal plants reached to US$ 853 million. Generally the trade has shown upward trend except for the year 1990 when it dipped slightly followed by again uprising trend from US$ 1.3 billion in 1995 to nearly US$ 1.4 billion, but subsequently decreased to US$ 1.1 billion in 1999. The six leading **importers** (volume wise) were **Hong Kong, Japan, Germany, USA, South Korea and France** during late 1990s. World trade in medicinal plants has now been put at over US$ 62 billion with annual average growth rate of 7 percent to reach US$ 5 trillion by 2050. The growth is fastest in the European countries (10%) and USA (20%).

Indonesian export figures for traditional medicines continue to rise dramatically. In 1993, total export value of essential oil was US$ 31.03 million with an annual growth rate 15%.

The average annual export of medicinal and aromatic plants from Sudan was worth US$ 10 million during 1995–1999. The export of plants for herbal teas was US$ 0.26 million and for perfumery, medicaments, insecticidal & fungicidal to European countries was worth US$ 4.5 million. The South African countries also traded about 20,000 tonnes of raw material from about 800 plants species worth about US$ 65 million annually.

Pakistan exported a significant volume of medicinal plants to the world market (about 200 tonnes from the Punjab & Sindh provinces). The present export volume of crude drugs from India stands at about 42,600 tonnes valued around US$ 30 million. The figure reaches US$ 90 million if the plant products are also included into the list. It is expected that it will jump from 6–8 times by 2005.

The Herbal based drug industry is growing at the rate of 7–15% annually. The Exim Bank report states that the medicinal plants related trade in India alone is approximately Rs. 5.5 billion and it estimates the global market for herbal medicine to be US$ 5 billion (expected to reach US$ 16 billion by 2005) and that China accounts for nearly 40% of this trade while India only 2%. According to the Exim Bank report, the export of Ayurveda and Siddha herbal products and services offer huge potential and the world demand for herbal products has been growing at a rate of 10–15% per annum. The report identifies supply side constraints such as "lack of standardization, lack of knowledge on international regulations governing the import of such products, etc." as well as demand dynamics in the overseas market, which inhibit India's export of herbal products and services.

INTERNATIONAL TRADE

Trade codes

The term worldwide trade applies to International trade in medicinal plants for which the raw materials have been coded under Standard International Trade Classification (STIC) and the **Harmonized Commodity Description and Coding System (HS) or Customs Cooperation Council Nomenclature (CCCN)**. For example CCCN code 1211, is widely accepted by the **World Trade Organization** (WTO) indicating the botanical drugs (plants or parts of the plants used primarily in perfumery, pharmacy or for insecticidal, fungicidal or similar purposes), then for specific drugs or single drug it is further sub-coded as given in the Table 2.1 & 2.2.

Worldwide trade in medicinal plants is being classified into three main categories i.e. the Liquorice roots (HS 1211.10), Ginseng roots (HS 1211.20) and other medicinal plants. Both the liquorice roots and ginseng roots are in high demand in International market and are therefore kept under separate category and all other medicinal plants species have been kept under one broad category (other medicinal plants).

Trade Centres

It has been observed that the sales of medicinal plants and their products is governed by the price levels prevailing in **Hamburg, New York & Osaka** and to a lesser extent in **Hong Kong, Paris, Marsilles, Basel, St. Gallen London & Amsterdam**. The world's leading trade centre in medicinal plant materials is **Hamburg**, the most important **exporting countries** to Hamburg are Albania, China, Egypt, France, Greece, Hungary, India, Netherland, Poland and Zaire.

Table 2.1. SITC and HS or CCN codes for major botanical drug groups in International Trade

HS or CCCN Code	Commodity	SITC, Rev. 3 code
1211.00	Plants and plant parts of a kind used primarily in perfumery, in pharmacy, or for insecticidal, fungicidal, or similar purposes.	292.40
1211.10	Liquorice roots	292.41
1211.20	Ginseng roots	292.42
1211.90	Others including pyrethrum, tonquine beans, mint linden, verbena, Origanum vulgare and Salvia officinalis	292.49

Table 2.2. Sub-categories of CCCN codes 1211.20 and 1211.90

HS or CCCN	Code	Description
1211.20.00.00		Ginseng root
	20	Cultivated ginseng root
	40	Wild gingseng root
1211.90.00.00		Other medicinal plants
		Mint leaves:
	20.00	Crude or not manufactured
	40.00	*Others:*
	40.20	• Herbal teas and herbal infusions (single species, unmixed)
	40.40	• Others
	60.00	• Tonka beans
	80.00	• Other substances having anaesthetic, prophylactic or therapeutic properties and principally used as medicaments or as ingredients in medicaments:
	80.10	• Coca leaves
	20	• Psyllium seed husk
	30	• Others
	40	• Basil
	50	• Sage

Hong Kong, Germany, Japan & Singapore are the highest **importing countries** in medicinal plants trade with estimated share of 18.3, 12.5, 10.2 and 8.4% respectively of the total import of medicinal plants. These countries either use the plant materials for their own traditional medicine or re-export them after value addition. As per the literature survey reports **Germany, Bulgaria and Poland** are having the largest market in the world for **herbal medicines** with the annual sale about US$ 1.2 billion representing nearly 25% of the national pharmaceutical market. The botanical retail market inclusive of herbs and medicinal plants in USA has total sales estimated at approximately US$ 1.7 billion annually.

The **world trade** of medicinal plants is estimated to be **US$ 62 billion** with the major share of European Union as 45%, Asia 10.8% and Japan 9.8%. **India's** share in the global export market is just 0.5%.

The world production of the **essential oils** is dominated by **Brazil** (40%), **USA** (20%) and **India** (15%) but when compared for the quality it is highest for USA (26%), followed by India (21%) and Brazil (8%). But on the other hand, India's share in world export of essential oils and perfumery materials is merely 0.4%. This situation exposes our position on the front of value addition. The plants cultivated for essential oils production in India are mainly of *Mentha* spp., *Cymbopogon* spp., *Ocimum* spp., *Pelargonium graveolens*, *Tagetes species*, *Vetiveria zizanioides* and *Rosa* spp. In recent years the essential oil of *Lavandula officinalis*, *Pelargonium graveolens* and *Pogostemon patchouli* are imported.

Among the importers of drug, **Hong Kong is at the top** with import volume around 77,250 tonnes (US$ 133.7 million) followed by Japan with approximate volume of 43,500 tonnes (US$ 114.5 million), Germany with 42,800 tonnes (US$ 96.25 million) and USA with 35,000 tonnes (US$ 96.25 million). These assessments of international trade in medicinal plants include plants and their parts like roots, tubers, wood, bark, leaves, flowers, fruits and seeds.

In view of the phenomenal increase in demand of herbal drugs, the concerned medicinal plants have been indiscriminately over exploited leading to scarcity or endangerment of many valuable plant species. In India more than 90% plant species used by the industry are collected from wild and over 60% of the collection involve destructive harvesting. According to an estimate over half a million tonnes of the raw materials are indiscriminately collected from the wild, mostly following destructive harvesting procedure and thus about 165,700 hectares forest being clear-felled each year. Hence, alarming situations have resulted into short supply, high prices, forced import, or substitution and adulteration of crude drugs.

Convention on International Trade in Endangered Species (CITES) of wild fauna and flora already has been notified by over 130 countries, which regulate the International trade of the threatened species. Following Indian medicinal plants are included in the appendices of CITES.

Saussurea costus, Aquilaria malacensis, Dioscorea deltoidea, Rauwolfia serpentina, Cibotium baromtez, Podophyllum hexandrum, Pterocarpus santalinus, Nardostachys grandiflora, Picrorhiza kurroa and *Taxus wallichiana.*

Following is the list of threatened (endangered) medicinal plants not included in the appendices of CITES (Table 2.3).

In India first official step to regulate trade in endangered medicinal plant species by Govt. of India was taken in the year 1994 [vide public notice 47 (PN) 92–97 dated 30th March 1994] by which around 56 medicinal plants entities were banned for export purpose. Under this law no one is allowed to export the drug in original form but only derived products permitted to be exported.

Table 2.3. Endangered Medicinal Plants of India

Aconitum spp.	*Gastrochilus longiflora*
Adhatoda beddomei C.B. Clarke	*Gentiana kurroa* Royle
Angelica glauca Edgew	*Ilex khasiana*
Aquilaria malaccensis Lam.	*Inula racemosa* Hook.
Arnebia benthamii (Wall. ex G. Don) Johnston	*Luvunga scandens* (Roxb.) Buch.-Ham. ex Wight
Aristolochia bracteolate Lam.	*Meconopsis aculeata* Royle
Atropa acuminata Royle ex Lindl.	*Nardostachys grandiflora* DC.
Berberis spp.	*Nepenthes khasiana* Hook.
Chlorophytum spp.	*Nothapodytes nimmoniana* (J. Graham) Mabb.
Colchicum luteum Baker	(= *Nothapodytes foetida* (Wight) Sleumer)
Commiphora wightii (Arn.) Bhandari	*Panax pseudoginseng* Wall.
[= *C. mukul* (Hook. ex Stocks) Engl.]	*Przewalskia tangutica* Maxim.
Coptis teeta Wall.	*Picrorhiza kurroa* Royle ex Benth.
Crateriostigma plantagineum Hochst.	*Podophyllum hexandrum* Royle
Curcuma caesia Roxb.	*Rauwolfia serpentina* Benth. ex Kurz.
Dactylorhiza hatagirea D. Don	*Saussurea gossypiphora* D. Don
Dioscorea deltoidea Wall. ex Griseb.	*Swertia chirayita* (Roxb. ex Fleming) H. Karst.
Ephedra gerardiana Wall. ex Stapf	(= *S. Chirata* (Wall.) C.B. Clarke
Ferula jaeschkeana Vatke	*Taxus wallichiana* Zucc.
Fritilaria roylei Hook.	*Valeriana jatamansi* Jones

MAJOR IMPORTING-EXPORTING REGIONS AND COUNTRIES

Major Importing Regions and Countries

Europe, USA and Japan are the biggest **consumer markets** of medicinal plant materials. Europe, Germany, France, Italy and Spain are the major markets for medicinal herbs. Germany dominates the European trade in medicinal plants as it dominates the European market for phytopharmaceuticals. During 1991–1997 about 46,000 metric tonnes of botanicals were imported annually from more than hundred countries into Germany, amounting to about US$ 142 million. One-third of the material was re-exported as finished products primarily to Western Europe and USA.

In North America, USA is an important market for medicinal plants. In 1988, the annual turnover of the plant-derived pharmaceutical industry in the USA was US$ 10 billion. The herbal product industries in 1994 was US$ 1.6 billion at retail sales. In the US market the health products are the fastest growing sector and demand for medicinal plant material is significantly high. The major part of the material is sourced from Europe (Eastern Europe) and Asia. Over the last decade, the demand in North America for medicinal plants from Latin America, China and India has increased significantly.

The major importers of medicinal plants in Asia are Hong Kong, Japan, Singapore and Malaysia. The volumes of material used in the traditional systems of medicine, particularly in Asia are of great concern while considering the demand for medicinal plants. China also imports significant volumes of medicinal herbs apart from being largest producer and exporter of medicinal herbs.

Hong Kong, Japan, USA and Germany were the major importers of this commodity with annual average import volumes about 74,000; 57,000; 51,000–72,000 and 46,000 metric tonnes respec-

tively during 1991–1997. Among others, the leading importers are Republic of Korea, France, Pakistan, Italy, Singapore, China, UK and Spain.

Major Exporting Regions and Countries

The trade in medicinal plants not only takes place from developing to urban industrialized countries, but also among developing countries. For instance, there is a major trade from the Himalayas, including Nepal to India and beyond, mostly for use in herbal medicine (notably Ayurvedic medicine). The volume of this trade is unknown, because it is believed that the greater part of it passes through unofficial channels. Among developing countries China is the leading exporter of plant drugs having exported an average about 140,000 metric tonnes during 1991–1998. India is the second largest exporter and has exported on an average about 1/4th of the volume exported by China during the same period.

Among the major exporting countries, top twelve are :

- Germany,
- Singapore,
- Egypt,
- Chile,
- USA,
- Morocco,
- Mexico,
- Pakistan,
- France,
- Thailand,
- Singapore, and
- Hong Kong

Singapore & Hong Kong are the main reexporters of medicinal plants to the world market.

China's total output of medicinal plants from both cultivated and wild harvested sources was estimated to about 1.6 million metric tonnes. In comparison, Germany produces relatively small volume of 40,000 metric tonnes. Ayurvedic and Unani herbs are also traded in large quantities and over a very wide geographical area. For example in 1992, estimated 4,117 metric tonnes were exported, largely to Bangladesh, Japan, Pakistan, Saudi Arabia, US and United Arab Emirates.

WORLDWIDE TRADE OF THE SPECIFIC DRUGS (As Per AICTE Syllabus)

LIQUORICE

Liquorice of medicine and commerce is derived from sweet roots of various species of *glycyrrhiza*, a genus which contains about twenty species, among them five are confined to Europe and others are native of South-East Europe and South-West Asia as far as Persia. Liquorice extract was known in times of Dioscorides and appears to have been in common use in Germany during middle ages.

A widely used species is *Glycyrrhiza glabra*, a herbaceous, perennial, native to the Mediterranean region, the near East, Central Asia, as well as western Siberia. Among other highly exported species are *G. uralensis* is native to western to Eastern Siberia, as well as across Central Asia to Mongolia; *G. echinata* are grown in an area extending from the Balkanes across Asia minor to South-Eastern Russia and Western Siberia; and *G. pallidiflora* native to the Far East and China.

Its cultivation is done in Italy, Southern France & Spain and also in Central Asia, Australia and Brazil but the widely growing liquorice also continued to be exploited to a large extent.

Until 1870 Spain produced practically the entire world supply of Liquorice. As per the Internatio-

nal Trade Centre information during 1994–1997, USA was the leading importer of Liquorice roots with annual average **import volume of about 17,887 metric tonnes**, valuing to about US$ 10.5 million. The main source countries were China, Afghanistan, Pakistan, Azerbaijan and Turkmenistan. In 1996 European countries imported 6000 metric tonnes of roots, almost all from Asia. Main source countries were Azerbaijan, Turkmenistan, Afghanistan, Iran and Pakistan. Afghanistan exports liquorice roots mainly to the USA, Japan, France and India with an Annual export value of US$ 4.2 million. The Europe exports of liquorice roots amounted to 2,700 metric tonnes only, more or less evenly directed to North America, Africa and Asia. France dominates the import trade in Europe.

As per the information from trade sources, **Turkey is the biggest exporter of liquorice**. About 3,040 metric tonnes was exported in 1991; 1,684 in 1992, 1,350 in 1993; 1,140 in 1994; 1,560 in 1995 and 1,730 metric tonnes in 1996. In addition to the liquorice roots, Turkey also exports liquorice extracts to USA, Egypt, Italy, France and Israel.

Spain also exports liquorice but the quantities involved are much less. It is mainly obtained from wild stock and also from cultivation.

GINSENG
(*Panax ginseng*)

Ginseng obtained from the roots of *Panax ginseng* (Araliaceae) and has honoured place in Chinese medicine for the last 2000 year.

Ginseng is of two types:

- White ginseng, and
- Red ginseng.

White Ginseng

It is prepared by removing the outer layers, followed by drying in sun.

Red Ginseng

It is obtained by first steaming the root, followed by artificial drying and then sun drying.

Grading

Roots are graded on the basis of size and quality of drying, the best quality are wrapped in silk followed by cotton and paper. The wrapped drug is stored in container containing quicklime.

Geographical Distribution

It is produced in China, Korea and Siberia. The drug ginseng in considerable quantities are also derived from *P. quinquefolium* and exported from USA and Canada through Hong Kong.

Ginseng contains mixture of both **steroidal and pentacyclic** triterpenoid saponins. This drug is used for the treatment of general anaemia, diabetes, gastritis, sexual impotence and for general ailments which arise with the onset of old age and in recent the drug has become popular remedy particularly for the improvement of stamina, concentration, resistance to stress and disease (adaptogenic).

Ginseng products are available as OTC products either for oral administration or for cosmetic preparations in the US market. Ginseng has gained third position in Herbal sale, with the retail sale more than US$ 60 million in the year 1999–2000.

The annual **world trade** in ginseng roots is in between 3,500–4,100 metric tonnes. **Major exporter is China followed by Korea, USA, Canada and Japan**. More than 60% of the world production of ginseng is produced in Canada from cultivation of American ginseng roots (*Panax quinquefolium*) and it exports almost 90% of its production to overseas.

The USA is the second largest producer of American ginseng and fourth in the terms of all ginseng supply It represents about 30 percent of total American ginseng production.

Hong Kong is the major importer of American ginseng. About 84% of all American ginseng is imported from Canada. China and USA were the second and third at 10% and 2% respectively. In 1998, about 1,299 metric tonnes of ginseng roots were imported from Canada. More than 80% of the **American ginseng** is re-exported to China from Hong Kong, thus the China is the ultimate user of American ginseng. Other markets for American ginseng are Singapore, Taiwan, Malaysia and the member countries of the Association of Southeast Asia Nations (ASEAN).

The USA also imports good quality of wild ginseng. On the basis of information available about the world trade in ginseng, USA importation values during 1990–1996 were 208 metric tonnes of wild ginseng from China; 59 metric tonnes from South Korea, 34 metric tonnes from Mexico and 19 metric tonnes from other countries including Canada. *P. quinquefolia* or another ginseng species export from the USA or elsewhere to Canada for processing and subsequently exported to USA is prohibited.

The amount of wild American ginseng, harvested and exported has remained almost constant as the wild crafted ginseng fetches higher price. Wild crafted ginseng, being considered to be of superior quality in comparison to cultivated ginseng. According to the United States Fish & Wild Life Services (USFWS) in 1996, about 64 metric tonnes of wild ginseng was harvested in the USA. Out of which 46 metric tonnes was exported to Hong Kong and smaller amount was exported to Taiwan (3.6 metric tonnes), Singapore (2.7 metric tonnes), Malaysia (769 kg) and Canada (459 kg).

It is among the major botanical drugs of US foreign trade. It is cultivated in North Central Wisconsin and about 90% of the US cultivated drug is produced and supplied by Wisconsin.

England (Biggleswade), Holland, Germany and France (Champagne Distt.) have also started cultivation of commercial quantity of ginseng but on small scale.

Best quality and expensive one is obtained from Korean roots.

DIOSGENIN

Diosgenin is the major raw material used in the synthesis of corticosteroids, sex hormones and anti-fertility compounds. Out of the steroid drug precursors diosgenin accounts for 60% of the total steroidal product of the world. Present world requirement of steroidal drug for pharmaceuticals in terms of diosgenin is huge, equivalent to about 10,000 tonnes of dioscorea tubers per annum. It is estimated that about 60% of all steroidal drugs are derived from diosgenin. Much of the **world's production** has come from **Mexico**, where tubers of *D. composita* (barbassco), *D. mexicana* and *D. floribunda* mainly harvested from wild plants are utilized.

The total annual requirement of diosgenin by pharmaceutical industries of our country is about 450 tonnes, while the total production of diosgenin in India is about 100 tonnes, the rest of the requirement is met through import in the form of diosgenin and drug intermediates. The synthesis of diosgenin is not being commercially feasible for the production of steroidal drug and hence the pharmaceutical industry has to resort to natural source for the procurement of this raw material as the present rate of dioscorea tubers in Indian market is Rs. 10/kg and diosgenin content varies from 3.8–4.6% at the time of sprouting and 3.8% at the flowering stage and 4.0% during the fruiting stage. Tubers weigh anything up to 5 kg and some species tubers have been recorded to reach weights as high as 40–50 kg.

PLANTS CONTAINING LAXATIVE

Plant laxatives and purgatives may be classified according to their mode of action.

1. *Agar, psyllium and ispaghula :* Hydrophilic colloids which function as bulk producing laxatives.
2. *Bran :* An indigenous vegetable fibre which absorbs water and provides bulk.
3. *Senna leaves and fruit :* Contains anthraquinone derivatives which is hydrolysed in the bowel to stimulate Auerbach's plexus in the wall.
4. *Cascara, rhubarb, aloe* – as senna.
5. *Castor oil :* Contains glycosides which on hydrolysis yields ricinoleic acid, irritant to the small intestine.

Constipation is a common problem of Western and European countries because of protein rich diet. On an average, India exports 15000 tonnes of **Plantago**; 10,000 tonnes of **Senna** and 5000 tonnes of **Rhubarb** annually. Trade in plant laxative increases by over 8–10% every year. **India is the sole supplier of** *Plantago ovata* **seeds and husk (Psyllium) in the International market.**

AGAR

It is the dried colloidal concentrate from the decoction of various red algae (*Gelidium pterocladia* species, both belonging to Gelidiaceae, order Gelidiales) and Gracilaria (Gracilariaceae order Gigartinales). Agar is obtained from Japan (*Gelidium amansii*), Korea, South Africa, both Pacific and Atlantic Coasts of USA, Chile, Spain and Portugal. About 6800 tonnes are produced annually of which 1/3rd world supply of Agar is produced by Japan. The genus Gelidium provide about 35–40% of the total world supply.

PSYLLIUM (flea seed)

Psyllium is the dried, ripe seeds of *Plantago afra* (*P. psyllium*) *P. indica* (*P. arenaria*) and *P. ovata* (Plantaginaceae) used in medicine. National formulary includes all three species under the name Plantago seed. The BP describes seeds of *Plantago afra* and *P. indica* under the name (title) Psyllium and the husk of *P. ovata* seeds are included under the name of Ispaghula husk.

The seeds of *Plantago afra* and *Plantago indica* are known in commerce as Spanish or French psyllium. The seed of *Plantago ovata* are known as blonc psyllium, ispaghula.

The seeds are used for laxative purposes due to the mucilage contents present in the epidermis of the testa.

As per the information available on the International trade in medicinal plant, it is reported that during 2001-02, India exported about 20,000 tonnes of psyllium husk and 5000 tonnes of seed, valued in Indian Rupees about 1620.28 million and about 165.20 million, respectively.

BRAN

Bran consists of the coarse outer coat or hull of wheat grain, *Triticum aestivum* Linn. (Gramineae) technically it comprises the pericarp, the inte);guments and the nucleus of the seed.

Bran contains about 26.7% of dietary fibre. The therapeutic value of bran (crude fibre) is in the treatment of certain gastrointestinal disorders, such as constipation, appendicitis and haemorrhoids and is also recommended as preventive measure for cardiovascular disorders.

World supply of the bran is made by USA, Australia, China and India.

SENNA

The commercial drug consists of dried, green leaves and shells of nearly dried and ripe pods of *Cassia acutifolia* Delile and *Cassia angustifolia* vahl, belonging to Leguminosae.

It is a well known drug in the Unani system of medicine and has been included in I.P., U.S.P.

and B.P. as a purgative. The drug from India is known as **Tinnevelly senna** and that from Arabian countries is known as **Alexandrian senna**. Presently it is used both in the Ayurvedic and Allopathic systems of medicine and is also a household medicine.

Senna is an erect shrub, upto 1.8 m in height, highly drought resistant and may be suitable for desert. It is largely cultivated on a marginal land in 10,000 hectare both as rain-fed and irrigated crop, mainly in Tamil Nadu (Tirunelvelli, Ramanathapuram, Tiruchchirapalli and Madurai District and to a lesser extent in Salem District). It is also cultivated in Andhra Pradesh, Karnataka and Maharashtra. It is also found occuring wild in Cuddapath District of Andhra Pradesh and Bhuj District of Gujarat. Trials conducted at Jammu, Rajasthan and Delhi have given encouraging results of cultivation.

The leaves, pods and roots contain rhein, chrysophanol, emodin and aloe-emodin. Two active anthraquinones, sennosides A and B (optical isomers) have been isolated from leaves and pods. Besides these sennosides presence of sennosides C, D and G has also been reported.

The chief **centres of trade** in India are Tuticonin, Madurai, Mumbai and Calcutta. **India is the major supplier of the leaves and pods as well as the glycosides to the world market**. Approximately 75% of senna product in India is exported. The most important markets are Germany, Japan, Zechoslovakia, USA, Hong Kong, Spain, Italy, France and United Arab Emirates. In 1987-88, India had exported about 6000 tonnes valued about 35 lakh rupees. Presently, India export is more than 10,000 tonnes of drug @ Rs.50.00 per kg.

CASCARA BARK
[Cascara sagrada (sacred bark)]

Cascara is the dried bark of *Rhamnus purshi-*

anus DC (Frangula purshiana DC) A. Gray. ex. J.C. Cooper (Rhamnaceae).

It is collected from wild tree 6–18 m high, growing on the pacific coast of North America (British Columbia, Washington & Oregon). **Although cultivation is started in Western Canada, USA and Kenya but not of much success.**

The bark is collected in the month of April to the end of August by giving longitudinal incision about 5–10 cm apart on the trunk of the tree and dried in shade. But for the commercial supply, the bark is cut into small uniform fragment and dried in shade. The medicinal bark should be one year old although it is no longer BP requirement but even then, it appears to increase in medicinal value and price on storage for about 4 years (due to hydrolysis or other changes, which make the drug more tolerable). It improves the quality of the bark.

Cascara contains about 6–9% anthracene derivatives, which are present both as normal O-glycosides and as C-glycosides (cascarosides A, B, C and D) in addition to these primary glycosides it also contain aloin but it is reported that cascarosides (primary glycosides) are more active, where as free anthraquinone and dimers have little purgative activity. The cascarosides have sweet and more pleasant taste than the aloin.

Cascara bark is used as purgative like senna in action, in the form of liquid extract or elixir or as tablet prepared from a dry extract.

In these days anthracene derivative (emodin) is significantly produced by cell suspension culture from *Rhamnus purshianus* by having 12 hours light/dark cycle, illumination set up in the laboratory.

RHUBARB

Rhubarb (Chinese Rhubarb) is the dried underground parts of *Rheum palmatum* L. (Polygo-

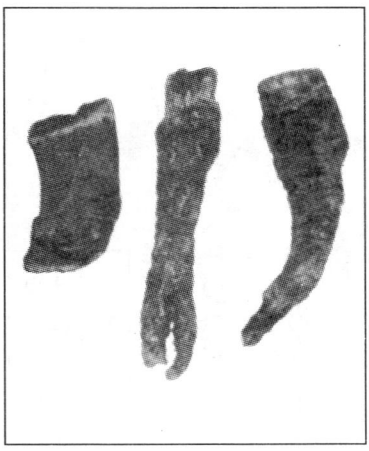

RHUBARB *(Rheum officinalis)*
(for colour, see Plate 1, Fig. 1)

naceae) or *R. officinalis* or hybrids of these species or mixture of these.

The drug is obtained both from wild and cultivated trees grown in high plateaus of Asia from Tibet to South-East China.

The drug contains anthraquinone (e.g. chrysophanol, aloe emodin, emodin, rhein and glucorhein).

This drug is not fit to be used for chronic constipation as it causes purgation followed by an astringent effect.

ALOE

Aloe vera is used as a natural laxative (helps to produce easier bowel movements). The total world business of aloe is estimated to be US$ 214 million for which **India is the pivotal** and major supplier. Indian market rate for aloe leaves is Rs. 30/kg to 35/kg.

RAUWOLFIA

Rauwolfia drug consists of air dried roots of *R. serpentina* L. (Apocyanaceae). The roots are stout upto 40–45 cms long, 2–2.5 cms in diameter, tortuous; surface slightly wrinkled, rough and coarse with longitudinal marks; sometimes

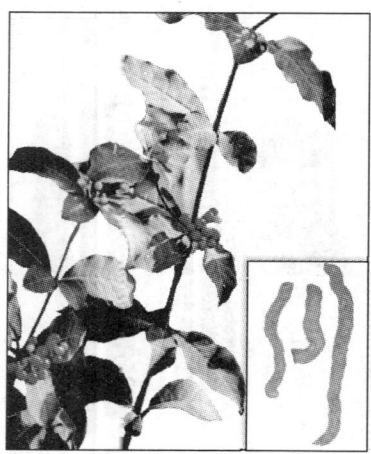

RAUWOLFIA (*R. serpentina*)
(for colour, see Plate 1, Fig. 2)

branched; fracture short and irregular. The roots are odourless and very bitter. *Rauwolfia* is official in Indian Pharmacopoeia (I.P.), as per the I.P. standards the roots should be collected from 3 to 4 years old plants; they should contain alkaloids 0.8%; and foreign matter 2.0%. As per British Pharmaceutical Codex reserpine (alkaloid) content should not be less than 0.15 percent. Besides the root, its liquid extract, the dried extract and tincture are official in Indian Pharmacopoeia.

Rauwolfia belong to a large genus of shrubs or under shrubs or occasionally tree distributed in tropical Asia, Africa and America. Five species are recorded in India, of these *R. serpentina* has become well known as a medicinal plant.

For centuries the drug *Rauwolfia* has been used in Ayurvedic system of medicine in India. But since last decade, the major alkaloid reserpine has been recognized in the allopathic system of medicine, in the treatment of hypertension and as tranquillizer. Major part of the commercial supply of the drug is used in USA and European countries **supplied from India, Pakistan, Ceylon, Burma and Thailand.** Major supplier of the *Rauwolfia serpentina* is India, which holds almost **a world monopoly**, has been threatened with over exploitation of wild resources of the plant. The

Government of India had now imposed ban on the export of crude drug, in order to conserve the natural growth from indiscriminate exploitation. This step resulted in an immediate shortage of *R. serpentina* rhizome and roots in the world market. Other species, which are being used as substitute possible source of reserpine are : *R. tetraphylla* in America and *R. vomitoria* in Africa.

Rauwolfia serpentina is an erect, evergreen perennial under shrub 15-45 cms high; with tuberous soft tap roots; bark is pale brown corky with irregular longitudinal fissures; leaves in whorls of three, large (7.5–17.5 cm × 4.4–6.6 cm) elliptic lanceolate or obovate, acute or acuminate dark green above, pale green below; flowers, white or pinkish cyme inflorescence; fruits drupe, obliquely ovoid, purplish black.

It is widely distributed in the sub-Himalayan tract from Punjab eastward to Nepal, Sikkim and Bhutan, in Assam, in the lower hills of gigantic Eastern and Western ghat and in some of the parts of Central India. Although *R. serpentina* is widely distributed; but its occurrence is sporadic. The growth of the plants is scattered. **The commercial supply from India is available from the states of Uttar Pradesh, Tamil Nadu, Kerala, Karnataka and Maharashtra.**

Reliable data on exact quantity of *Rauwolfia* roots **exported** from different states of India or quantity of drug being consumed by pharmaceutical industries is not available. Whatever information is available, they all are only approximate estimates. The areas and the annual output known are – Vishakhapatnam 20–22 tonnes; Assam 400-500 tonnes, Buxa and Cooch-Bihar in West-Bengal 80–100 tonnes; East Bartar and Bindrawagarh in Madhya Pradesh 5–10 tonnes, from other areas drug is not available for commercial purposes.

The roots are usually marketed (@ Rs.100.00/ kg) under the names of their origin and are designated as Assam, Bengal, Bihar, Dehradun, Himalayas, Coastal plain, Malabar and Ceylon types. Only small fraction of drug is consumed by the Indian pharmaceutical firms and the remaining part is exported. The important places for marketing are Delhi, Amritsar, Saharanpur, Calcutta and Mumbai. Major part of the drug exported from India is to Europe, U.S.A., Japan and Germany.

The supplies in recent years have fallen short of demand due to the restriction imposed by the Government of India. Hence, *Rauwolfia* alkaloids are exported annually instead of roots.

Rauwolfia vomitoria Afzel (African snake root) is in the list of International Trade of African Medicinal Plants.

DIGITALIS (Foxglove leaves)

Digitalis consists of the dried leaves of *Digitalis purpurea* and *Digitalis lanata* (Scrophulariaceae).

D. *purpurea* is commonly found in England and produced commercially in Holland. *D. lanata* is indigenous to Central and South-Eastern Europe. It is also cultivated in Holland, Eucador and USA.

The glycosides of digitalis (Cardenolide group) mainly act on the cardiovascular system increasing the excitability of cardiac muscle. As per the survey reports from trade sources most of the digitalis glycosides originate from European countries mainly the Federal Republic of Germany and Switzerland and they export throughout the world. The total volume of **World trade** in Digitalis is estimated to 1000 tonnes per annum. An average of 22.4 million prescription prescribed digitalis for heart failure patients per annum with digoxin being used are 40.8 million prescriptions in 2002 in United States.

All of the requirements of digitalis glycosides for pharmaceutical industries in India come from imports. During 1978–79, about 33 kg of digoxin worth Rs. 1,25,500 was imported into India from UK but in the year 1981–82 report indicated that

only 1 kg of Digoxin worth Rs. 17,267 was imported from France. Although India imported the crude drug in earlier days but now India is self sufficient for the supply of pharmaceutical industry and even India is in the position **to export crude** drug to Australia, Saudi Arabia, Canada, Kenya, Oman, Sri Lanka. India exported 10,993, 13,267 and 2,000 kg of drug valued at Rs. 1,84,837, 2,37,605 and 52,936 during 1988–89, 1990–91 and 1992–93 respectively.

Prospectus for cultivation and trade of digitalis in developing countries is limited as sufficient supplies are not available. However, it can be grown in developing countries for internal demand, as it is an essential drug.

No real competition to natural digitalis glycosides is yet available in the world market.

PODOPHYLLUM (Podophyllum/resin)

Podophyllum (Podophyllum rhizome, May-apple root, wild mandrake).

It consists of the dried root and rhizome of *Podophyllum peltatum* (Berberidaceae), a perennial herb common in moist shady places in Virginia, North Casolina, Tennessee and Indiana.

Indian Podophyllum

It consists of dried rhizome and root of *Podophyllum hexandrum* Syn. *P. emodi* (Berberidaceae) a perennial herb found in Tibe*, Afghanistan and the Himalayan area of Pak;stan and India. In India, it is found in the inner range of Himalaya from Kashmir to Sikkim, at altitude of 3000 to 4,500 m. Indian podophyllum is classified into three or four varieties, viz. var. *hexandrum*, var. *axillaris*; var. *bhootanesis* and var. *jaesehbei*.

The rhizome and roots of the plant are obtained

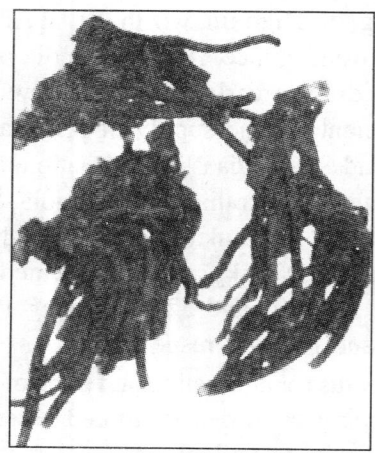

PODOPHYLLUM (*P. hexandrum*)
(for colour, see Plate 1, Fig. 2.3)

from wild source growing throughout the Himalaya, especially from the Central Himalaya.

Rhizome is irregular tortuous, knotty, about 2–5 cm, long and 1.2 cm thick some what flattened dorsiventrally; upper surface is characterized by the presence of 3 or 4 cm shaped scars; colour is externally yellowish brown to earthy brown with characteristic odour and taste is somewhat bitter and acrid.

The dried rhizome and root of *P. hexandrum* (Indian podophyllum) are official in I.P. and form the source of medicinal resin. According to B.P.C., the roots form a large proportion of Indian drug and are mainly detached from the rhizome. The official podophyllum contains not less than 8% resin, commonly used as a purgative but in recent years, the resin podophyllin and its active principle, podophyllotoxin, have received considerable attention for their antitumor nercotizing properties. The percentage of active principle (podophyllotoxin) is lower in concentration, i.e. resin (2–8%). It contains about half the amount of podophyllotoxin as that of Indian podophyllum.

Podophyllin is an amorphous powder, light brown to greenish yellow or brownish grey colour, with a characteristic odour and bitter and acrid taste. On exposure to light or temperature above 25°C, it becomes darker in colour. It is considered to be cholagogue, purgative alterative, emetic and a bitter tonic. It is drastic but slowly acting purgative producing copious watery stools; it may cause much griping and therefore given in conjunction with belladonna and hyoscyamus. It can also be used in cytological work like colchicine. It is also used in veterinary medicine as cathartic for dogs and cats. Podophyllin ointment is used in animals to remove warts. During recent years, podophyllin had acquired special importance for the possible use in controlling some forms of cancer.

Podophyllotoxin and α and β-pelatins have high potency in inducing damage in sarcoma 37 and in variety of other tumours including adenocarcinoma, carcinoma and melanoma.

The rhizome and roots of the plant have been suggested as a source for the preparation of quercetin.

Major part of the Indian drug is obtained from wildly growing plant, particularly in Jammu and Kahmir, Himachal Pradesh and part of Uttar Pradesh. Its collection is very difficult from high altitude; hence the cost of collection is very high while the American podophyllum is available at cheaper rate. Moreover the Indian podophyllum samples are not uniform in quality because of variation in elevation, climatic conditions and collection done by unskilled workers. The annual supply is not sufficient enough to meet the requirement of pharmaceutical industry and there is a fear of further depletion in the natural growth being slow regeneration of the herb. Steps are being taken to cultivate the plant in suitable places under forestry conditions to assure more sustained supply of uniform quality material. Most of the **world supply** is obtained from *Podophyllum peltatum* supplied by North Carolina and Indiana.

CINCHONA

Cinchona bark is obtained as dried stem bark in the form of quills from different species of Cinchona *C. succirubra*; *C. calisaya*, *C. ledgeriana* and *C. officinalis* or their hybrids (Rubiaceae). The cinchona trees are indigenous to Columbia, Ecuador, Peru and Bolivia. The former importance of cinchona bark and its alkaloids in the treatment of malaria has been lessened by the introduction of synthetic drugs, but it remains of great economic importance and salts of quinine and quinidine are included in most of the pharmacopoeia. At the time of Second World War, cinchona had great importance in the world trade, being the only source for anti-malarial quinine and related alkaloids. At that time 95% of world quinine supply came from **Java**. At present 90% of total cinchona bark is produced in **Indonesia, Zaire, United Republic of Tanzania, Burundi, India, Kenya, Guatemala, Peru, Ecuador, Bolivia, Rwanda, Sri Lanka, Columbia and Costa Rica**. World production of quinine has fallen considerably since 1950 due to the competition from synthetic drugs. Annual world production of quinine and its alkaloids is estimated about 850 tonnes. India produces only 15–20 tonnes annually. Besides inland trade, quinine salts are also **exported** to Italy, UK, Germany and USSR (Table 2.4). The price of Cinchona bark in Indian market is Rs. 65/kg and of quinine sulphate USP – Rs. 2700/kg. Quinine sulphate NF – Rs. 4000/kg and quinine hydrochloride NF – Rs. 3000/kg.

TROPANE ALKALOIDS

Plants of the Family Solanaceae produce tropane alkaloids. The plants are Henbane, (*Hyoscyamus niger*), Thorn apple (Datura spp. *Datura stramonium*), deadly nightshade (*Atropa belladonna*).

Tropane alkaloids also occur in Erythroxylaceae and Convolvulaceae.

The principle alkaloids of medicinal importance in this group are (–) hyoscyamine, its more stable racemic form are atropine and hyoscine (scopolamine).

Leaves of *Duboisia myoporoides* (Solanaceae) contains 2–4% of total alkaloids with about 60% hyoscine and 30% hyoscyamine and are the main source of tropane alkaloids in the world. Duboisia sp. have considerable prospects for replacing or at least supplementing Atropa, Datura and Hyoscyamus; as source of hyoscine and hyoscyamine which is used throughout the world extensively in medicine. **Commercial cultivation** of *Duboisia* is done only in Australia, mainly in Queensland area, from where it is exported to European countries for further processing and export to USA. The total **world trade** in tropane alkaloid is estimated to be of 580 tonnes the **major supplier** is Australia through Europe and next is the Egypt. New York market price of scopolamine hydrobromide USP is Rs. 46000/kg.

Table 2.4. Export of Cinchona Alkaloids (Qty in Kg; Val in Rs.)

	1983–84		1984–85		1985–86		1986–87		2001-02	
	Qty	Val	Qty	Val	Qty	Val	Qty	Val	Qty	Val
Quinine sulphate	700	1,110,840	–	–	1,060	1,046,291	2,638	2,089,198	4,600	115,00,000
Quinine hydro-chloride	5,303	5,656,327	500	227,000	4,600	21,152,901	7,450	371,289	17,880	75,096,000
Other derivatives of Quinine	600	264,550	–	–	170	132,845	–	–	–	–

TAXOL

The anti-cancer drug taxol extracted from the bark of the 100 year old Pacific Yew, *Taxus brevifolia* (Taxaceae), a slow growing shrub/tree found in the forests of North-West Canada (British Columbia) and the USA (Washington, Oregon, Montana, Idaho and North California). The drug was approved by the FDA for the treatment of refractory ovarian cancer in December 1992 and was introduced in the world market in January 1993 by Bristol-Myer's Squibb Company (BMS) operating under a Corporation Research and Development Agreement (CRADA) with National Cancer Institute (NCI). It was approved for treatment of breast cancer in 1994 and now it is in transition from second line to first line therapy.

The bark from about three matured (100 year-old) trees is required to provide one gram of taxol and a course of treatment may need 2 grams of the drug. Current demand for taxol is in the range of 100–200 kg per annum. The worldwide trade of taxol reached to US$ 1.92 billion in 2002.

Taxol® was registered as a trademark. Accordingly, the generic name Paclitaxel has been assigned to the compound.

In **India** *Taxus wallichiana* is found in Khasia

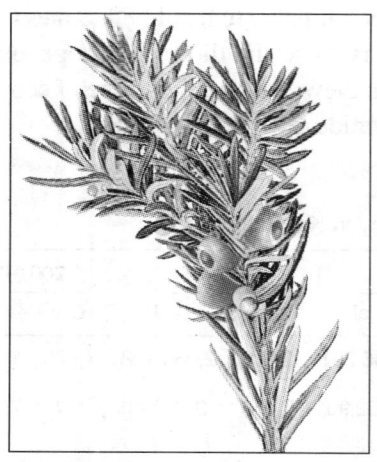

TAXUS *(T. wallichiana)*
(for colour, see Plate 1, Fig. 4)

hills and Himalayas above the height of 5000 feet in Sikkim, Meghalaya and Manipur.

PAPAIN

Papain is a protein-cleaving enzyme derived from Papaya latex. *Carica papaya* latex (Cucurbitaceae) native of **Tropical America, perhaps in Southern Mexico and neighbouring Central America.** At present it is cultivated practically all over the tropical and subtropical countries of the world particularly in Sri Lanka, India, Philippines, East and Equatorial Africa, South America and West Indies.

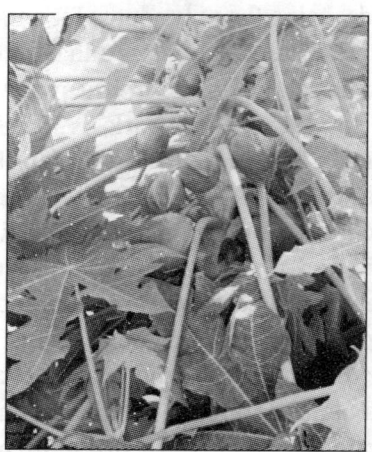

PAPAIN *(Carica papaya)*
(for colour, see Plate 1, Fig. 5)

Papain is a significant export item for Tanzania, Uganda, Zaire, Sri Lanka, Thailand and India. Japan imports the raw papain latex and treats it with potassium metabisulfate to make it in powder form and then exports. Zaire was the principal producer and exporter of papain in the world in 1971–1973.

The East African Countries Kenya, Uganda and Tanzania have been the major source of supply of papain to the world market for the past several years particularly Uganda.

The principal importing countries of Papain are

USA, Japan, Belgium, UK and France other importing countries include West Germany, Denmark, Sweden, Italy and Spain. It is reported that almost all the best quality of papain finds its way eventually to United States where it is refined and formulated into papain formulation/preparation. These formulations are used domestically in United States or re-exported to all over the world. During last decade the US bought about 15.6 to 20 thousand metric tonnes per annum of papain, which was about 232 million dollars annually.

Other major importer countries of papain are Belgium, UK and France. The main share of the Zaire exports going to Belgium.

Export of papain from India has been increased from near 212 kg in 1972–73 to 10877 kg up to 1983 followed by further increase at the rate of 10% per annum and in 1999–2000 it was 18.365 tonnes to the value of Rs. 1.5 million.

VALERIAN

Valerian consists of the rhizomes, stolons and roots of *Valeriana officinalis* L. (Valerianaceae).

It is a genus of perennial herbs or under shrubs of about 250 species occurring in India up to 1.5m in height, found in some localities in Kashmir

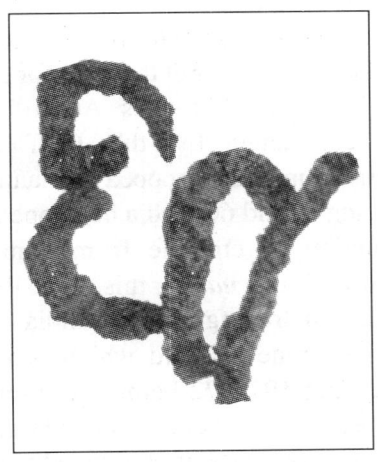

VALERIAN (*V. officinalis*)
(for colour, see Plate 1, Fig. 6)

at altitudes of 2,400–2,700m. Out of 250 species only three namely *Valeriana hardwickii*, *V. officinalis* and *V. jatamansi* or *V. wallichii* are considered important.

The dried rhizomes and roots of *V. jatamanshi* have been recognized as Indian valerian in IPC.

The herb is a native of Europe and North & South-West Asian countries. It has been grown on commercial scale for the drug valerian chiefly in several European countries. It is also cultivated in USA as ornamental plant.

Valerian grows well in all ordinary soils but prefers rich, heavy loam soil well supplied with moisture.

The drug as found in commerce consists usually of the entire or sliced erect rhizome, which is dark yellowish-brown externally, about 1 inch long, 1/2 inch thick and gives off numerous slender briffle roots from 2.5–4 inch long. Whilst short slender lateral branches (stolons) are also occasionally present. The root stock which is sometime crowned with the remains of flowering stems and leaf-scales is usually firm, horny and whitish or yellowish internally, but old specimens may be hollow.

The drug may also consists of small undeveloped rhizomes about 1/4 inch long crowned with the remains of leaves and bearing short tender roots.

The roots of valerian are of similar colour to the erect rhizome, about 1/10 inch thick striated longitudinally and usually not shriveled to any great extent.

The drug has strong and characteristic camphoraceous odour and slightly bitter taste. On drying drug develops disagreeable odour, which is due to chemical changes in the composition of volatile oil present in the drug.

The drug contains volatile oil (0.5–1.0%) present in the sub epidermal layer of cells in the root. The oil is of complex composition, chiefly consisting of valeric acid and bornyl esters of formic, acetic, butyric and isovaleric acid with small amount of pinene, camphene, terpineol two unidentified alcohols and a sesquiterpene. The drug also contains alkaloids, chatinine, valerine and pyridine bases.

It is used for the treatment of hysteria, hypochondriasis, as antispasmodic and CNS depression and other emotional states.

The oil is used as tonic and stimulant in certain medicinal preparations. It is also used in perfumery as it blends well with other oils such as lavenders methyl ionone, cedar-wood derivatives, quinoline derivatives and isocyclocitrol etc. It is also used in tobacco-flavouring and in beer or root beer flavouring.

The juice of the fresh roots is recommended as narcotic in insomnia and as an anticonvulsant in epilepsy.

Anticonvulsant effect of valerian was first reported by Fabius Calumna in 1592, as he had cured himself from the disease with it.

It is also recommended in the treatment of cardiac palpitations.

India is the **major supplier** of valerian to the world's market along with Belgium, France, the fomer U.S.S.R. and China.

Indian valerian (*V. wallichii*) is official in Pharmacopeia grows in Himalayan region.

Valeriana officinalis roots are also being exported from Poland to US Coast at the rate of US$ 2.45–2.75/kg.

IPECAC
(Cephaelis ipecacuanha)

Ipecac is derived from the dried rhizome and roots of *Cephaelis ipecacuanha* or *C. acuminata* (Rubiaceae) *Cephaelis ipecacuanha* in commerce known as Rio or Brazilian ipecac and is cultivated mainly in Brazil, whilst *C. acuminata* Karsten, known in commerce as Cartagena, Nicaragua or Panama ipecac, comes principally from Columbia and Nicaragua. Most of the commercial ipecac is now derived from *C. acuminata*. Ipecac is an age old remedy of South American Indians for the treatment of dysentery. It is also an ingredient of Dover's powder, where ipecac content functioned as diaphoretic drug containing 2.0–2.5% of alkaloids the principal ones being emetine and cephaeline.

The total production of Ipecac in the world was approx. 100 tonnes during 1991-92. The chief producing countries of *C. ipecacuanha* are Brazil (Matto Grasso) and India and of *C. acuminata* are Costa Rica, Nicaragua, Columbia and Panama. Principal suppliers to **world markets** are Nicaragua, Costa Rica and Brazil. Comparatively small quantities are exported by Columbia and Panama. **Main importing countries** are USA, West Germany, France, Switzerland, UK and Japan (Surveyed by the GATT). From this it was noted that the total exports amounted to 89 tonnes in 1970 against 61.5 in 1967 an average annual increase of 13.2%. These countries absorbed over 50% of the total export tonnages and most of the remainder going to Belgium and the Netherlands. Export of Ipecac from Nicaragua, Costa Rica and Brazil, during 1971 was 29.7 tonnes, 26.8 tonnes and 15.9 tonnes respectively with annual increase of 14%.

Imports of ipecacuanha roots into the UK, which is largest importer of this drug for the period 1961–1971 was 31.23 tonnes. According to the surveys conducted by the GATT import particularly from Brazil dropped substantially. The reason being in mid 60s India developed method of production of emetine from domestically cultivated *C. ipecacuanha*, this radically altered the traditional trading pattern. India has been exporting emetine alkaloid which had reached highest during 1971–72 being more than Rs. 7 lakh. As per the export data available from 1969–70 to 1974–75 exports of emetine alkaloids was declined due to the availability of synthetic emetine since 1968. Then number of other drugs like metronidazole, a synthetic product marketed under the name of 'Flagyl' along with some other similar preparations which had also captured 50% of Indian market in respect of amoebiasis and cough expectorant etc; thus demand for emetine salt was declined.

Since 1970 the bulk of ipecacuanha roots on the world market was of *C. acuminata*, chiefly supplied by Nicaragua and Costa Rica.

3

Indian Trade in Medicinal and Aromatic Plants

INTRODUCTION

The export of medicinal plants and herbs from India has been quite substantial for the last few years. India has a large endemic flora. There are more than 80,000 medicinal plants known and nearly 180 plant derived chemical compounds have been developed as modern pharmaceuticals, which are included in the Pharmacopoeia of India. The domestic Ayurvedic market is estimated to be US$ one billion and is growing at the rate of 15–20% annually. India has been the major supplier of medicinal plants in the world market until 1977, when it was kept to second position by South Korea with export worth only Rs. 16 crore during 1978–79. The quantum of export had dropped to almost half of the what it was in 1976–77 when India exported medicinal plants worth around Rs. 29.8 crores. The items of export value were opium, psyllium husks and seeds, Vinca rosea, kuth roots and senna leaves and pods. At present the annual trade of Indian medicinal plants is estimated to be 37,200 tonnes valued around US$ 93,540,272.00 which is expected to be increased to US$ 629,194,624.00 by 2005. During 1980s, India was the largest supplier of medicinal plants to the world market with the supply of 10,555 metric tonnes of medicinal plant

material and about 14 metric tonnes of plant derived products and their derivatives. The annual turn over was around US$ 300 million. In 1995 Psyllium husk, seeds and senna were the main export items from India. During 1998–99 India exported psyllium husk worth US$ 19.6 million and senna leaves worth. India also exported finished Ayurvedic and Unani medicine during the year 2000–01. It exported medicine worth around US$ 128 million to various countries including USA, Germany, Russia, UK, Hong Kong and Malaysia.

The global herbal industry is estimated to be US$ 50 billion annually and growing at the rate of 5.5–6.5% annually. The Indian contribution to the global industry is around at the rate of 10% only. One of the important items of export, covering approximately 80% of the world requirement, is a proteolytic enzyme, papain mainly manufactured in Maharashtra from raw papaya fruits. The commercial production of pectin from thalmus of sunflower is also carried out at Jalgaon in Maharashtra.

India is one of the few countries in the world where essential oil industry was developed at a very early stage. The essential oils, perfumes and flavours have been associated with Indian civilization for several thousand years. Because of its vast area and a variety of soil and climate, essential oil containing plants of all types can be grown in one or the other parts of the country. India produces essential oils from wild and commercially grown plants in appreciable quantities such as palmarosa, citronella, calamus, cardamom, celery seed, cedarwood, dill, ginger, lemon grass, vetiver and rose oil. The annual production of coriander is about 2,43,000 tonnes, which constitute approximately 80% of the world demand. About 30% of global demand in cardamom and 15% in saffron are met by India. The annual production of saffron is approximately 150 tonnes.

The most significant export is of the Sandalwood oil, for which country is the major producer, exporting approximately 50–60 tonnes to the world market. India is leader in the production of menthol as mentha oil steadily expanded in the last decade during the year 2000–01, India exported about 3,870 tonnes of mint oil worth **about Rs. 1.26 billion. India is also leader in the production and export of high value perfumes (attars) for the world market.**

The domestic market of Indian traditional system of medicine comprising of Ayurveda, Unani, Siddha and Homeopathy has been reported to the tune of approximately Rs. 5000 crores only and India is at present exporting herbal medicines and materials to the value of about Rs. 550 crores only. In the domestic market the Ayurvedic medicines accounts a major portions about 85% as compared to Unani, Siddha and Homeopathy system. The total patent and proprietary medicines of these systems are manufactured by over 9500 licensed pharmacies/herbal manufacturing units spread all over India.

With the development of phytochemical industry in India, domestic requirement for various medicinal plants grew considerably. Consequently the Govt. of India has adopted restrictive export policy in respect of those crude drugs which were indiscriminately exploited in the forest. Consequently the export of *Rauwolfia, Podophyllum, Indian rhubarb, Dioscorea, Kuth, Jatamansi, Atropa acuminata, Artemisia brevifolia, Berberis, Colchicum, Ephedra gerardiana, Gentiana kurroa, Picrorhiza kurroa, Swertia chirata, Valerian wallichii,* etc. However with the due permission from the Chief Conservator of Forest or officer authorized by him; the material of plantation or of nursery origin certificate, can be exported.

These medicines are mainly consumed within the country and some of these are also exported to the Middle East. Major destination countries are USA, Nepal, Japan, Sri Lanka, Russia, Germany, Italy, Nigeria and UAE and according to the survey reports, Sri Lanka, Egypt, Bangladesh and Mauritius are the countries having maximum export potential.

The major pharmaceuticals exported from India in the recent years were isabgol, vinca extract, senna derivatives, castor oil in dehydrated form, beta ionone, papain, berberine hydrochloride and opium alkaloids.

India's export of essential oil during last few years has shown the erratic trends. The sandalwood oil share is more than 50% in the total export, the USA accounted for major share of exports of this item followed by USSR. Similar position with mentha oil, the cheaper quality being exported by China. India is also exporting volatile oils to France, Japan, Sudan, Federal Republic of Germany and Switzerland. The other important items of export value are cardamom oil, lemon grass oil, palmarosa oil, pudina oil, peppermint oil, clove oil, geranium oil, Vetiver oil and Lavender oil.

Some of the medicinal plants, whose domestic and international market potential is very high, have been identified. These are:

- *Aconitum ferox* (Vatsnabh);
- *Aconitum heterophyllum wall* (Atis)
- *Allium sativum* (Garlic);
- *Andrographis paniculata* (Kalmeg);
- *Asparagus racemosus* (Satavari);
- *Azadirachta indica* (Neem);
- *Berberis aristata* (Daru haridra);
- *Commiphora wrightii* (Guggul);
- *Crocus sativus L.* (Saffron)
- *Nardostachys jatamansi* (Jatamansi);
- *Phyllanthus amarus;*
- *Emblica officinalis* (Amla);
- *Garcinia cambogia* (Kokum);
- Gymnema sylvestre (Gymnema)
- *Holarrhena antidysenterica* (Kutaj);
- *Ocimum tenuiflorum L* (Holy basil);
- *Picrorhiza kurroa* (Kutuki);
- *Plantago ovata* (Isabgol);
- *Saraca indica* (Ashoka);
- *Saussurea costus* (Kuth);
- Solanum nigrum (Black nightshade)
- *Tinospora cordifolia* (Guduchi),
- *Withania somnifera* (Ashwgandha).

EXPORT POTENTIAL

Indian phytopharmaceutical products

Indian phytopharmaceutical products which are in demand in the international market for their quality and potency.

Artemisinin – This is sesquiterpene lactone obtained from herb *Artemisia annua*, family Asteraceae, effective in treating malaria including cerebral malaria.

Berberine hydrochloride and berberine sulphate – This is benzyl isoquinoline alkaloidal salt obtained from Berberis spp. viz. *B. Aristata*, *B. vulgaris*. It is used as tonic astringent, febrifuge, hepatic dysfunction, diabetes and in gastroenteritis.

Colchicine – This is a yellowish benzyl tetra hydroisoquinoline type alkaloid, obtained from many species of *Colchicum (e.g. C. luteum, C. speciosum)* and also from genera *Androcymbium, Gloriosa, Iphigenia, Littonia and sandersonia*. It is use to relieve gout and rheumatic problems.

Diosgenin, Hecogenin and Solasodine – These are natural steroidal sapogenins, obtained from *Dioscorea* species (e.g. *D. deltoidea, D. maxicana, D. compositae and D. floribunda);* *Agave* spp. and *Solanum* spp. respectively – used in various hormonal preparations including birth control pills.

Ephedrine – It is a protoalkaloid obtained from various spp. of *Ephedra* (Ma-huang) and may also be prepared by synthesis. It is used for the relief of asthma and hay-fever.

Hyoscine and Hyoscyamine – These are tropane alkaloids obtained from *D. stramonium var. tatula, Hyoscyamus niger* and *H. muticus* used as Sedative in preoperative medication before the induction of anaesthesia and in ophthalmic practice to dilate the pupil of the eye.

Morphine, Codeine and Papaverine – These are the opium alkaloids obtained from the latex of *Papaver somniferum*. It is used as a pain killer (morphine) and anti–tussive (codeine).

Psoralen – This is furanocumarin obtained from *Psoralea corylifolia*. It is used in leucoderma and skin problems.

Quinine and Quinidine – These are quinoline alkaloids obtained from various spp. of *Cinchona bark* – used as Anti-malarials.

Reserpine, Ajmalicine – These are the indole alkaloids obtained from *Rauwolfia serpentina* – used to treat hypertension and as a vasodilator.

Rutin – This is yellow colored crystalline flavonol glycoside obtained from buckwheat

[*Fagopyrum esculentum (Polygonaceae)*]. It is included in dietary supplements and claimed to be benefit in treating conditions characterized by capillary bleeding.

Sennosides A & B – This is anthraquinone glycoside obtained from *Cassia senna* and is used to treat habitual constipation.

Taxol (Paclitaxel) – This is diterpene ester obtained from Taxus species (e.g. *T. brevifolia and T. wallichiana; Taxaceae)* used as anti-cancer agent.

Xanthotoxin – This is furanocoumarin obtained from *Ammi majus* and *Heracleum candicans* – used in leucoderma and other skin problems.

Indian Medicinal Plants used in Cosmetic and Aromatherapy

Following is the list of few Indian medicinal plants, which are in demand in the domestic as well as international market being useful in herbal cosmetic and in aromatherapy.

- *Aloe vera* (Kumari),
- *Rosa damascena* (Rose),
- *Pelargonium graveolens* (Geranium),
- *Matricaria chamomilla*,
- *Ocimum basilicum* and *O. sanctum*,
- *Lawsonia intermis* (Mehandi),
- *Hibiscus rosa-sinensis* (Japa),
- *Mesua ferrea* (Nag-Keshar),
- *Mentha arvensis* (Mint oil),
- *Mentha piperita* (Peppermint oil),
- *Eucalyptus globulus* (Eucalyptus oil)

Indian Medicinal Plants in Crude Form

The list of Indian medicinal plants having export potential in the **crude form** as well as their phyto-pharmaceutical products.

- *Aconitum* spp. (Vastsanabh),
- *Acorus calamus* (Vacha),
- *Adhatoda vasica* (Vasa),
- *Berberis aristata* (Daruhaldi),
- *Cassia senna* (Senna),
- *Colchicum luteum* (Colchicum),
- *Hedychium spicatum* (Kapur Kachri),
- *Heracleum candicans* (Kaindal),
- *Inula racemosa* (Pushkarmool),
- *Juglans regia* (Akhrot),
- *Juniperus* spp. (Aarar),
- *Plantago ovata* (Isabgol),
- *Picrorhiza kurroa* (Kutki),
- *Podophyllum hexandrum* (Bankakri),
- *Punica granatum* (Anar),
- *Rauwolfia serpentina* (Sarpagandha),
- *Rheum australe* (Revandchini),
- *Swertia chirata* (Chirata),
- *Valeriana wallichii* (Tagar),
- *Zingiber officinale* (Adrak)

List of medicinal plants which are on the Europe and USA export list.

- *Aloe* spp. (Aloe),
- *Allium sativum* (Garlic),
- *Centella asiatica* (Gotukola, Mandukparni),
- *Cimcifuga racemosa* (Black cohosh),
- *Echinacea* spp. (Echinacea),
- *Eleutherococcus senticosus* (Eleuthero),
- *Ginkgo biloba* (Ginkgo);
- *Hydrastis canadensis* (Goldenseal),
- *Hypericum perforatum* (St. Johnswort),
- *Mentha piperita* (Peppermint),
- *Panax* spp. (Ginseng),

- *Plantago ovata* (Psyllium);
- *Piper methysticum* (Kawa),
- *Serenoa repens* (Saw palmetto),
- *Silybum marianum* (Milk thistle),
- *Vaccinium murocarpon* (Cran berry),
- *Valeriana* spp.

Among them following are being produced in India

- *Aloe barbadensis*,
- *Centella asiatica*,
- *Hypericum perforatum*,
- *Mentha piperita*,
- *Panax pseudoginseng*,
- *Plantago ovata*,
- *Silybum marianum*,
- *Valeriana* spp.

SPICES

Spices form an important ingredient of culinary preparations in the tropics. They are added to the food in minor quantities to alter the taste and flavour of the preparation. Though they do not contribute to the energy content of the diet, they help to increase the digestion of the diet by enhancing the secretion of the digestive enzyme in the alimentary tract and by increasing the perspiration. There are **four major groups** of active constituents present in the spices, responsible for all these properties:

 (i) Volatile oils,
 (ii) Phenolics,
 (iii) Alkaloids, and
 (iv) Sulphur containing compounds.

Volatile oils

Volatile oils are sweet-smelling liquids and they emit fragrance to the food and they are also slight bitter in taste thus they help to enhance the secretion of digestive enzyme in the alimentary tract. All spices belonging to the Apiaceae (Umbelliferous fruits and their leaves) and the Lamiaceae (leafy spices) are rich in volatile oils. Since the oils are lost on cooking, these spices are mostly added as condiments.

Phenols

Phenolics component contribute to the taste, colour and flavour of a number of spices. The phenols present in spices are simple in structure mostly containing single aromatic ring, e.g. gingerols (ginger), phenolic amines are the pungent principles (capsaicins) in red pepper and phenylpropenes are present in cloves (eugenol) and fennel (anethole).

Alkaloids

Alkaloids are the largest group of nitrogenous natural organic compounds but only a few spices belonging to the genus Piper contain them. Alkaloid present in this genus are of piperidine type.

Sulphur Compounds

Spices such as mustard, onion and garlic owe their pungency and characteristic odour to sulphur containing compounds. These compounds are present in the form of glucosinolate (mustard seed) and are volatile with an offensive odour (onion, garlic and *Asparagus*).

EXPORT OF SPICES FROM INDIA

Following is the list of spices being exported from India to East Asia, United States, West Asia, European Community and Africa, UAE, Singapore, Germany, France, Canada, Sri Lanka, Japan, Malaysia, Russia, Bangladesh, Pakistan, Saudi Arabia and Netherlands.

1. Ajowain	7. Fennel
2. Black pepper	8. Garlic
3. Cardamom	9. Ginger
4. Chilli	10. Long pepper
5. Clove	11. Mint
6. Cumin	12. Turmeric

Although other countries like China, Brazil, Thailand etc. also started export of spice, but even then the demand for Indian spices is not being affected.

The trend in the spice trade from the country has been steadily increasing. At presently India is exporting spice in the tune of 300 million kg per annum earning about US$ 240 million, with the increase in volume-wise about 14%, while the increase in value-wise is only approximately 2% in the comparison of previous years (Table 3.1).

Table 3.1. Export trend for spices from India

Sr. No.	Year	Quantities (tonnes)	Value (Rs. in lakh)
1.	1967-68	52.195	2717
2.	1977-78	91.354	15492
3.	1987-88	78.374	30708
4.	1997-98	229.534	150780

The history of Indian spice is very old, as there are evidences of India having trade of vegetable drugs and spices with Greece even before Alexander's invasion in 327 BC. India's glory for the land of spice and perfumery attracted foreigners (French, British, Arab, Portuguese and Dutch). Portuguese invaded India and controlled over the spice trade of the country. They were taken over by Dutch, who exploited spices of India for many years. Later the British Empire took over and shared most of the world spice trade with Holland. Arabs had taken the spice products from southern India and established a strong trade with Europe.

Even after independence, spices have continued to be the main attraction of international trade in India. The Government of India had established separate board as "Spice Board of India", for promoting the spice trade which control their production and quality. Besides, the Spice Board, Indian Institute of Spices Research (IISR) was established at Calicut in 1986, which is responsible for providing latest biotechnology for the more production of spices.

Southern states of India remained the main centre of region of spice production. Even today, Southern states of the country produce most of the spices.

At present Kerala tops in the production of black pepper, cardamom and ginger, while producing substantial quantities of long pepper and turmeric. Andhra Pradesh has monopoly in the production of turmeric and chillies. More than half of the country's chillies and turmeric production is produced by the State of Andhra Pradesh alone. Currently about 50 million tonnes of chillies were produced by the Andhra Pradesh.

PRODUCTION OF SPICES

1. Ajowain

Ajowain is widely cultivated on commercial scale in the state of Rajasthan, Madhya Pradesh, Andhra Pradesh, Gujarat, Maharashtra and Uttar Pradesh. Rajasthan is producing as much as 8500 tonnes of ajowain annually.

2. Black pepper

Black pepper grows widely in South Western India. Kerala alone is producing 90% black pepper and is having about 19 million hectares of land under cultivation of this crop. It is also cultivated in Tamil Nadu and Karnataka and to some extent in Assam and Pondicherry.

3. Cardamom

Cardamom is produced by Kerala, Karnataka and Tamil Nadu. Kerala produced more than 6000 tonnes of small cardamom in 1999–2000.

4. Clove

Clove is cultivated in the states of Kerala, Tamil Nadu and Karnataka and to some extent in Andaman and Nicobar Islands. India imports, considerable amount of clove from Tanzania and Singapore. India also import clove oil from France, United Kingdom, Netherland and Tanzania.

5. Cumin

Cumin is mainly cultivated in **Rajasthan, Gujarat, Madhya Pradesh and Uttar Pradesh. Rajasthan** top in the production by producing about 80,000 tonnes of the cumin seeds. While Gujarat produce 65,000 tonnes annually while UP and MP produce only small quantity.

6. Fennel

Fennel fruits exist in different varieties with respect to shape, size and odour both in wild and cultivated states. Actually it is cultivated as a kitchen garden herb throughout India but the **commercial cultivation** is mainly taking place in **Rajasthan and Gujarat** but to a lesser extent in the states of **Karnataka, Uttar Pradesh and Punjab**. Presently Gujarat state produce more than half of the country's total production of about 31,000 tonnes.

7. Garlic

Garlic is native of the mountainous regions of Central Asia. It reached China then was carried to western hemisphere by Spanish, Portuguese and France.

In India garlic is cultivated in Madhya Pradesh, Gujarat, Maharashtra, Orissa and Uttar Pradesh and to lesser extent in the States of Rajasthan, Bihar, Haryana and Tamil Nadu.

8. Ginger

Ginger is under cultivation in India since time immemorial. **West Bengal** is the largest producer of ginger while the states of Tamil Nadu, Mizoram, Nagaland and Orissa produce considerable quantities of ginger. Nagaland produce ginger about 7000 tonnes from just 470 hectares of land.

9. Long pepper

Long pepper is mainly derived wildly from **Assam, West Bengal and Arunachal Pradesh.** Some quantities are also obtained from the forest of Kerala and Andhra Pradesh. India also imports long pepper from Nepal and Bhutan. Although its cultivation has also been started in some states like Arunachal Pradesh, Kerala and Annamalai hills of Tamil Nadu.

10. Turmeric

Turmeric is the major spice of India on the export list. It is cultivated in almost all parts of the country, especially the warmer parts.

India accounts for 43% of world trade in spices. The world's total production is estimated at 4,60,000 tonnes per annum worth at US\$ 1.8–2.4 billion. The main spices produced in India include chillies, turmeric, garlic, coriander, ginger, cumin, fenugreek, pepper, fennel and cardamom. The average export during 2000–01 in tonnes was highest for chillies (62000) followed by turmeric (35,500), pepper (20,250), Cumin (15,800), Coriander (13,700), garlic (11,600) and fenugreek (11,500). But in the terms of value in billion Indian Rupees, the pepper has the largest share (3.28) followed by chillies (1.95), cumin (1.18), turmeric (0.94) and cardamom (0.56). India also exported spice oils and resin amounting to around Rs. 3.64 billion. The yearly export figure from India was about 347.97, 295.45, 428.87 and 468.72 tonnes in the years 1996–97, 1997–98, 1998–99 and 1999–2000 respectively. India is the main producer of turmeric, ginger and pepper, having 90, 35 and 30% respectively of the total world's market.

The main drugs of import into India have been *Glycyrrhiza glabra* (Mulethi), *Pimpinella anisum* (Anise fruit), *Thymus vulgaris* (Hasha), *Operculina turpethum* (Turbud), *Cuscuta epithymum* (Aftimum vilaiyti), *Smilax ornata* (Ushba), *S. china* (Chobchini), *Lavandula stoechas* (Ustukhudus). In addition to the above mentioned crude drugs, following plant products are also being imported: pyrethrum, theophylline and theobromine alkaloids and their derivatives, ephedrine hydrochloride and papaverine.

List of medicinal plants which are being imported to meet the domestic market requirements.

- *Anacyclus pyrethrum* (Akarkara),
- *Borago officinalis* (Gauzoban),
- *Centaurea behen* (Bahman safed),
- *Cuscuta epithymum* (Aftimum vilayati),
- *Cydonia oblonga* (Bihidana),
- *Glycyrrhiza glabra* (Mulethi),
- *Lavandula stoechas* (Ustukhudus),
- *Operculina turpethum* (Turpeth),
- *Paeonia officinalis* (Udsaleeb),
- *Pimpinella anisum* (Anise),
- *Smilax chinensis* (Chobchini),
- *Thymus vulgaris* (Hasa),
- *Panax ginseng* (Ginseng)

Chapter

4

Plant-based Industry and Institutions involved in work on Medicinal & Aromatic Plants in India

INTRODUCTION

The demand for plant-based medicines, health products, pharmaceuticals, food supplements, cosmetics etc., is increasing in both developing and developed countries, due to the growing recognition that the natural products are non-toxic, have less side effects, easily available at affordable prices and sometimes the only source of health care available to the poor.

Global estimation indicate that over 80% of the world population can't afford the products of the western pharmaceutical industry and they have to rely upon the use of traditional plant-based medicines. Moreover as a part of strategy to reduce the financial burden on the developing countries, which spend 40-50% of their total budget on health. WHO currently encourages, recommends and promotes the inclusion of herbal drugs in national health care programmes because such drugs are easily available at a price within the reach of a common man and safer than the modern synthetic drugs.

In the last decade, it has been observed that the resurgence of interest in herbal drugs in the Western European countries has affected the growth of herbal industry in the world at the rate of 7-15% annually. In developed countries, the

resurgence of interest in herbal medicines has been due to the preference of many consumers for products of natural origin. In addition, manufactured herbal medicines from their countries of origin often follow in the wake of migrants from countries where traditional medicines play an important role. The growth in this sector in addition to medicine also has extended to the herb health food industry (nutraceuticals) and to cosmeceutical industry. The majority of leading companies specializing in herbal drugs are located in **Germany, France, Italy, Switzerland, China and India.**

India has been identified as one of the top twelve mega-biodiversity centres of the world with immensely rich flora of medicinal and aromatic plants occurring in diverse eco-systems. India has a long history of more than five thousand years as a supplier of medicinal and fragrant materials to the Western civilizations in Greece, Rome and Egypt. In the last century also (up to 1985) India remained a major supplier of **sandalwood oil and lemon grass oil in the world market products**.

The art of perfume making was first conceived and employed in the East, especially in India, Egypt, Persia and China. The Indian essential oil industry on commercial scale has begun with the production of 'Attars'. Actually 'Attars' essentially are flowers distillates, collected over sandalwood oil. The data on the production of Indian Attars are not available, because of the improper documentation and more over the production is scattered in different parts of the country and carried out on cottage scale.

During the last 50 years the commercial production of essential oils initiated and established in this country were from sandalwood, lemon grass, palmarosa, ginger, eucalyptus and oleo gum resin of turpentine, Mentha species (*M. piperita, M. spicata* and *M. arvensis*), Himalayan cedarwood oil, Jaborosa basil and many other like Jasmine flower extract and spice oil. However some of the traditional oils like sandalwood oil and lemon grass oil are showing downward trend.

The Indian medicinal plant-based industry faces many problems and is affected by number of factors which include absence of well defined policies/guidelines and strategies for promotion of cultivation and post harvest technology, standardization and marketing. The most alarming problem of the plant-based industry is the dwindling supply of plant materials from natural resources. A national policy on medicinal plants with a view to preserve endangered species and promoting cultivation of plants which are being extensively used by industry, will help in solving the major problems of the industry. Special attention is required on medicinal plants on which significant research leads have been obtained e.g.:

---

* *Acorus calamus* (Tranquilizer)
* *Albizia leback* (Immunomodulator)
* *Andrographis paniculata* (Antihepatotoxic)
* *Boswellia serrata* (Antihepatotoxic)
* *Boswellia serrata* (Antiarthritic)
* *Commiphora mukul* (Antihypercholesterolaemic)
* *Coleus forskohlii* (Cardiotonic)
* *Centella asiatica* (Brain tonic)

* *Phyllanthus amarus* (Antihepatotoxic)
* *Sida rhombifolia* (Anabolic)
* *Valeriana wallichii* (Tranquilizer)
* *Withania somnifera* (Adaptogen)

Indian industry is based on small family based units which are unable to compete at global level and need structural changes in production (size) and productivity (unit) through corporate entry in farming and utilization of technological innovation. There is a need to have separate marketing and development board for medicinal & aromatic plants and phytopharmaceuticals. Such board could interact with the growers and users industry to bring stability in their production, demand, price, quality and also to help in international trade.

In fragrance and flavour industry the major formulation manufacturers are located in **developed countries like USA, UK and Japan**. The major manufacturers for aroma chemicals are also located in developed countries. Low volume chemicals are generally made in the developing countries due to lower overheads. Bulk of the natural products are made in the developing or under developed countries. The world production of essential oils is estimated to be around 1.3 lakh tonnes annually valued at around US$ 1.5 billion and India's position is number two in value terms behind the US. The primary market for essential oils are the flavour and fragrance industries i.e. soft drink companies, food companies and perfume companies.

List of the institutions involved in plant-based industry are given in the Annexure I.

CLASSIFICATION OF MEDICINAL PLANT-BASED INDUSTRY

Medicinal plant-based drug industry can be classified into six categories:

(i) Plant drugs for Indian system of Medicine (traditional system) covering - Ayurveda, Unani and Siddha.

(ii) Over the counter, non-prescription products consisting of plant parts, extracts and galenicals.

(iii) Essential oils industry.

(iv) Phytopharmaceuticals.

(v) Natural health products.
- Health foods
- Nutraceuticals
- Recombinant proteins

(vi) Cosmeceutical industry.

MEDICINAL PLANT-BASED INDUSTRIES IN INDIGENOUS SYSTEM OF MEDICINE

Several traditional health care systems of medicine are being practised in Indian subcontinents. The most commonly used one are Ayurvedic, Siddha, Unani and Tibbi system of medicine. The Ayurvedic systems of medicine is practised in India and Nepal; while Unani and Tibbi in Pakistan. All alternative systems introduced at different stages co-exist with its indigenous systems of medicine in the multiethnic states of India.

There are many small manufacturing units using medicinal plants and thousands of Vaidyas preparing their own drugs from various plants. Herbal industry in India uses about 8000 medicinal plants; out of them, some of the important plants are enlisted in Table 4.1.

Following is the list of few medicinal plants, which are being frequently used in number of traditional herbal formulations.

FREQUENCY OF USE OF MEDICINAL PLANTS IN TRADITIONAL HERBAL FORMULATIONS

Terminalia chebula, T. bellirica, Emblica officinalis (Amla)	219
Glycyrrhiza glabra (Mullethi)	141
Piper longum (Pipali)	135
Adhatoda vasica (Vasaka)	110
Withania somnifera (Ashwagandha)	109
Cyperus rotundus (Mastak)	102
Tinospora cordifolia (Guduchi)	88
Berberis aristata (Daruharidra)	65
Holarrhena antidysenterica (Kutaja)	59
Boerhavia diffusa (Punarnava)	52

In India, up to several decades ago, the medicines used in indigenous systems of medicine were generally prepared by the practising physician themselves. In recent decades, this practice has been largely replaced by the establishment of organised indigenous drug industry. It is estimated that at present there are about 25,000 licenced pharmacies of Indian system of Medicine and nearly about 700,000 registered practitioners of Ayurveda, Siddha and Unani medicines are available. Presently about 1000 single drugs and about 3000 compound formulations are registered. Similarly Siddha, Unani and Amchi (local version of Tibetan) systems of medicine utilize as many as 600-800, 700-800 or 500-600 medicinal plants respectively. However exact quantification of the usage of individual plant material in the traditional system of medicine is not possible as no reliable data exists.

Development in Herbal Medicine Industry

Herbal medicines are the finished, labeled medicinal products that contain active ingredients from aerial or underground parts of plant or other plant materials, or combination thereof, whether in the crude state or as plant preparations. Plant materials include juices, gums, fatty oils, essential oils and any other substances of this nature. Herbal medicines may contain excipients in addition to the active ingredients. Medicines containing plant material combined with chemically defined active substances, including chemically defined, isolated constituents of plants are not considered to be herbal medicines.

Table 4.1. Some important medicinal plants used by the Indian Herbal Industry

Plant Name	Common Name	Plant Part	Estimated Consumption (tonnes)
Aconitum heterophyllum wall. ex Royle	Ativish	Root	20
Acorus calamus L.	Vacha	Rhizome	150
Aloe vera (L.) Burm.	Aloes	Leaf	200
Anacyclus pyrethrum (L.) Link	Akkarkara	Fruit	50
Andrographis paniculata (Burm. f.) wall. ex Nees	Kalmegh	Aerial part	250
Asparagus racemosus Willd.	Shatavari	Root	500
Bacopa monnieri (L.) Pennell	Brahmi	Whole plant	700
Berberis aristata DC.	Daruhaldi	Root	500
Cedrus deodara (Roxb. ex D. Don) G. Don	Deodar	Heart wood	200
Chlorophytum borivilianum L.	Safed musli	Root	25
Cinnamomum zeylanicum Blume	Dalchini	Bark	200-300
Commiphora wightii (arn.) Bhandari [= C. mukul (Hook. ex Stocks) Engl.]	Guggal	Gum resin	500
Crocus sativus L.	Kesar	Stigma	5
Cuminum cyminum L.	Jeera	Fruit	-
Cyperus rotundus L.	Nagar motha	Rhizome	150
Eclipta alba (L.) L.	Bhringraj	Aerial parts	500
Elettaria cardamomum (L.) Maton	Cardamon	Seed	60
Embelia ribes Burm. f.	Vidanga	Fruit	200
Glycyrrhiza glabra L.	Mulathi	Root	5000
Hedychium spicatum Buch. Ham.	Kapurkachri	Rhizome	400
Hemidesmus indicus (L.) W.T. Aiton	Anantmool	Root	200
Holarrhena pubescens Wall. ex G. Don [= H. antidysenterica (Roxb. ex Fleming) Wall. ex A.DC]	Kurchi	Bark	150
Justicia adhatoda L.	Vasaka	Leaf	500
Mucuna pruriens (L.) DC.	Kaunch beej	Seed	200
Myristica fragrans Houtt.	Jaiphal	Fruit	500
Nardostachys grandiflora DC.	Jatamansi	Root	200
Phyllanthus emblica L. [= Emblica officinalis Gaertn.]	Amala	Fruit	10000
Picrorhiza kurroa Royle ex Benth.	Kutki	Root	200
Piper cubeba L.	Cubeb (Kankol)	Fruit	150
Piper longum L.	Pipramul, Long pepper	Fruit	200
Piper nigrum L.	Black pepper	Fruit	150
Plumbago zeylanica L.	Chitrak	Root	500
Pueraria tuberosa (Roxb. ex Willd.) DC.	Vidarikanda	Root	200
Saraca indica L.	Ashoka	Bark	1200
Senna alexandrian Mill. [= Cassia angustifolia Vahl.]	Senna	Leaf & pod	1000
Strychnos nux-vomica L.	Kuchla	Seed	1000
Swertia chirayita (Roxb. ex Fleming) H. Karst. [= S. chirata (Wall.) C.B. Clarke]	Kirata or Chirayita	Whole plant	300
Syzygium aromaticum (L.) Merr. & L.M. Perry	Clove or Laung	Flower bud	150
Syzygium cumini (L.) Skeels	Jaman beej	Seed	300
Trachyspermum ammi (L.) Sprague ex Turrill	Ajwain	Fruit	200
Terminalia bellirica (Gaertn.) Roxb.	Bahera	Fruit	500
Terminalia chebula Retz.	Harar	Fruit	500
Tinospora cordifolia (Willd.) Miers	Guduchi	Stem	1000
Valeriana jatamansi Jones [V. wallichii DC.]	Tagar	Root & Rhizome	150
Withania somnifera (L.) Dunal	Ashvagandha	Root	500
Zingiber officinale Roscoe	Ginger	Rhizome	500

Exceptionally, in some countries herbal medicines may also contain (by tradition) natural organic or inorganic active ingredients which are not of plant origin.

The annual turnover of Indian herbal industry was estimated around about US$ 300 million in 1995. In 1997-98 the export value of Ayurvedic and Unani medicine was about US$ 27.7 million; in 1998-99 again went up to US$ 31.7 million; in 1999-2000 of the total turnover of US$ 48.9 million of Ayurvedic and herbal products, the major OTC products contributed about US$ 25.5 million and the ethical formulations around US$ 13.8 million and the classical Ayurvedic formulations remaining US$ 9.6 million.

List of few manufacturers (Govt. of India survey record) is given in the Annexure II & III.

Non-Prescription Production (OTC) Consisting of Plant Parts, Extracts and Galenicals

The direct utilization of plant material is a feature of traditional medicines not only in the developing countries but also in Europe and USA. Europe has a long history of research and processing of botanical extracts and has strict regulations, established quality control procedures and details of clinical data to support the products. Overall, the European market is as well regulated as the drug industry and many of the compounds sold in USA as dietary supplements are marketed as drugs in other countries.

Herbal formulation on health food shops viz. decoctions, tinctures, galenicals and total extracts of plants also form a component of many pharmacopoeias of the world. The current trend of medicinal plant-based drug industry is to procure standardized extracts of plants as raw material, for which, they are trying to establish their own Research and Development unit as per the guide line issued by WHO.

The objective of these guidelines, therefore, is to define basic criteria for the evaluation of quality, safety and efficacy of herbal medicines and thereby to assist national regulatory authorities, scientific organizations and manufacturers to undertake an assessment of the documentation/submission/dossiers in respect of such products. As a general rule in this assessment, traditional means which are in long term use as well as the medical, historical and ethnological background of these products shall be taken in account. The assessment shall also take into account a description in medical/pharmaceutical literature or similar sources, or a documentation of knowledge on the application of a herbal medicine without a clearly defined time limitation.

Herbal and related extracts will see the strongest growth based on expanding scientific evidence of health benefits and rising popularity of alternative medicines. Widely perceived health benefits among consumers will drive demand for herbal and related extracts up by ten percent annually.

Following Govt. Institutions are involved in the standardization of raw material as well as formulation.

Government of India has set up Pharmacopoeial Committees for Ayurveda, Siddha, Unani and Homeopathy systems. The Pharmacopoeial Laboratory for Indian Medicines (PLIM) and the Homeopathy Pharmacopoeial Laboratory (HPL) at Ghaziabad are providing the technical back up to these committees. At present about 178 monographs are ready for publication. The Pharmacopoeia Committee has also published two volumes of Ayurvedic Formularies of India consisting of 635 formulations. The Siddha Pharmacopoeia Committee has brought out seven volumes containing standards of 910 drugs.

The Unani Pharmacopoeia Committee has published one National Formulary of 441 formulations of Unani medicines. Now 45 monographs on single Unani drugs have been published. The Homeopathy Pharmacopoeia Committee has brought out 7 volumes containing standards of 910 drugs.

Essential Oil Industry

The essential oil industry was traditionally a cottage industry in India. After independence, during the last 55 years, a number of industrial companies have been established for a large scale production of essential oils, oleo-resins and perfumes (Aroma-therapy). The essential oils from plants being produced in India are more than 500 tonnes accounts for 90% of world production.

The following is the list of Indian aromatic medicinal plants from which essential oils are being produced on large scale:

Ajowain oil, celery oil, citronella, cedarwood, devana oil, Eucalyptus, lemongrass, Mentha species, geranium, lavender, palmarosa, patchouli, rose oil, orange (cold pressed), jasmine, vetiver, coriander, sandalwood and pine trees.

In India the production of turpentine oil and the resin from pines is well-established industry; having annual production about 35,000-40,000 tonnes annually. Another big well established oil industry is of mentha oil, from *Mentha arvensis*, Eucalyptus oil (*E. globulus*) and lemon oil from the discarded orange and lemon peel from which limonene is isolated.

Annual world production of limonene is about 75,000 tonnes and Brazil is the biggest producer in the world market. It is the by product of citrus industry though turpentine oil and Eucalyptus oil also yield limonene but the best economically cheap raw material is the discarded orange and lemon peel which is being used by Brazilian Phytochemical Industry.

During the year 2000-01, India exported, 3,875 tonnes of mint oil valued at Rs. 1.26 billion, lemon grass, citronella, palmarosa, vetiver and rose oil are the main essential oils produced in the country.

India also produces jasmine concentrate, which is of high value product in the perfumery.

Phytopharmaceuticals

Before independence, plant-based phytopharmaceutical industry in India was confined only to Quinine from Cinchona in the three state-owned factories. The very first industry was established by British Government at Mungpoo in Darjeeling. During the past fifty five years, bulk production of plant-based drug has become major part of Indian pharmaceutical industry. Following is the list of the phytopharmaceuticals which are produced in India:

Morphine, codeine, papaverine, thebaine, emetine, reserpine, quinine, quinidine, digoxin, caffeine, hyoscyamine, berberine, colchicine, rutin, vinblastine, vincristine, brucine, strychnine, ergot alkaloid, senna glycosides, diosgenin, plant laxatives, podophyllotoxin resin and citral.

Phytopharmaceuticals for which technology has been developed by Govt. Institution, for the large scale production include *L.* **dopa from mucuna beans, ajmaline and ajmalicine from** *Rauwolfia serpentina* **and** *Catharanthus roseus* **roots and 18 β-acetyl glycyrrhetic acid from** *Glycyrrhiza glabra*.

Indian Institute of Chemical Technology (IICT), Hyderabad has developed methods for **etoposide & teniposide** production; and CIPLA is now producing it on commercial bases. National Chemical Laboratory, Pune developed the method for **vincristine** (VCR) and **vinblastine** (VLB) production and CIPLA has further improved the production technique and they are the third largest manufacturer of VCR and VLB in the world.

Natural Health Products Industry

In these days the interest in herbal medicine is on rise, not only in the phytodrugs but also in natural health products. which include, health foods, nutraceuticals and personal care products.

Health Food

Health food are the food products supplemented with herbal ingredients. Vitamins, minerals and nutrients or ingredients isolated from plants. They have physiological benefits and reduce the risk of chronic diseases.

Nutraceutical

Nutraceutical is a latest term for health food, first innovated by Stephen Deffice, founder of the Foundation for Innovation in Medicine of New Jersey, USA. The word **nutraceutical** is an amalgamation of the term **"nutrition"** and **"pharmaceutical"** or it can be more correctly defined as parts of a food that have a medical or health benefit including the prevention and treatment of disease. The three main constituents, which make-up nutraceuticals are **herbal and related extracts, vitamins, minerals and nutrients.**

Antioxidant and herbal teas also form an important part of the nutraceuticals market. The leading **antioxidant phytochemicals in demand are Vitamin A, C and E; carotenoids and flavonoids.**

The US demand for nutraceuticals increased from US$ 830 million in 1987 to US$ 1.7 billion in 1996 and was expected to reach US$ 4.5 billion in 2005.

Japan is the third largest producer of nutraceuticals in the world and largest in the Asia pacific region. About half of all patents for nutraceuticals have been developed in Japan.

Nutraceuticals are the most progressing sector for health food and pharmaceutical industry based on plants. Many functional food/nutraceutical companies are part of larger food or pharmaceutical industries. A number of large food and

pharmaceutical companies, such as Abbott Laboratories, Smithkline Beecham, Glaxo, Ledrle, Dabur, Himalayas, Zandu pharmaceuticals, Allen laboratories and Aimil pharmaceuticals are also manufacturing nutraceuticals. Recently Ranbaxy Pharmaceutical Industry has also started its herbal research and development units.

Herbal Cosmetics and Personal Care Products

Cosmetic and personal care products containing natural products have rapidly growing trend in the market. Beginning in the early 1990's, cosmetic manufacturers began to use the term cosmeceuticals to describe the OTC skin care products. Claiming therapeutics benefits, the cosmeceutical products contain phytoconstituents in the extracts form or in the purified form such as α-hydroxy acids, vitamins, antioxidants and emollient oils rich in vitamin A and E. The items, which are on more demand in cosmetics and coppicing industry are Aloe extracts, botanical extracts, plant acids/ enzymes and essential oils.

Botanical extracts are canola (*Brassica napus*); chamomile (*Matricaria chamomilla*) dry extract, marigold (*Calendula officinalis*) dry extract, echinacea (*Echinacea* supp.), bilberry (*Vaccinium myrtillus*) dry extract, pumpkin seed (*Cuccurbita pepo*) lipophilic extract, ivy (*Rhus toxicodendron*) soft extract, peruvian bark (*Cinchona succirubra*) fluid extract; ginkgo (*Ginkgo biloba*); *Centella asiatica* (leaf extract of *Centella asiatica*); hawthorn (*Crataegus* spp.) and willow herb.

PRODUCTION AND UTILIZATION OF MEDICINAL PLANTS IN INDIA

Herbal industry in India uses over 800 medicinal plants. Most of the plant material used by more than 9000 manufacturing units is produced in the country. India, with its rich and long culture of using medicinal plants, has herbs for almost all human ailments. More than 80% of the medicinal plants required by the industry are collected from wild; only 20% of the plants species are cultivated. Following is the list of few important plants cultivated in India (Table 4.2).

While only for the following plants, technology for cultivation and processing is available (Table 4.3).

It is very difficult to collect the exact data of volume of consumption, production of medicinal plants and their phytochemical constituents as the trade operates through a complex chain consisting of unskilled collectors, small merchants, middlemen

Table 4.2. Some important medicinal plants cultivated in India

Aloe vera (L.) Burm.	*Mucuna pruriens* (L.) DC.
Asparagus racemosus wild. & A. adscendens Roxb.	*Papaver somniferum* L.
Bacopa monnieri (L.) Pennel	*Phyllanthus emblica* L. [= Emblica officinalis Gaertn.]
Catharanthus roseus (L.) G. Don	*Piper nigrum* L.
Centella asiatica (L.) Urb.	*Plantgo ovata* Forssk.
Cephaelis ipecacuanha (Brot.) Tussac *Chlorophytum* spp.	*Saussurea costus* (Falc.) Lipsch. [= S. lappa (Decne.) C.B. Clarke]
Cinchona ledgeriana (Howard) Bern. Moens ex Trimen	*Senna alexandrina* Mill. [= Cassia angustifolia Vahl]
Crocus sativus L.	*Solanum khasianum* C.B. Clarke
Mentha spp.	*Withania somnifera* (L.) Dunal

Table 4.3. Technology sources of some medicinal plants in India

Plant Source	Product	Technology source
Solanum khasianum C.B. Clarke	Solasodine	RRL-Bhu, RRL-Jmu, RRL-Jor
Dioscorea composita Hemsl. *Dioscorea floribunda* M. Martens & Galeotti	Diosgenin	RRL-Jmu, RRL-Jor
Catharanthus roseus Inn. G. Don	Vinca alkaloids	CIMAP-Lkw
Artemisia annua L.	Artemisinin	CIMAP-Lkw, RRL-Jmu, Cx-Pal
Eucalyptus youmanii Blakely & McKie & *Eucalyptus macrorhyncha* F. Muell. ex Benth.	Rutin	RRL-Jmu
Ammi majus L.	Xanthotoxin	CIMAP-Lkw
Tanacetum cinerariifolium (Trevir.) Sch. Bip. [Pyrethrum]	Pyrethrum	CIMAP-Lkw
Hyoscyamus muticus L.	Hyoscine	CIMAP-Lkw
Duboisia myoporoides R. Br.	Tropane alkaloids	CIMAP-Lkw
Atropa acuminata Royle ex Lindl	Atropine	CIMAP-Lkw
Matricaria recutita L.	Chamomile oil	NBRI-Lkw, CIMAP-Lkw
Taxus baccata L.	Taxol	RRL-Jmu
Claviceps purpurea Tul.	Ergot alkaloids	CIMAP-Lkw, RRL-Jmu

RRL-Jmu　　：Regional Research Laboratory, Council of Scientific & Industrial Research (CSIR), Jammu, Jammu and Kashmir
RRL-Jor　　：Regional Research Laboratory, CSIR, Jorhat, Assam
RRL-Bhu　　：Regional Research Laboratory, CSIR, Bhuvaneshwar, Orissa
CIMAP-Lkw ：Central Institute of Medicinal and Aromatic Plants, CSIR, Lucknow
NBRI-Lkw　：National Botanical Research Institute, CSIR, Lucknow.

and large trading houses at regional and international markets. In number of places, collection of the medicinal plants is being done through illegal way and as a result companies and traders are hesitant in giving the true information about the total trade or consumption. The practice is in contrast with the required standards of Good Manufacturing Practice (GMP) of herbal medicine products. According to which the manufacturing units have to keep the detailed history sheets of raw material, beginning from its point of origin to type of treatment that it has undergone during the process of transportation in the company, their storage and production procedure.

Over 70% of wild collections are destructive as they involve root, rhizome, whole plant, bark, wood or stems with the result even a most abundant resource can become exhausted by simply not following good collection practice. For example *Phyllanthus emblica* Linn. (*Emblica officinalis* Geartn) fruit is extensively used in the Indian system of medicine. The plant is commonly and abundantly available in the forest of Madhya Pradesh but the collector instead of collecting the fruits, they chopped off branches and even fell tree to make quick collection which resulted in reduction of plant population to an extent that it becomes part of the list of **endangered species** in the state e.g. *Rauwolfia serpentina* Benth in the state of Gujarat and Maharashtra; *Santalum album* L. in the state of Tamil Nadu, Karnataka, Orissa and Kerala.

CINCHONA BARK

Cinchona bark consists of dried, stem and root bark, obtained from various species, races and hybrids of Cinchona belonging to family Rubiaceae; indigenous to Colombia, Ecuador, Peru and Bolivia.

The followings are the official species:

1. *Cinchona succirubra*,
2. *Cinchona calisaya*,
3. *Cinchona ledgeriana* and
4. *Cinchona officinalis* and their hybrids.

Production

1. Cultivation and collection

Collected from wild as well as cultivated source.

Indonesia and India are important producers of Cinchona, high percentage of total crop is now collected from plantation in Tanzania, Kenya, Gutemala and Bolivia. The annual world production of quinine and its alkaloids is estimated about 1080 tonnes. India produces 20-30 tonnes annually.

In India, it is cultivated in Nilgiri and Annamalai hills (Tamil Nadu) and in Darjeeling (West Bengal).

The bark should contain not less than 6.5% of total alkaloids, 30-60% of which consist of quinine type alkaloids.

Cinchona production is highly specialised technique of tropical agriculture. An acid soil, rainfall and altitude are important factors in the production of good quality of bark with high percentage yield of alkaloids.

Propagation is done both by vegetative means as well as from seeds.

1. *Grafting technique :* Young *Cinchona ledgeriana* scion are grafted on *Cinchona succirubra* root stock, to get tree with the production of bark rich in the quinidine (alkaloid).
2. *Seed propagation* need careful treatment before propagation to avoid disease attack (stripe canker).
3. *Vegetative technique :* It is practised in West Bengal only while in Tamil Nadu both vegetative and seed propagation methods are employed.

2. Suspension culture (Tissue culture)

Production of Cinchona alkaloids by in vitro culture

of *C. ledgeriana* has also been reported. Quinine and quinidine proved to be the major alkaloids in leaf and root organ suspension culture.

Production of Phytochemical Constituent of Cinchona

Quinine is obtained from dried bark of *Cinchona calisaya, Cinchona ledgeriana, Cinchona officinalis* and *Cinchona succirubra*.

The bark is collected (by coppicing method) from branches and trunk of the cinchona tree. The bark so obtained is dried in sun light shade (not direct sun light) and by artificial heat (not more than 65°C) while drying, care should be taken to avoid mold or fermentation.

For the collection of root bark, plant to be uprooted and bark is separated manually.

Govt. institution – Govt. quinine factory at Mungpoo, Darjeeling (W.B.) and Cinchona at Annamalai, Tamil Nadu; the former contributing about two-thirds of the total production in India. The Cinchona Department of Tamil Nadu contributes about 1500 kg of quinine sulphate annually to the National Malaria Eradication Scheme (NMES).

A considerable number of alkaloids have been characterized in Cinchona bark, four of which (30-60% of the total alkaloidal content) are quinine, quinidine, cinchonidine and cinchonine. Quinine is usually the major component but the proportion of four alkaloids varies according to species or hybrid.

Production technique of quinine alkaloid is shown in the schematic diagram Fig. 4.1.

Utilization

Cinchona bark and its alkaloids are used for various ailments in different parts of the world. Its properties can be briefly described as - analgesic, anaesthetic, antiarrythmic, antibacterial, antimicrobial, antiparasitic, antipyretic, antiseptic, antispasmodic, antiviral, astringent, bactericide,

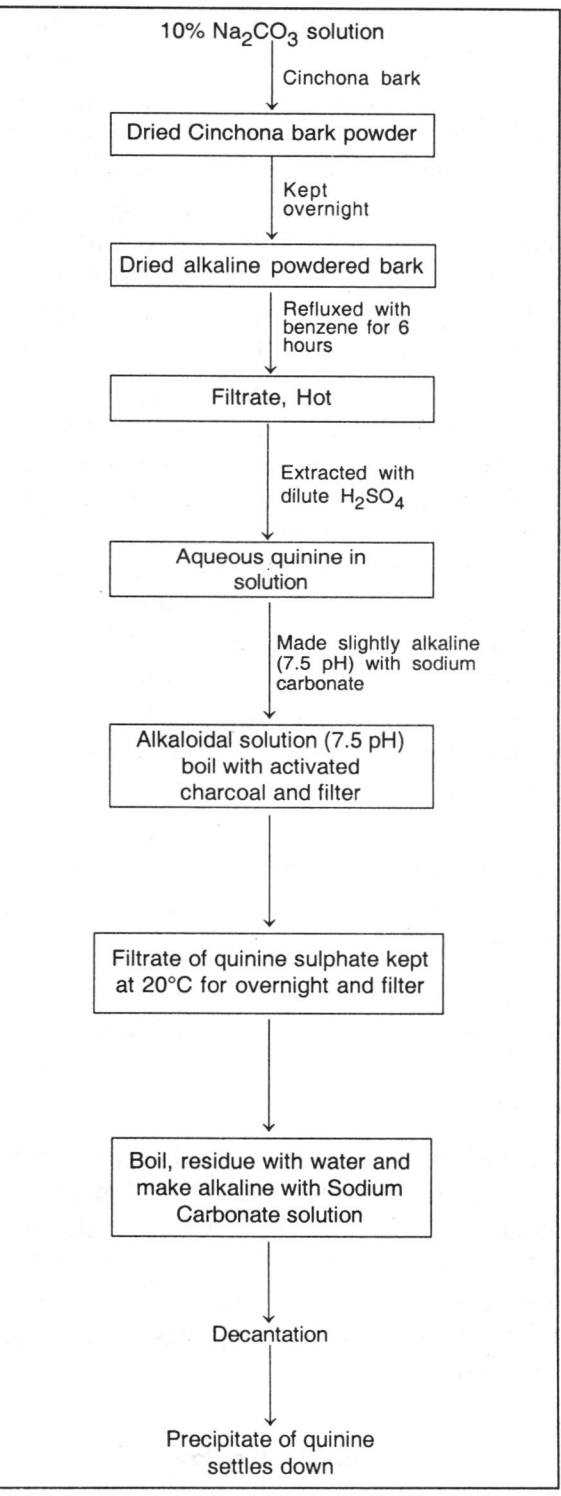

Fig. 4.1. Production technique for Cinchona alkaloid.

nervine tonic and stomachic, appetiser, anticramp, and for haemorrhoids and vericose vein treatment.

Quinine is very effective in the treatment of malaria as it kills the malarial parasites in the human blood. It has become a prophylactic measure for prevention of malaria. Although synthetic quinine is available but there is no substitute of natural quinine for certain types of malaria, e.g. chloroquine resistant malarial fevers caused by *Plasmodium falciparum*. It is administered, intravenously in cerebral malaria.

In Venezuela, cinchona is also recommended for the treatment of cancer. Cinchona and its alkaloids, particularly quinine, have been used for many years as an analgesic in common colds, cough, influenza and headache. It is also recommended for amoebic dysentery, atonic dyspepsia and infestation of pinworm. It is prescribed in labour cases for strengthening uterine contraction.

Recent use for quinine drugs is in treatment of noctural leg cramps and muscle spasm for which dose given is 400 mg daily for 2 weeks.

Quinine sulphate is one of the basic ingredients of Unani medicine for fever due to elephantiasis.

Cosmetics

Extract of cinchona is used in hair tonic, for stimulating hair growth and to check oilyness of hair.

Food

Quinine hydrochloride and sulphate are listed in Food Chemical Codex and are used extensively along with red cinchona extracts as a bitter tonic; water and alcoholic bitters. (Maximum limit 0.0028%). Cinchona extracts are also used in frozen dairy desserts, candy, baked goods and condiments.

OPIUM POPPY

Opium poppy (*Papaver somniferum* L.) is an

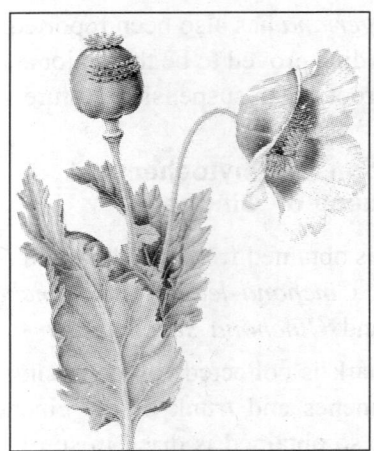

OPIUM POPPY (*P. somniferum*)
(for colour, see Plate 1, Fig. 7)

annual herb 50-150 cm high, with white, pink, red or purple flowers. Seeds range in color from white to a slate shade that is called blue in commercial classifications. It is native to South Eastern Europe and Western Asia. The species are cultivated extensively in many countries, including Iran, Turkey, Holland, Poland, Romania, Czechoslovakia, Yugoslavia, India, Canada and many Asian, Central and South American countries.

OPIUM

Opium is the dried latex obtained by incision from the unripe capsules of *Papaver somniferum* Linn. (Papaveraceae) and dried or partly dried by heat or spontaneous evaporation known in commerce as raw opium.

Production

In India, poppy plant (*P. Somniferum* var. album) is cultivated under licence. **Indian opium** is considered as the only legal source of opium to many countries including United State of America and Britain. Seed are sown in month of November to March in fairly rich loamy soil having pH 4.5–8.5. The plant grows best in rich, moist soil and tends to be frost sensitive. Young seedling are thinned out 15-30 cm apart. Flowers appear after one and half month to two months of seed sowing. Collection of latex is to be done from April to June.

Production of Latex (Opium)

Latex containing several important alkaloids is obtained from unripe (one to three weeks after flowering) capsules.

The incisions are made in the afternoon with an instrument known as a "nushtar" (the incision should not penetrate into the interior of the capsule otherwise latex will lost). The latex, which is at first white, rapidly coagulates and turns brown on exposure. Early in the next morning, the partly dried latex is scraped off with an special instrument (Charpala). Several cuts are given to each capsule at the interval of 2–3 days. After collection, the latex is placed in a tilted vessel so that the dark unwanted fluid might drain off and on exposure to air the opium (purified latex) acquires a suitable consistency for packing. It becomes hard and brittle on further storage. This dried mass is called **opium**. It has characteristic odour and bitter taste and of variable consistency, should contains not less than 9.5% of morphine.

Opium contains water (10-15%); sugars (10-20%) as well as organic acids: meconic acid, lactic, fumaric and oxaloacetic acid and most of the active principles are alkaloids (10-20%). The total yield of alkaloids is dependent on light, temperature, plant species and the time of harvest. About thirty alkaloids are reported, among these six alkaloids are major in quantity are grouped into two groups:

(i) **Morphine and related alkaloids**, which contain a structural nucleus related to Phenanthrene.

(ii) **Papaverine group of alkaloids**, which contain benzylisoquinoline nucleus or its derivatives.

The **poppy seeds** and **fixed oils** (that can be expressed from the seeds) are not narcotic, because they develop after the capsule has lost the opium yielding potential. The ripened capsules are collected and dried in open and seeds are removed by beating.

The average yield of the opium is 28–30 kg/hectare and of the seeds is about 50-60 tonnes per hectare. The opium collected by this way is either exported or some of the part is further processed at Government Opium Alkaloid Factory Gazipur (UP) and Govt. Opium Factory, Neemuch (MP).

Morphine Group (Phenantherene)

Morphine, thebaine and codeine are the major ones in this group. These occur in the opium to the extent of 9-12% morphine, 0.8-2.5% codeine and 0.1-1% thebaine.

Papaverine Group (Isoquinoline alkaloids)

The major one in this group is papaverine (0.5-1.5%), noscapine (4-8%) and narceine (0.1-0.7%).

Morphine

Morphine (the free base) unlike most other alkaloids in their free base forms, is only sparingly soluble in chloroform and nearly insoluble in ether or benzene. Its solubility in various solvents differs rather markedly from the solubility of codeine and this solubility difference can be utilized in their separation/production.

Papaverine

Papaverine is a weak base, behaving as tertiary amine. It is insoluble in water, slightly soluble in cold alcohol or ether and soluble in chloroform.

Noscapine

Noscapine (commonly called **narcotine**) is a

weak monoacidic tertiary base. It is nearly insoluble in water, sparingly soluble in cold alcohol or ether and readily soluble in benzene, acetone or ethyl acetate. It is insoluble in cold alkali or ammonia but soluble in hot alkali. It forms unstable salt with acids and these salts are dissociated by water. When boiled with dilute acids noscapine is hydrolysed to op anic acid and hydrocotarnine.

Narceine

Narceine occurs in opium as such, but it can be prepared from **noscapine**. It behaves as a weak monoacidic tertiary base. It yields well-crystallized salts such as hydrochloride, picrate and aurichloride. Narceine dissolves in ammonia and in solution of alkali hydroxide forming crystallizable metallic derivatives. It also esterifies with alcohol in the presence of hydrogen chloride.

Production of Phytoconstituents

Separation of major alkaloids from opium.

Mainly on the basis of the solubility properties described above six major alkaloids may be isolated from opium by a procedure represented by schematic outline shown in Fig. 4.2.

Utilization of Poppy

Poppy is one of the most important medicinal plants. Traditionally, the dry poppy was considered an astringent, antispasmodic, diaphoretic, expectorant, hypnotic, narcotic and sedative. Poppy has been used against toothache and coughs.

Poppy seeds are used as a condiment with baked goods and pastries for their nutty odour and flavour. **Poppy oil** is widely used as an edible cooking oil. The oil is also used in the manufacture of paints, varnishes, and soaps. **Poppy plants** are also important as ornamental plants in flower gardens.

Opium is used in the production of morphine, codeine, other alkaloids and deodorized forms of opium. Morphine is the raw material from which heroin is obtained.

Pharmacological Properties

Opium alkaloids have characteristic simultaneous depressing and exciting effect on the central nervous system. As the series ascends in the order, morphine, papaverine, codeine, narcotine and thebaine, the narcotic action diminishes and power of reflex stimulation increases.

Narcotine and papaverine relax intestinal muscles in contrast to **morphine and codeine**, which increases their tone. This action contributes to the greater constipating effect of opium as compared with that of morphine. The pure alkaloid has the advantage that it is absorbed more readily, can be given hypodermically with greater accuracy of the drug.

Utilization of Opium

Opium is official in Pharmacopeia of several countries. Now-a-days whole opium is not in use but derivatives of opium are used in pharmaceutical industry as antidiarrhoeals, antispasmodic and antitussive formulations.

- Opium is used in aromatic powder of chalk for intestinal use in diarrhoea.
- Opium tincture and camphorated opium tincture are used in dosage forms for the treatment of cough.
- Opium with lead in suppositories dosage form is used to relieve rectal and pelvic pain.
- Opium with gall (tannins) in the ointment dosage form is employed in the treatment of haemorrhoids.
- Opium is employed externally in liniments and the tincture is added to lotion preparation.

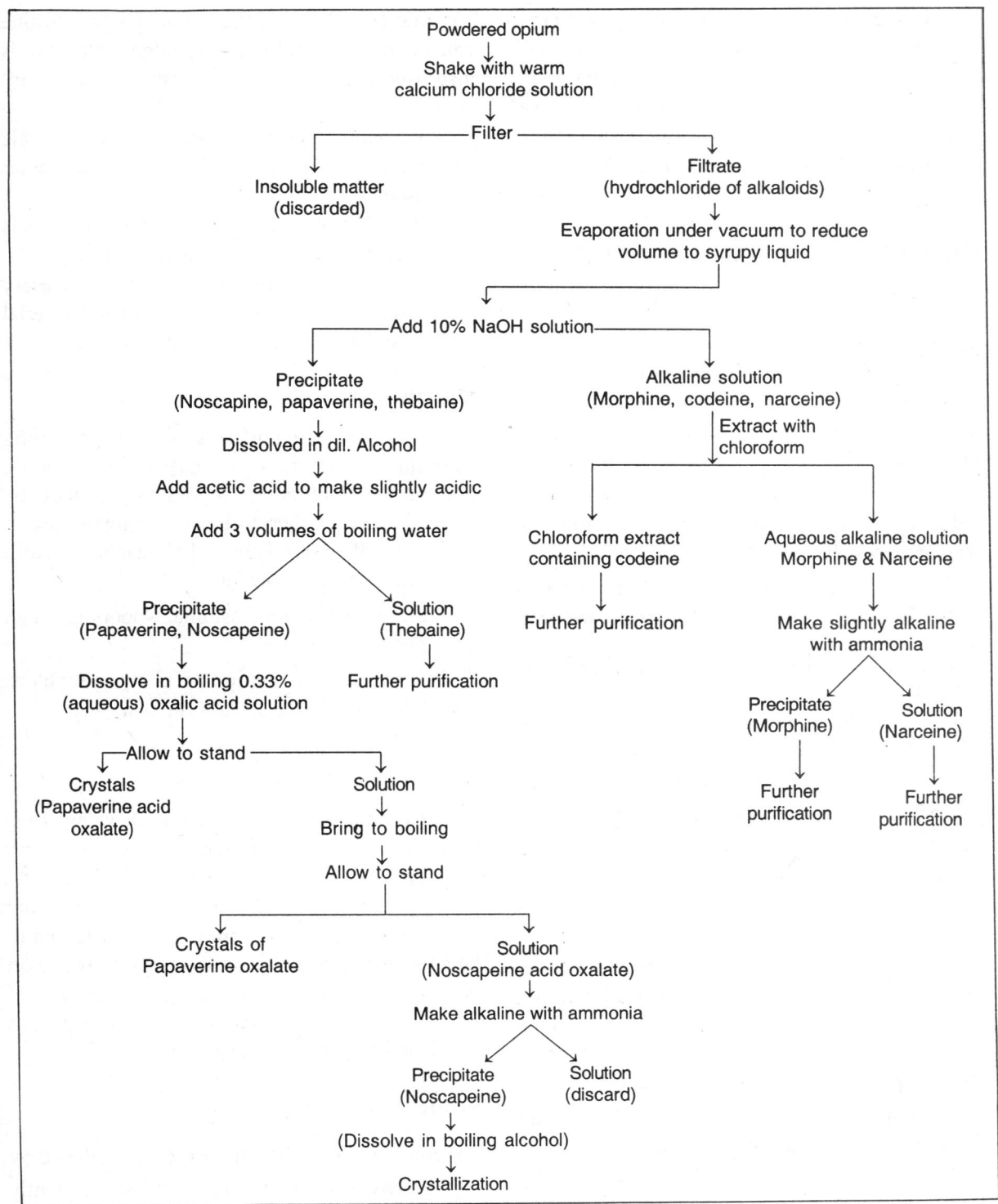

Fig. 4.2. Production of phytochemical constituents of Opium.

- Opium is used in veterinary practice as sedative expectorant and as antispasmodic in the treatment of diarrhoea and dysentery. The hypnotic and sedative effect is not well marked in animals except in dogs with the toxicity of nausea and vomiting in higher dose (not calculated properly).

UTILIZATION OF OPIUM ALKALOIDS

Morphine

Morphine alkaloids are employed/used to relieve pain, anxiety and sleeplessness but it is invaluable in the treatment of biliary or renal colic, severe trauma, internal haemorrhage, myocardial infarction and in congestive heart failure.

As a sedative to respiratory centre it has special value in the treatment of cardiac asthma and whooping cough.

It is used in the treatment of cold, rheumatism and influenza in the form of Dover's powder.

Note: Morphine should be used with care under the direct supervision of the physician because it is a habit forming drug.

Codeine

It is widely used for the relief in irritating cough e.g. in tuberculosis and is recommended in insomnia due to incessant coughing.

It is used to relieve the pain in the patient suffering from the pain of cancer and in head trauma.

It is also used as a sedative in the patient of mental disorders. Since the codeine addiction is rare (rather it is sometimes recommended for morphine addict) it has great advantage over morphine. It is excreted through kidney.

Codeine is administered as phosphate in the form of tablet dosage form or linctus.

Papaverine

It is used as an antispasmodic, in the treatment of spasmic conditions of the stomach and intestine caused by hyperacidity and duodenal ulcers. It is also used in the treatment of asthma and biliary colic.

- Papaverine hydrochloride is smooth muscle relaxant, dose orally 150 mg; intramuscular 30 mg.
- A 10% solution of papaverine sulphate is used for anaesthesia in **conjunctiva**.
- It is used in the treatment of coronary artery disease, pulmonary and peripheral arterial embolism and in Raymaud's disease.

Narcotine

To eliminate misunderstanding and wrong connotation the name **noscapine** is given in pharmaceutics literature. It possesses no narcotic properties and is therefore called a **narcotine**. It is used in allaying cough and headache, because of its antitussive properties.

It is also used in mild asthma, whooping cough and spasm of intestine.

It is available in syrup and chewable tablets. Usual dose is 15 mg up to 4 times a day.

ERGOT (Fig. 4.3)

Ergot is the common name for *Claviceps purpurea*, a parasitic fungus, which infects rye grass. The fungus replaces ovary of the rye plant with its own biological material and a hard mycelial mass known as a **sclerotium**. It is considered to be an example of a mycotoxin because the toxin produced are formed by a fungus. Ingestion of the sclerotia is poisonous to both plants and animals and is known cause of **ergotism**.

Production of Ergot

For commercial supply, the Ergot is produced by

(i) **Cultivation** of rye plant and subsequently infecting with the fungus, and

(ii) **Saprophytic production**.

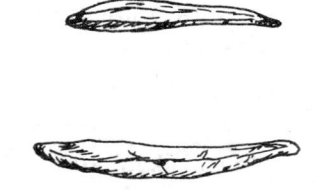

Fig. 4.3. Ergot (*Claviceps purpurea*).

Controlled field cultivation on rye is the main source of the crude drug. The most important cultivators are Czechoslovakia, Hungary, Switzerland, and former Yugoslavia.

For natural way of production; the rye plant *Secale cereale* (Host) are **devoted** to its cultivation. Different selected strains of *Claviceps purpurea* are used for the production of the alkaloids ergotamine, ergocristine or ergocornine and ergocryptine. The various other known species of this fungus are *C. microcephala*, *C. nigricans* and *C. paspali*, which can produce **Ergot**. Commercially, ergot of rye is becoming less important and currently U.K. dealers trade mainly in the ergot of wheat.

Procedure (Harvesting)

The rye (*Secale cereale*; Family Gramineae) plants are infected with suspension of **conidospore** as a spray in the spring or early summer by the **ascospore** of fungus at the base of young ovary, where in damp weather they find sufficient moisture to germinate.

In the early infection, the fungus secretes a sticky substance from young florets, which is subsequently replaced by the hardened fungal mycelial mass, the **sclerotia**. The sclerotia can be described as a long (1-5 cm) structure with tapering ends. They are often deep-purple to blackish in color and are the resting stage of the fungus. At the end of a growing season, the sclerotia fall to the ground where it remains on or in the soil. In the spring, sclerotia remaining on the surface of the soil germinate and form 1-60 stalks. Each stalk tip develops into many

perithecia, each with many **asci**. Each ascus in turn has **8 ascospores**, which are capable of infecting ovaries of other plants after dispersion by the wind or insects. The fungus in the ovary forms a **sporodochia**, which in turn produce **conidia** which exude a sticky substance, sometimes referred to as **honeydew**. The honeydew is very attractive to insects and thereby creates a nice dispersal mechanism for the fungus. A schematic of the life cycle of *Claviceps purpurea* is shown in Fig. 4.4.

Saprophytic production technique

The saprophytic process of production was initiated in Japan by Prof. Abe. In this method various strains of Ergot are used depending upon the type of ergot alkaloid to be required e.g. *C. paspali* gives **clavine** and simple **lysergic acid derivatives** which can be further converted into peptide alkaloids (Ergot alkaloid). For nutrition of cultures of fungus specific nutrients are used and fermentation is carried out in large fermenters at a temperature range from 20-30°C and at pH 4.5-6.3. The fermentation process take place from 7-21 days. The isolation, separation and purification of simple lysergic acid and derivatives is done by usual method given in the Fig. 4.5.

Note : The saprophytic production is much in practice in these days because the percentage yield of alkaloid is higher than the natural sclerotia.

Utilization of Ergot

Whole ergot preparation are traditionally used in labour to assist delivery and to reduce post-partum haemorrhage but in the present days the whole ergot has been replaced with the isolated ergot alkaloids.

Production of Phytoconstituents of Ergot

Ergot contains number of alkaloids, which can be divided broadly into two types:

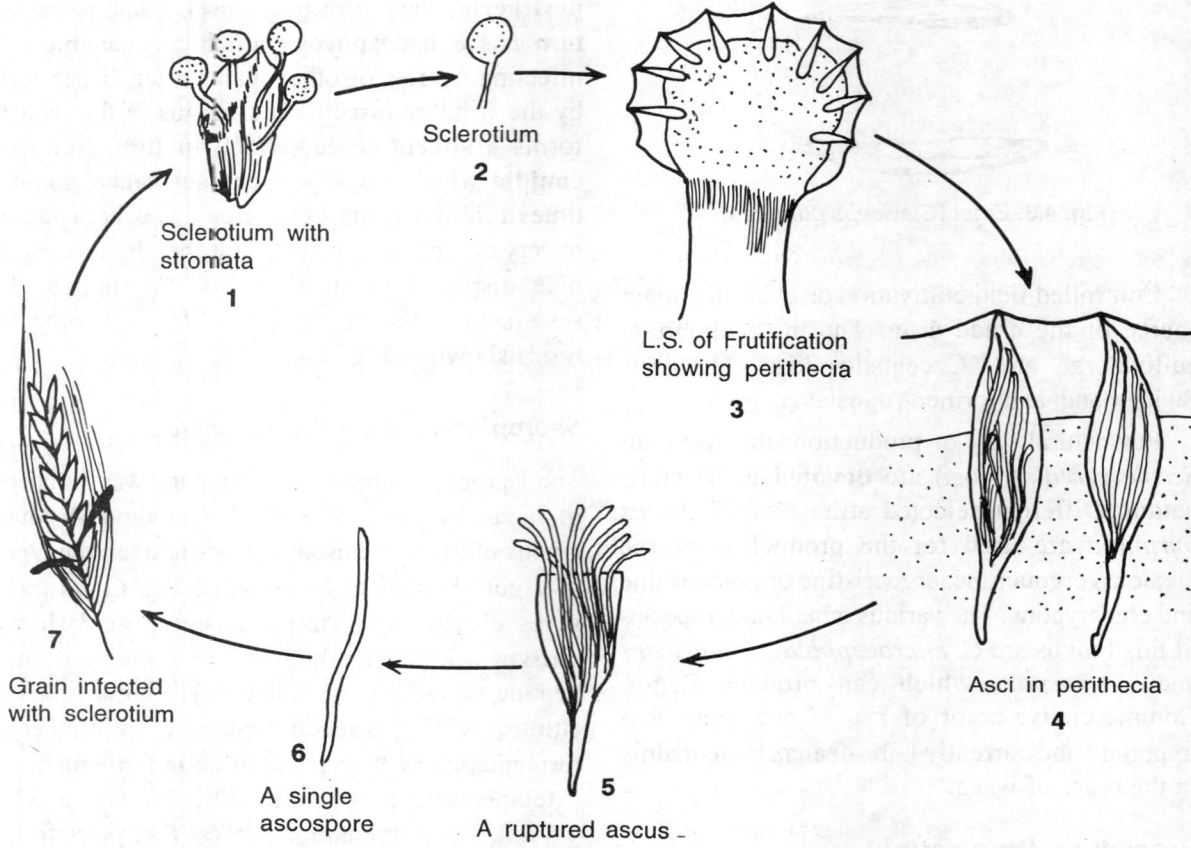

Fig. 4.4. Schematic diagram of life cycle of Ergot (*Claviceps purpurea*)

- *Clavine type :* These are derivative of 6, 8 dimethyl-ergoline and have been extensively studied in culture of the mycelium of the ergot fungus.

- *Peptide type :* Water insoluble (lysergic acid derivative). These are pharmacologically active alkaloids. Each active alkaloid occurs with an inactive isomer, obtained from isolysergic acid.

There are mainly six pairs of alkaloids reported:

L-Rotatory

1. Ergometrine group or (Ergonovine group)	Water soluble
2. Ergotamine group	Water insoluble
3. Ergotoxine group	

D-Rotatory

1. Ergometrinine, ergosinine
2. Ergocristine
3. Ergocryptine
4. Ergocornine

EXTRACTION PROCEDURE FOR TOTAL ALKALOIDS FROM ERGOT

Powdered ergot is extracted with petroleum ether to make it free from fatty material. The defatted ergot powder is moistened with ammonia solution, dried and then extracted with chloroform (or ether). The chloroform extract (Alkaloidal solution) so obtained is shaken with 0.2 N sulphuric acid (H_2SO_4) or 2% tartaric acid solution. The acidic solution made alkaline with ammonia and extracted with chloroform, till the complete exhaustion of alkaloid. The chloroform extract washed with water and dried over anhydrous sodium sulphate. Chloroform removed from the dried chloroform extract by distillation, the residue thus obtained will be pure total alkaloidal residue (Fig. 4.5).

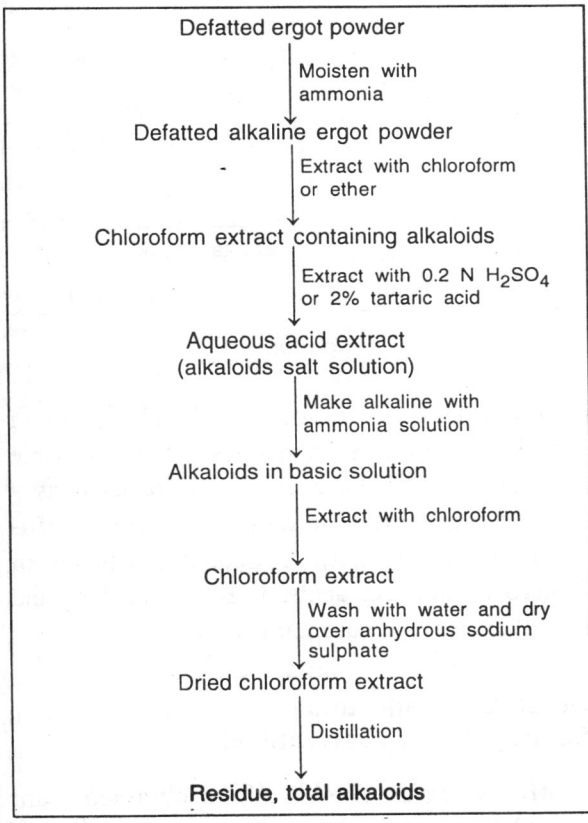

Fig. 4.5. Total ergot alkaloids extraction procedure.

Production of Individual Alkaloids from Ergot Powder

The procedure for the production of Ergometrine (Ergonovine), Ergotamine and the constituents of ergotoxine are summarised below and also given in the form of schematic diagram (Fig. 4.6, 4.7 & 4.8).

Methylergometrine

Methylergometrine maleate (injection solution). It is used intramascularly for obstetric emergencies for its oxytocic properties and is administered during the final stages of labour and immediately following child birth, especially if haemorrhage occurs, to check the extra bleeding because of its vasoconstriction effects. It is also used after caesarean sections, after abortion by suction or curettage, and for uterine atony after giving birth.

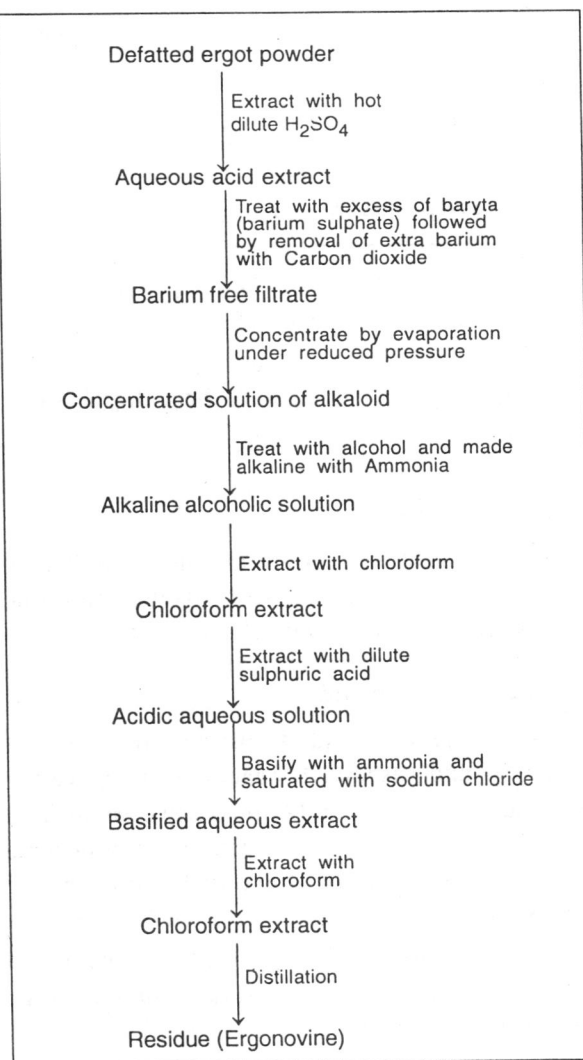

Fig. 4.6. Production procedure for Ergonovine (phyto-constituent of ergot).

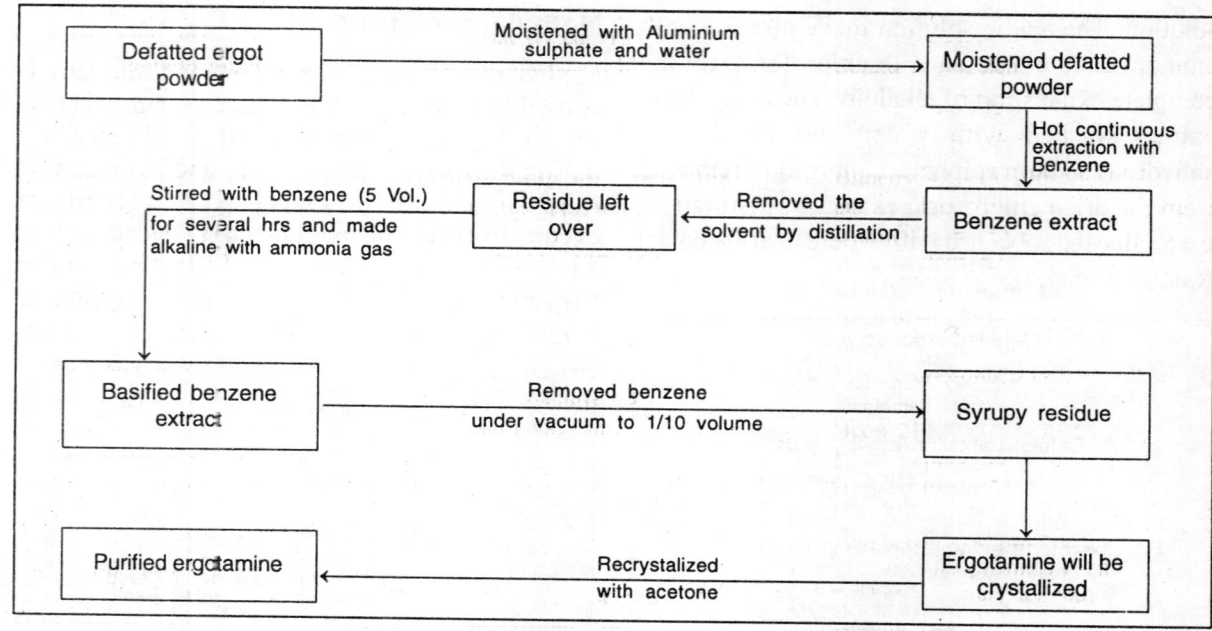

Fig. 4.7. Ergotamine production from the defatted ergot powder.

In specialized hospital wards, this alkaloid is used for diagnostic purposes or to evaluate certain treatment.

ERGOTAMINE

It is used orally or rectally in combination with caffeine in the treatment of acute migraine headache and related vascular headache.

Dihydroergotamine

It is also recommended for the treatment of migraine and vascular headache, to improve the symptoms of venous and lymphatic vessel insufficiency. It is also used in the treatment of orthostatic hypotension. It should be avoided in pregnant or breast-feeding women.

Dosage form: Orally (tablet, capsule or solution form), injection and spray solution dosage forms are available.

Dihydroergotoxine - Dihydroergocristine

Dihydroergocristine mesylate is available under various dosage forms, for oral administration (solution, tablet or single dose lyophilisate and capsule containing microgranules) and an injectable solution both of these alkaloids are used as a corrective treatment of **senile cerebral insufficiency** (memory loss), to treat the sequelae of cerebro-vascular accidents, dizziness in elderly and retinal disorder of vascular origin.

Other Synthetic and Semisynthetic Derivatives

Methysergide (INN) : It is obtained from methylation of the indole nitrogen atom of methylergonovine. It is used in adults in the treatment of migraine and facial pain of vascular origin.

2-Bromo-α-ergocryptine (Bromocryptine) : It results from the bromination on the carbon atom which is α- to the indole nitrogen atom. This compound is indicated in the following:

1. **Prolactin - secreting adenomas :** Clinical consequences of hyperprolactinemia : Severe disturbance of the menstrual cycle, sterility, galactorrhea and in men, gynecomastia and impotence.

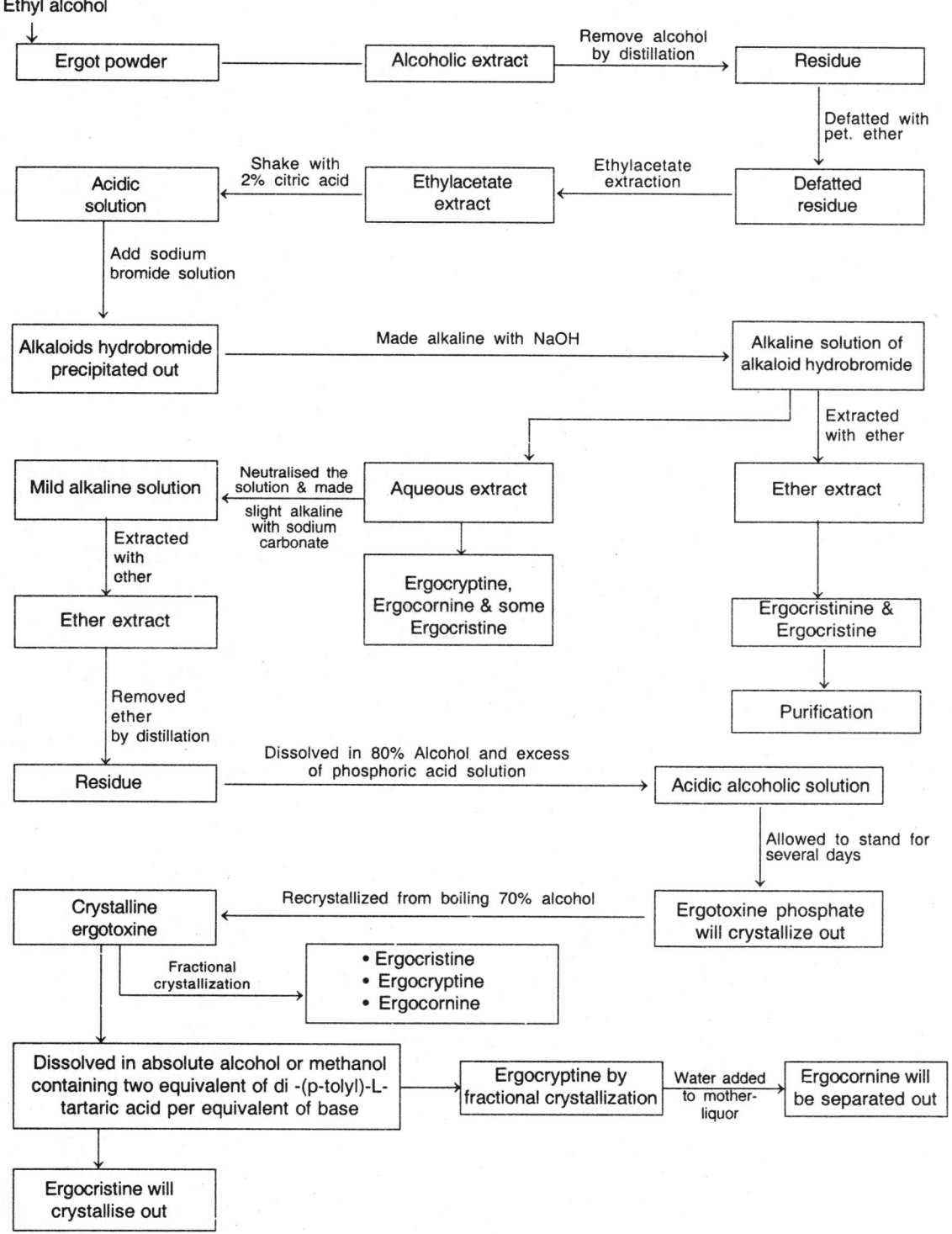

Fig. 4.8. Procedure for the isolation (production) of Ergotoxine group from Ergot powder.

2. **Inhibition of lactation :** Prevention and inhibition of physiological lactation for medical reasons, immediately after delivery (ablactation) or a long time after delivery (weaning).

3. **Treatment of parkinsonism :** This drug alone or in combination with levodopa used to decrease the doses of each drug and delay the onset of fluctuation in efficacy and abnormal movements.

LISURIDE

Lisuride maleate is a synthetic derivative of the **8α-aminoergoline** type compound; used in the treatment of parkinsonism, alone or in the combination with levodopa.

DIGITALIS

Digitalis (Purple foxglove leaves) consists of the dried leaves of *Digitalis purpurea* and *Digitalis lanata* belonging to family Scrophulariaceae. It required to contain not less than 0.3% of total **Cardenolides** calculated as *digitoxin* [digitoxigenin-(digitoxose)$_3$].

D. purpurea is an erect biennial, rarely perennial herb, 45-105 cm high; having alternate leaves 10-40 cm long and 4-15 cm wide, ovate, lanceolate to broadly ovate and petiolate. They are grayish-green in color with serrate or dentate margin. The flowers are pinkish-purple with deeper purple spots. The plant is widely distributed and cultivated throughout Europe. It is indigenous to the United Kingdom and grown there as an ornamental plant. It has also been cultivated in Egypt, temperate Asia (Japan, India) and North America. Commercially produced in Holland.

D. lanata leaves are used as a source of the glycosides digoxin and lanatoside C. It is a perennial or biennial herb about 1m high. The leaf are alternate and sessile, generally 20-30 cm long and up to only 4.5 cm wide. The margin is entire, the apex is acuminate and the veins leave the midrib at a very acute angle. The flowers are yellowish-white with or without purplish network. The plant is indigenous to Central and South Eastern Europe. It is also cultivated in Holland, Ecuador and USA. Its cultivation on trial basis is taken place in many countries including asian countries.

About 100 tonnes of plant material is required annually to meet the world demand.

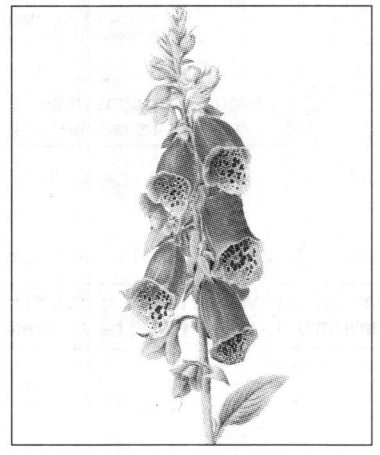

DIGITALIS (*D. purpurea*)
(for colour, see Plate 1, Fig. 8)

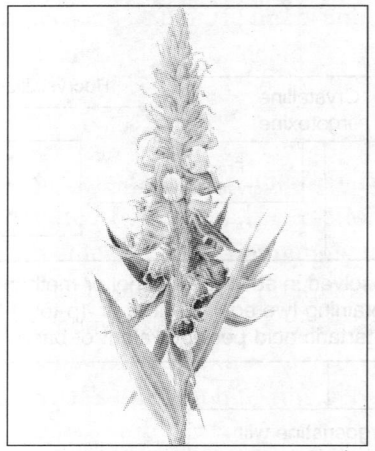

DIGITALIS (*D. lanata*)
(for colour, see Plate 1, Fig. 9)

Apart from *D. purpurea* and *D. lanata* other species which contain cardiac glycosides are: *D. dubia*, *D. ferruginea*, *D. grandiflora*, *D. lutea*, *D. nervosa* and *D. thapsi* but these species are not of much importance from commercial point of view.

D. purpurea was introduced in India as an ornamental plant but being medicinally important, it was successfully, grown on experimental scale at a number of places along with *D. lanata* at Dehradun, Chakrata (old UP) Ranikhet and Kalatop (HP) Nilgiris, Baramula and Jammu (J&K), West Bengal, Himachal Pradesh and hilly area of Tamil Nadu. As these areas have potential for the growth of digitalis plant, to fulfill the requirement of pharmaceutical industry.

So far India could not established successful large scale cultivation because of lack of processing facilities and limited demand. Therefore major demand of the pharmaceutical industries is being met from import.

Cultivation

Cultivation of Digitalis plant is done by **seed propagation**. It requires well-drained sandy, mild acidic soil for *D. purpurea* and alkaline soil for *D. lanata* but both plants require semi-shady places. It is a warmth loving plant. The growth and the glycosidal content are maximum between 20-30°C. At lower temperature both, growth and biogenesis of glycosides are affected.

It is produced commercially in Holland and Eastern Europe. Digitalis plant is grown from seeds, after being soaked in water at 30°C for two days to hasten germination. Seeds are sown directly into the field in the month of October-November, and weeding in the month of April-May following spacing at approximately 30 × 45 cm apart.

For the collection of the digitalis leaves either first or second year leaves are permitted by the Pharmacopoeia. Best time of cutting the leaves **is early afternoon in the month of June-August** in order to obtain maximum glycosides concentration. Cutting of the entire plant 10-15 cm above the ground is suggested. In the case *D. lanata* cutting of rosette leaves 2-3 cm above the soil in autumn gives the maximum leafage and cardenolide contents.

After collection, the leaves should be dried as rapidly as possible at a temperature of about 60°C and subsequently stored in airtight container protected from light. Moisture content should not be more than 6%.

The fresh leafage yield of 15.5-16.0 tonnes/hectare has been reported at Solan (HP) and Kodalkanal (TN) respectively but under the agroclimatic conditions of the upper Shillong (Meghalaya), 100 tonnes/hectare yield of digitalis herb has been reported.

Cell and organ culture technique for production of cardenolide glycoside.

It has been reported that the green tissues appear to be requisite and **green hairy roots produced by light exposure** give a 600 fold increase in cardenolide accumulation, over the roots cultivated in dark. In the case of *D. lanata* the reports are discouraging as both cell and hairy root culture have proved to be disappointing as a source of cardio-active glycosides.

Isolation Technique

As prescribed in B.P. : The drug is pulverized and extracted with 50% ethanol at low temperature, followed by the addition of lead acetate solution to remove the impurities, the precipitates are removed by centrifugation, the cardiac glycoside present in the supernatant are extracted with chloroform, the chloroform extract is evaporated under vacuum and the residue (cardiac glycoside) left behind is further purified by chromatography.

Utilization

D. purpurea and *D. lanata*, leaves contains cardio-active glycosides of which **digoxin** is most important *D. lanata* is more potent than *D. purpurea*, hence the leaves of *D. lanata* are preferred raw material for the manufacture of digoxin and other glycosides.

The glycosides of digitalis are used to increase the force of myocardial contraction (the positive ionotropic effect) resulting in complete emptying of the ventricles, without increasing the rate in congestive heart failure. As a result of depression of conduction in the bundle of HIS, the atrio-ventricular conduction time is increased, resulting in an extended P-R interval on the electrocardiogram. Arising from their vagus effects, the digitalis glycosides are also used to control supra-ventricular (atrial) cardiac arrhythmias; hence clinically it is used in the treatment of various cardiac arrhythmia such as atrial premature beats, atrial fibrillation and supra-ventricular tachycardia.

Digitalis leaves are used in the manufacture of **digoxin, digitoxin**. But digitoxin is the most potent and most cumulative of the digitalis glycoside. **Digoxin** is stable in an aqueous solution at pH 7 but in acidic pH it is hydrolysed to digoxigenin. For urgent digitalization, oral administration of prepared (powdered) digitalis may be given. Otherwise digoxin is particularly valuable for rapid digitalization and in the treatment of atrial fibrillation and in congestive heart failure, it is excreted more rapidly than the other digitalis glycoside, hence it is less cumulative.

Digoxin is also employed in the treatment of animal heart failure.

ISPAGHULA (ISABGOL)
(*Plantago ovata Forsk*)

Commonly known as **Blonde Psyllium** or **Indian plantago** in commerce. It belongs to genus Plantago, which is one of the three genera comprising of family Plantaginaceae.

The name **ispaghula** is a Persian word consisting of two parts **"Isap"** and **"ghol"** meaning horse car, referring to its characteristic boat shaped seeds. **Plantago** in Latin meaning is **"sole of the foot"** and refers to the shape of the leaf.

Psyllium in **Greek** wordly meaning is **flea**; the name refers to color, size and shape of seeds.

Plantago ovata is indigenous to the Mediterranean region and west Asia, extending to Sutlej, Sind and West Pakistan.

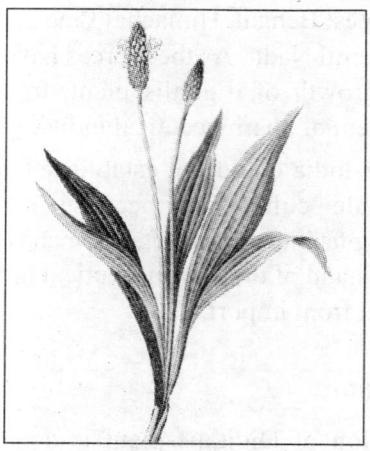

ISPAGHULA (*Plantago ovata*)
(for colour, see Plate 2, Fig. 1)

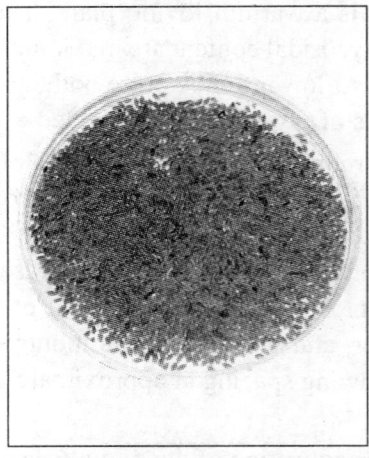

ISPAGHULA (*Plantago ovata* seeds)
(for colour, see Plate 2, Fig. 2)

Plantago, has only two species, namely *P. ovata* and *P. psyllium* (French Psyllium), are cultivated for their seed husk, which is used in pharmaceutical and cosmetic industries. Seed husk of *Plantago ovata* is superior in terms of swelling qualities and colorlessness.

Production

Initially the plantago seeds were used to be collected from wild source. As the wild source depleted and the demand for the seeds supply had increased, the plants were brought under cultivation. India holds monopoly in the world trade of Psyllium. **More than 90% of the Indian produce is exported and earning runs into crores. Total production is about 98000 tonnes of seeds.**

At present the Gujarat state acquired the place of dollar-earner in ispaghula production. About 16,000-20,000 hectares of land in Mehsana and Banaskantha district is being used for ispaghula cultivation. New areas in the districts of Kutch, Jamnagar, Ahemdabad, Rajkot, Junagarh, Bhavnagar and Kaira have also been brought under cultivation for ispaghula crop. It is also cultivated in small areas of Sirohi (Rajasthan), Rewari (Haryana), Sasaram (Bihar) and to a very small extent in Uttar Pradesh, but the produce is not of superior quality and is being consumed locally.

Cultivation

Plantago ovata is a short-stemmed annual herb, which attains a height of 30-40 cms. It grows well in warm temperate regions. In India the crop is grown in the winter. In general, cool and dry weather is favourable for the crop.

Cultivation is done by **seed propagation**. Good quality of seeds are selected, treated with tetramethylthiuram disulphide or any other mercurial seed dressing mixed with fine sand or sieved farm yard manure. The seeds are· sown by broadcasting in well-tilled dry sandy soil of pH 7.2-7.9 with about 0.8 kg organic carbon and 280 kg potash per hectare but low in phosphate. Irrigation is to be done at an interval of 7-8 days after germination, and about 6-7 total irrigations are sufficient.

Flowering starts two months after sowing and the crop is ready for harvesting in March or April. Plants are cut with the help of hand sickles 15 cm above the ground, heaped and dried for 2 days and then threshed in the threshing yard. Seeds are collected and winnowed repeatedly to separate out the undesirable plant parts. Seeds collected after thrashing the harvested plants, are transported to factories/mills for processing. The main factories are located at **Palampur, Sidhpur and Kakosi**. The seeds are passed through sieving pans to separate out dust particles, shrivelled and deformed seeds. The remaining seeds are passed through grinding mills. The grounded seeds materials is again sieved and winnowed to separate out the husk from the coarse remains of the kernel. The kernels are passed through screens of 30, 40, 60, 70, 80 and 100 mesh to separate it out into products of different fineness, such as ordinary shell (broken shell), flat husk and powdered husk.

The husk obtained from different milling vary in quality and are kept separate and mixed in different proportion on the basis of the quality in demand.

The factories engaged in the processing of Isabgol husk are mainly concentrated in **Banaskantha and Mehsana District of Gujarat**. The important centres are Sidhpur, Unjha Patan and Palampur.

Utilization

Plantago ovata seeds contain mucilage, fatty oils, large quantities of albuminous matter and pharmacologically inactive glycoside known as **aucubin**.

Seeds of ispaghula were noticed early by the

western practitioners and were adopted into Indian pharmacopoeia in 1868. The Persian physician **Alhervi**, prescribed its use as early as 10th century for the treatment of chronic dysentery and intestinal fluxes. Seeds are demulcent and mildly astringent. Astringency is increased by roasting.

Plantago seeds and seed husk are recommended for the following uses:

1. The seed husk has property of absorbing and retaining the water. On account of this property the seeds husk is utilized in the treatment of **chronic dysentery** and for the demulcent property of the seeds, it is used in the ulcerated surface of the intestinal mucosa.

2. In indigenous medicine the seeds are considered **cooling and diuretic**, and are recommended in febrile conditions and in the infections of kidneys, bladder and Urethra.

3. Crushed seeds made into **poultice** are applied to rheumatic and glandular swelling.

4. The seed husk are used in **reducing the serum cholesterol level**. The *P. ovata* oil contain linoleic acid, (responsible for reducing the cholesterol level) is reported to be more potent than sunflower (recommended for reducing serum cholesterol level). Its therapeutic value is increased when prescribed along metronidazole. As per the clinical data available the dose of 10 g isabgol every day for a month reduces the serum cholesterol level by 9.6% and triglyceride level by 8.6%.

5. The seeds decoction with honey is used to treat sore **throat and bronchitis**. Chilled decoctions is recommended as **eye drops**. Water decoction is used locally for all types of skin blemishes.

6. **Isabgol jelly** useful as a substitute for agar-agar; can be obtained by treating the husk with hot caustic soda solution and subsequent neutralization.

7. The husk has been found to act as a **good** binder and **disintegrant** in compound tablet.

8. The mucilage of the seed coat **provide protective coating** to the inner wall of intestine and protects it against the irritant action produced by the irritant particles present in the food. The mucilage also **absorbs the toxin** if present in the gut and help in excreting them out from the body. It acts as a lubricant in the large intestine. The seed husk can be given alone or in combination with powdered anhydrous dextrose, sodium bicarbonate and citric acid etc.

9. It may serve as **stabilizer in ice-cream**, filler for wheat starch and additive in chocolate etc.

10. Some of the leading pharmaceutical companies like M/s. Parke Davis and M/s. J.B. Williams are marketing the seed husk, supplement with fruit fragrance under different trademark named as **"Siblin"** and **'Sirutan'** respectively and are prescribed as laxative.

11. The Central Drug Research Institute (CDRI), Lucknow has developed sweet palatable, flavoured granules and fine powdered preparation of Isabgol marketing under the name of **"Ligafin"**, Laxative. The CDRI, Lucknow has also developed **Isapatent sticks** from Isabgol for use in termination of pregnancy (MTP) and are marketed under the brand name Isabgol (dilex-C) tent. This device is quite safe, cheap and quick in action in comparison to age old laminariatent made from sea weeds.

The seeds of *P. ovata* soaked in water are recommended for treatment of Cancer.

12. The seeds and husk mucilage is also used in **textile** and **cosmetic industry**.

13. A product of Psyllium i.e. "Isabgol-Gola" is recommended as **cattle feed** without any side effects.

DIOSCOREA

Dioscorea is one of the largest plant genera known, containing 600-800 species (Diosco-reaceae) and numbers of these are cultivated for their large starchy tubers commonly known as **Yams**. About 15 species are reported to contain steroidal sapogenin, chiefly **diosgenin**.

Most of the world production of diosgenin is met with Central American species; *D. floribunda* and *D. composita* both growing wild in Central America.

In **India** *D. deltoidea* and *D. prazeri* occurring wild in North West and North East Himalayas respectively are the natural source of diosgenin. *D. deltoidea* is found in India, Pakistan, Nepal and Bhutan extending to south Western China while *D. prazeri* occurs in Eastern India. Burma, and Northern part of Malaysia, Mexico, Guatemala, Costa Rica, India, China and some countries in Europe and Africa are the major Dioscorea producing countries.

Production of Dioscorea

Dioscorea deltoidea grows wild throughout North western Himalayas and extends from Kashmir, Himachal Pradesh, Darjeeling to Sikkim, Nepal

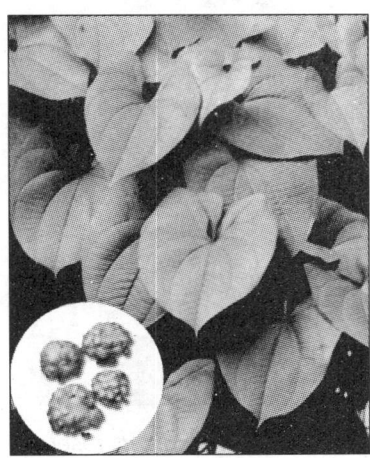

DIOSCOREA (*D. deltoidea*)
(for colour, see Plate 2, Fig. 3)

and Bhutan at an altitude ranging from 1000-3500 metres. In J&K it is widely distributed in the forest of Bhadarwah, Kishtwar and Doda (Jammu) and forest of Ovra (Pehalgam) Shikargarh, Kangan and Pirpanchal in Kashmir.

In Uttar Pradesh, it is available in upper reaches of hills and Jamuna valley, dry temperate regions of Uttarkashi and Chamoli in Garhwal and in Kumaon hills.

In the mountainous region of J&K, H.P. and Punjab, *D. deltoidea* grows better in the areas where annual rainfall varies between 100–200 cm and minimum temperature in winter goes below freezing point and the maximum temperature in summer does not exceed 32°C. It has also been observed that *D. deltoidea* grows generally on the Northern and Eastern slopes in shady but well drained conditions.

The total estimated demand of corticosteroids is about 10,000 kg whereas actual production is about 4000 kg. The synthesis of diosgenin not being commercially feasible for production of steroidal drugs, the pharmaceutical industry has to resort to natural source for the procurement of this raw material. The diosgenin percentage of *D. deltoidea* varies from 0.6-10.3%. Hence, *D. deltoidea* seems to be the best natural source of diosgenin, but it is too slow growing for adoption as a commercial crop.

Dioscorea is obtained both from wild and culti-vated sources. Dioscorea tubers can be grown from seeds propagation, but it takes long time for harvesting. Commercially it is economical to grow it from tubers. Its cultivation from tubers requires attention to correct the soil and drainage. Soil should be rich in humus with pH 6.8-7.2, free from weeds, virus, fungus and insect to result in healthy growth of tubers. Healthy tubers weighing about 50-70 gms in weight are selected, they are treated with fungicide and sown in nursery beds.

Tubers take four to five weeks time to sprout. After two to three months of growth, tubers are retransplanted into well manured, fungicide and insecticide treated soil. The tubers are placed at a distance of 30 × 60 cm, initially support (bamboo stakes or wire cages) is provided for the vines, which are weak. According to the species, the tubers reach maturity in 3-5 years and on average, yield 1-8% of the total sapogenin. They are collected after the leaves drop. The average production in the case of *D. floribunda* is 16-18 metric tonnes of tubers or approximately 500 kg of diosgenin per hectare.

In tubercles, **diosgenin** occurs as **dioscin**, closely related glycosides **gracillin** or both. **Dioscin** comprise two molecules of L-rhamnose and one molecule of *D. glucose*. **Gracillin** comprises two molecules of *D. glucose* and one molecule of L-rhamnose.

Production of Diosgenin

Fresh tubers are cut into small pieces and crushed, followed by fermentation for 4-10 days. The fermented mixture is then hydrolysed with mineral acid, filtered, washed and dried (sapogenin is water insoluble).

Another method is to cut the tubers into small pieces, dried, powdered and hydrolysis of dioscin is done by mineral acid, to liberate the **diosgenin**. After filtration, the insoluble fraction is neutralized, washed and extracted with a non-polar solvent (e.g. petroleum ether or toluene) which will extract **diosgenin**.

For the isolation of glycoside the following method can be adopted; the tubers are washed, dried, sliced and extracted with hot water or 95% ethyl alcohol for several hours. The alcoholic extract is concentrated under vacuum and the glycosides is precipitated with solvent ether or by lead acetate (in the case of acid saponin) followed by hydrolysis and extraction with petroleum ether, 40-60°C will isolate the diosgenin.

Utilization

Dioscorea is the major source for the production of diosgenin, which is the main raw material used in the synthesis of corticosteroids, sex hormones and anti-fertility compounds.

- Diosgenin accounts precursors for approximately 50% of the total steroidal products in the world.
- Dioscorea is also utilized for the treatment of rheumatic arthritis, in natural hormone replacement therapy. It is also used for the relaxation of muscles and to promote glandular balance in women. Wild yam is prescribed for the improvement of digestive system and as nerve tonic.

VINCA
(*Catharanthus roseus*)

Synonym : Vinca Rosea; Lochnera Rosea.

Common Name : Sadabahar, Sadaphul, Nayan tara, Rattanjot and Gul Feringhi.

Vinca (Catharanthus) is the dried whole plant of *Catharanthus roseus* G. Don (Apocynaceae). It is an erect, ever blooming pubescent herb or

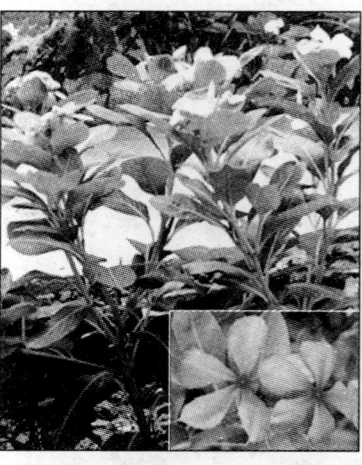

VINCA (*Catharanthus roseus*)
(for colour, see Plate 2, Fig. 4)

sub-shrub, woody at the base and 40-80 cm high. The plant is probably native to Madagascar but now cosmopolitan in the tropics and is widely cultivated as an ornamental. The flowers are normally violet, rose or white in color. Botanically, it is closely related to vinca minor Linn, the common periwinkle.

It is grown commercially for its medicinal uses in Australia, Africa, India and Southern Europe.

The species *Catharanthus roseus* (L) G Don has also been referred in the literature as *Vinca rosea* L and as *Lochnera rosea* (L).

The alkaloids isolated from the Catharanthus (Lochnera) species and from Vinca species are collectively referred to as the **vinca alkaloids**.

It has been reported that alkaloidal content of *C. roseus* varies considerably in different parts of the plant and from different localities. It has been reported that total alkaloidal content is more in the roots (0.15-1.795%) in some strains. The plant contains more than 100 alkaloids of **Indole group** out of which about 25 are of **dimeric** in nature. Two of the dimeric alkaloids; **vinblastine** and **vincristine** have been found to be used in the treatment of human neoplasm. Among **monomeric ajmalicine** (Raubasine) has been found to be used in the relief of obstruction of normal cerebral blood flow. In combination with Rauwolfia alkaloids it has been reported to be used to lower high blood pressures.

Due to the clinical importance of the plants, i.e. **oncolytic** dimeric (VC & VB) alkaloids (present in the leaves) and the **hypotensive** alkaloids (ajmalicine, present in roots), the plant *C. roseus* has found high place in commerce. The bulk of leaves, which were exported to USA and Hungary are now being processed for alkaloidal contents (Vineristine and Vinblastine alkaloids) in India by **M/s. Southern Herbals Bangalore**. The process of production of these two dimeric alkaloids is based on the technology provided by NCP Pune. For the production of **ajmalicine** (monomeric alkaloid) from roots of the plant, by the same company, method of production has been provided by RRL Jammu.

Production of Vinca

Cultivation

The plant is cultivated for its alkaloids. It is commonly grown in garden for beddings, borders and for mass effect. The plant blooms throughout the year and is propagated by seeds or by cutting. The plant can grow luxuriantly under a great variety of climatic and soil conditions except the highly alkaline or water logged soils. It prefers light, well-drained, sandy loam. A mild tropical climate and well distributed rainfall of 100 cm per annum sufficient to raise a commercial rain-fed crop.

The fresh seeds are sown with the onset of monsoon in late June in rows 10-15 cm apart in small beds and then irrigated immediately. The seedlings are transplanted at a distance of 30 to 45 cm. About 75,000 plants are sufficient for a hectare.

Harvesting

About 150 days after sowing the roots penetrate the soil up to 15-20 cm then develop lateral roots. Roots collection is done after one year, during this period, two stripping are obtained and third one at the time when whole plant is to be harvested. The harvested leaves are dried in shade and stored in gunny bags. In between the leaves harvesting, the plants are manured with 20 kg nitrogen per hectare to hasten the growth.

For harvesting the roots the plants are cut about 7 cm above the ground level. The roots are washed. The basal stem up to 10 cm long are dugged out and separated from roots, cut into pieces, dried and stored at normal storage condition till are in use (one to two years).

Yield - The total roots from an irrigated plant is about 2.2 tonnes/hectare.

The rain fed crop yield about 1-1.5 tonnes per hectare.

Plant Tissue Culture Technique for the Production of Vinca Alkaloids

New methods of biotechnology have also been developed for the production of vincristine and vinblastine through **shoots suspension culture** and have shown good results.

Ajmalicine, catharanthidine, serpentine, vindoline and yohimbine alkaloids have been produced by **Hairy root culture** obtained by infection with Agrobacterium rhizogenes.

The alkaloids **serpentine** and **ajmalicine** have also been produced in cell suspension culture of *C. roseus*. For large scale alkaloids production specific medium is employed (Zenk's medium)

most cell lines had shown maximum accumulation in 3rd to 5th week of the culture.

For **alkaloids isolation**, water is removed by freeze drying and alkaloids are extracted in the conventional manner. The studies show that the percentage of alkaloids **ajmalicine** and **yohimbine** per gram of cell weight increased with time and the optimum production at 3-4 weeks.

Production of Ajmalicine (alkaloid) (Fig. 4.9)

Regional Research Laboratory Jammu has developed a process on pilot plant scale for the extraction of **ajmalicine** and **serpentine** from *C. roseus*, to export a high value low volume

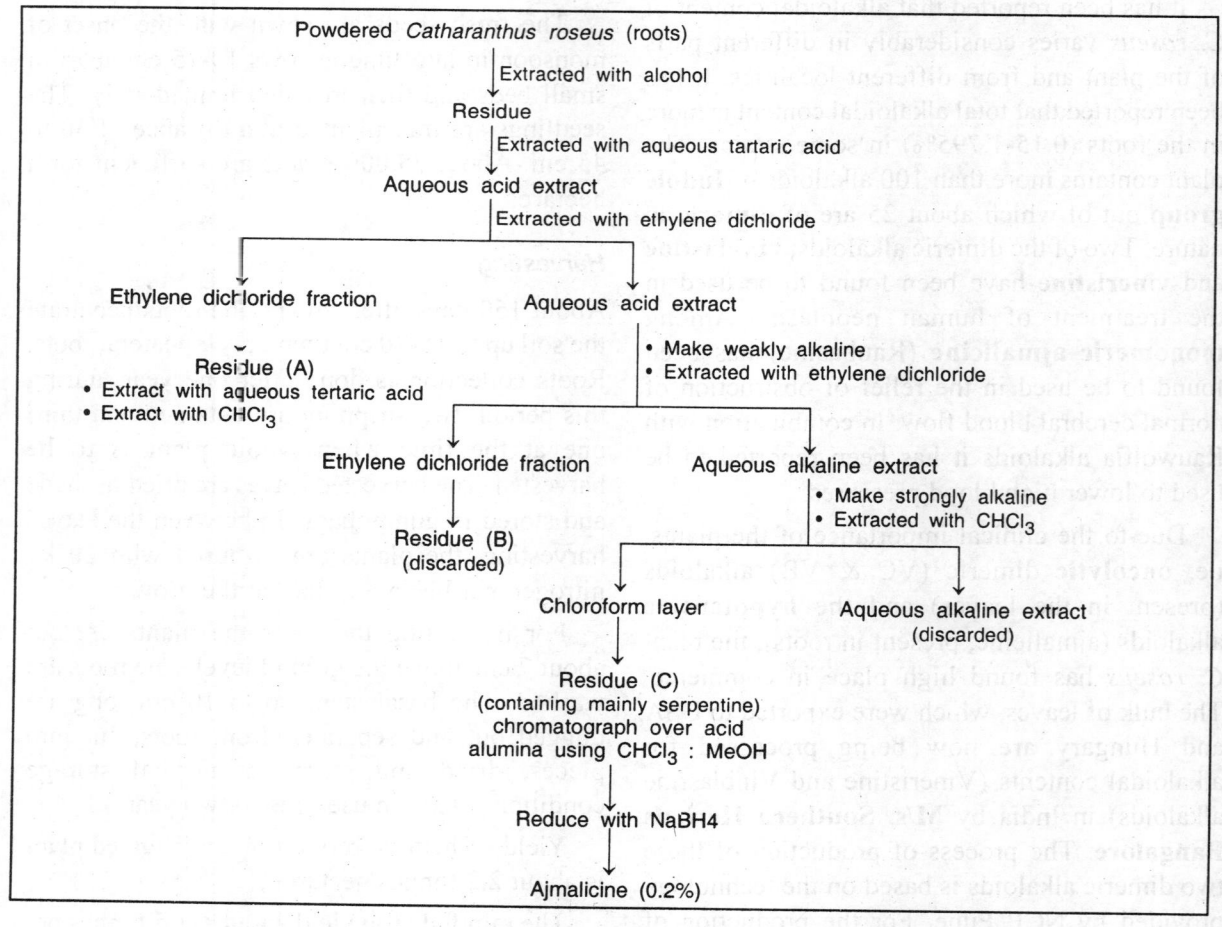

Fig. 4.9. Isolation of Ajmalicine from Catharanthuis roseus (Vinca) roots.

product ajmalicine instead of low value high volume product like root, which were exported to European countries. The RRL institute has also developed a technique of conversion of serpentine to ajmalicine and giving an overall yield of 0.15-0.2% depending upon the percentage of total alkaloids in roots (Fig. 4.9).

The extraction process of Vincristine and total Vinca alkaloids is given in the Fig. 4.10 & 4.11 respectively.

Utilization of Vinca (*C. roseus*)

The plant has been used as folk remedy for diabetes in natal and various other parts of South Africa and also in India and Ceylon. The juice of the leaves is used as an application for wasp stings. The roots were considered to be toxic and stomachic. However, the discovery of tumour inhibiting properties and the isolation of alkaloids useful as sedative and for hypertension had opened new avenues for the use of this plant.

Leaf alkaloids vinblastine, vincristine vindoline, vinleurosine and vincosidine have been shown to be effective in the treatment of neoplastic disease in animals and in man.

Vinblastine sulphate is a cytotoxic drug that arrests cell growth at the metaphase stage and used mainly for the treatment of Hodgkin's disease and other lymphomas and choriocarcinoma. Other conditions in which **vincristine sulphate** has produced remission are : lymphosarcoma, reticulum sarcoma, neuroblastoma,

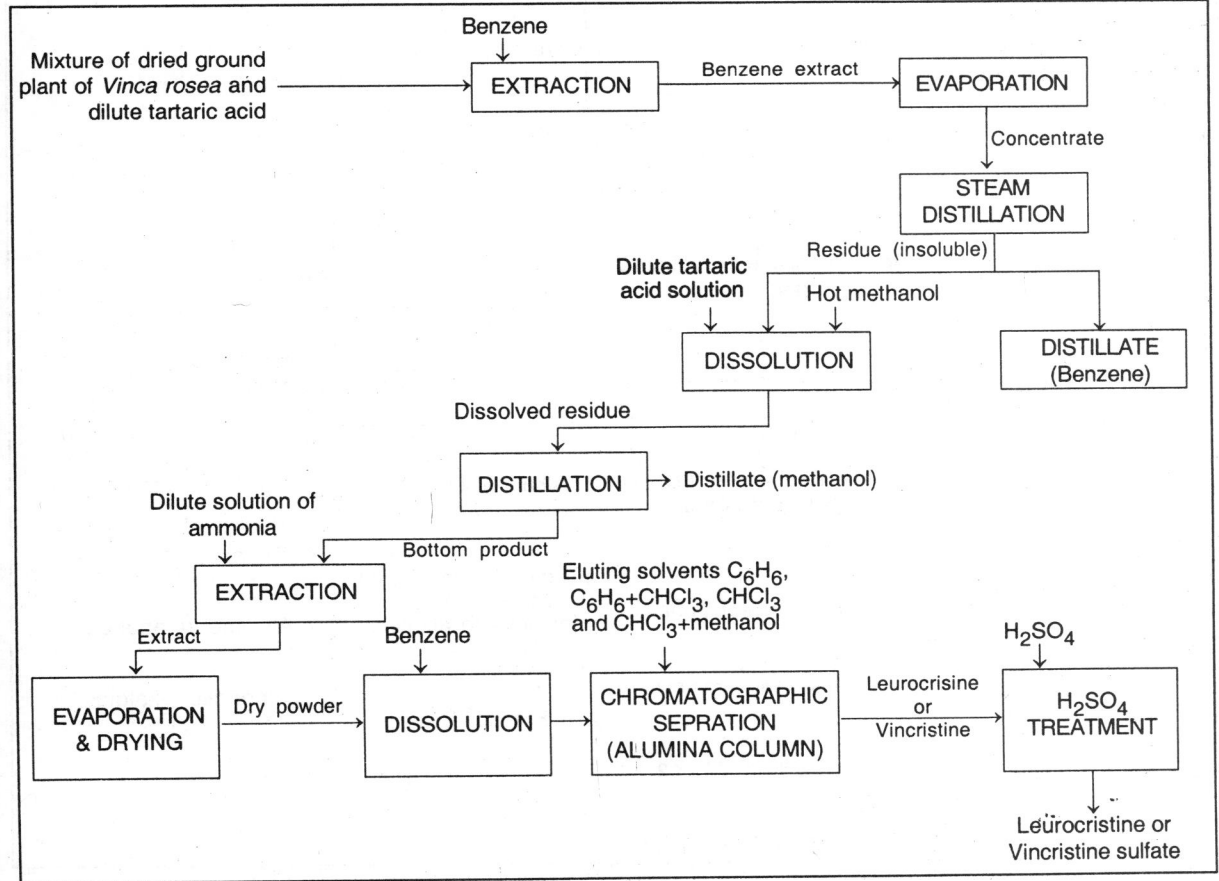

Fig. 4.10. Block diagram for Vincristine sulphate or Leurocristine sulphate.

wilm's tumour and tumour of breast, brain and lungs. The treatment should be given under the supervision of oncologist.

Root alkaloids : serpentine and ajmalicine are used in the treatment of high blood pressure.

In Jamaica, **tea of vinca** was used to treat **diabetes**. The alkaloids catharanthine, leurosine sulphate, lochnerine, tetrahydroalstoline and vindoline lower blood sugar levels.

Madagascar vinca (Periwinkle) has also been

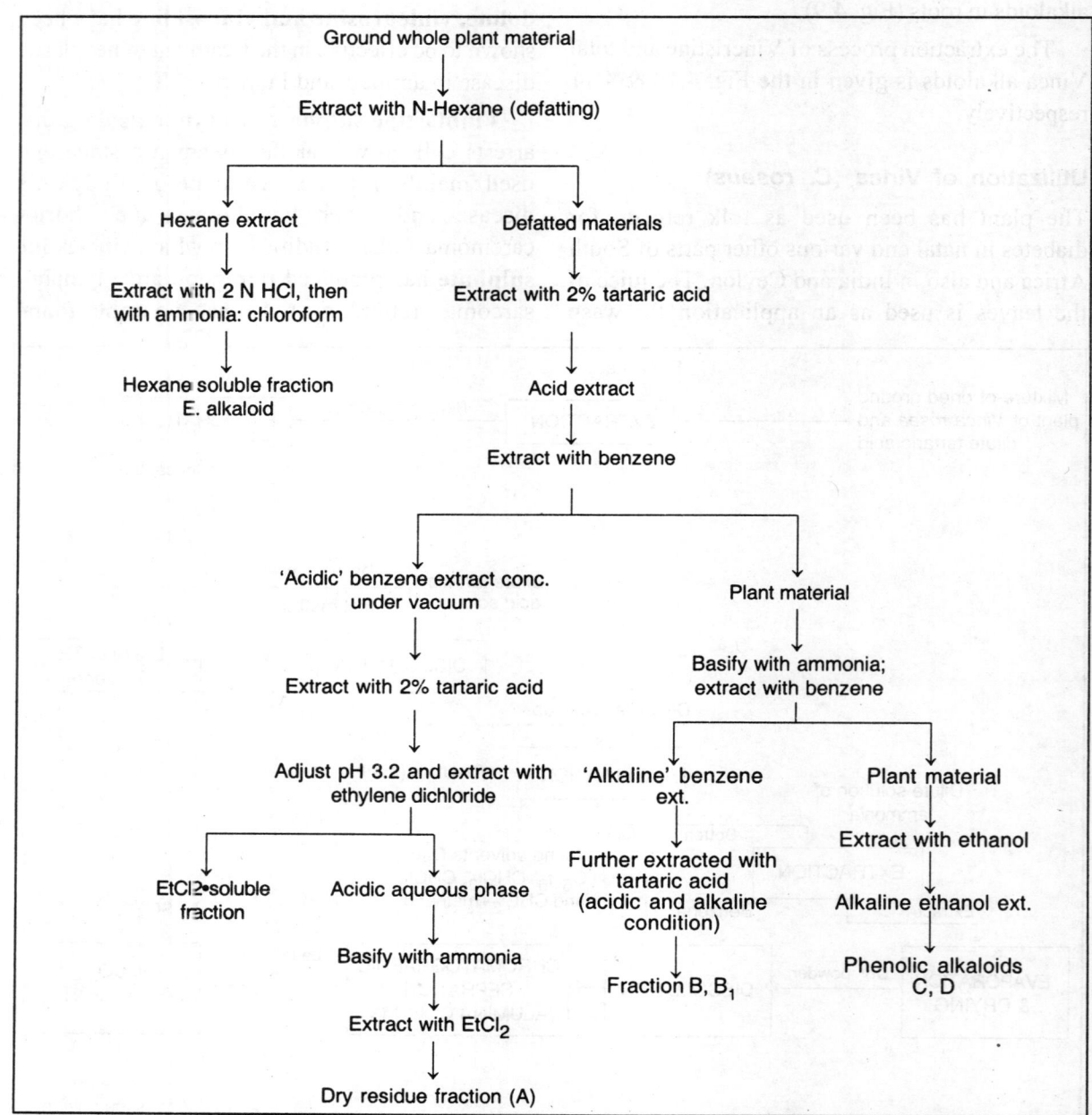

Fig. 4.11. Flow chart for extraction and separation of Vinca alkaloids (Svoboda's method).

used for centuries to treat diabetes, high blood pressure, asthma, constipation and menstrual problems. More recently extracts from Madagascar (periwinkle) have also shown to be effective in the treatment of various kinds of leukaemia, skin cancer, lymph cancer, breast cancer and Hodgkin's disease.

ALOE

Aloe is the solid residue obtained by evaporating the juice which drains from the transversely cut leaves of various species of Aloe (Liliaceae/Aloe-aceae) including *Aloe ferox* (Cape aloes), *Aloe barbadensis* (Curacao aloes) and *Aloe perryi* (Secotrine aloes).

The juice is usually concentrated by boiling and solidify on cooling.

It is hard and friable soluble in hot water, somewhat plastic in summer, and growing soft between the fingers, easily pulverizable and when reduced to powder, it is bright, golden color.

Production of Aloes

About 300 species of aloe are known, most of which are indigenous to Africa. Many have been introduced into the West Indies and Europe. It is

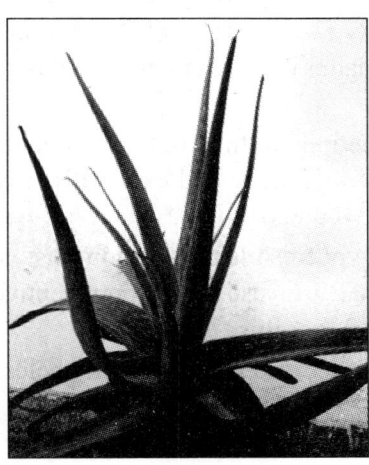

ALOE *(A. vera)*
(for colour, see Plate 2, Fig. 5)

also now cultivated in many parts of India, including North West Himalayan region; Alwar in Rajasthan, Satnapalli in Andhra Pradesh and Rajpiplain in Gujarat.

The aloes are typical xerophytic plants that have fleshy sessile leaves, usually have spines at the margins.

The plant is cultivated from root sucker, planted in row about 50 cm apart in dry climatic conditions. The plant can grow even in poor grades of soil. The leaves are harvested after two years of cultivation and subsequent collection can be continued annually for ten to twelve years, and after twelve years the plants are completely harvested by uprooting and replanted in the freshly prepared ground.

Leaf juice of aloes contains number of chemical compounds. It contains aloins, a small amount of volatile oil, resin, gum, emodin, anthraquinone derivatives, chrysophanic acid and traces of coumarins.

Cape aloes (shining aloes) is obtained from wild plants of *Aloe ferox* and its hybrids from South Africa and Kenya. The leaves are cut transversely in March and April and placed cut end downward in a shallow hole in the ground, which is lined with plastic sheet or more traditionally with a piece of canvas or a goat skin. After about 6 hours all the juice is collected and transferred to a drum or paraffin tin in which it is boiled for about 4 hours on an open fire. The product is poured while hot into tins, each holding 25 kg, where it is solidified and ready for export.

Cape aloe has a glossy or resinous fracture, a deep brown or olive color. Its odour is more powerful and unpleasant than the **Barbadensis aloes**. Its taste is peculiar and bitter and its powder is bright yellow having a greenish tint.

Aloe Barbadensis (USP), Barbadoes aloes

The variety is available in hard masses, orange

brown, opaque, translucent on the edges; fracture waxy or resinous, odour saffron-like, taste strongly bitter, when examined under microscope (alcoholic solution) exhibits numerous crystals.

Aloe socotrina USP (Socotrine aloes)

It is also available in hard masses, occasionally soft in the interior, opaque, yellowish-brown, orange-brown or dark ruby-red, translucent on the edges. Fracture resinous, somewhat conchoidal. Odour is fragrant, saffron like. **Taste** peculiar bitter.

Solubility : Almost entirely soluble in alcohol and in 4 parts of boiling water.

Microscopic Examination : It also exhibits numerous crystals when its alcoholic solution is examined under microscope.

Curacao Aloes

Curacao aloes is produced from cultivated plants of *Aloe barbadensis* from the West Indian Islands of **Curacao, Aruba and Bonaire**. The cut leaves are placed with cut end downwards on a V-shaped trough, the latter being inclined so that latex can led into a vessel. When sufficient juice has been collected, it is evaporated in a copper kettle. The temperature used is generally lower than in the case of Cape aloes, therefore the product is generally opaque. The products, which are semi-transparent may be known in commerce as **"Capey Barbadoes"**. The drug is exported to USA in cases, each holding about 58.5 kg.

Note: Socotrine and Zanzibar varieties are no longer official.

Aloe purificata (USP)

Aloes can be purified by using following Pharmacopoeial method of purification. Take one thousand grams (1000 gm) of aloe and two hundred cubic centimeter (200 cc) of alcohol. Heat the aloes by means of water bath until it is completely melted.

Then add the alcohol and having stirred the mixture thoroughly, strain it through a no 60 Sieve, (which has just been dipped into boiling water). Evaporate the strained mixture over water bath, constantly stirring (avoid overheating) until the thread of the mass becomes brittle on cooling. Lastly break the product (when cold) into pieces of a dull-brown or reddish brown or blackish brown depending upon the variety and having peculiar aromatic odour and packed in a well-stoppered container.

Utilization

- Aloe is a pharmaceutical aid for a compound benzoin tincture and a cathartic.
- Decoction of dried leaves is taken orally to induce abortion for sexual vitality.
- Hot water extract of dried entire plant is used as an emmenagogue, purgative, anthelmintic, stomachic, for liver enlargement, spleen enlargement and for piles treatment.
- Hot water extract of fresh plant juice is taken orally for the treatment of inflammatory amenorrhea and to increase menstrual flow.
- In USA, fresh leaf juice taken orally for stomach ulcers and used externally to heal wounds.
- In India fresh leaves are crushed and applied locally for guinea worms and orally to treat viral jaundice, it is taken twice daily for three days.
- Decoction of the root is taken orally for venereal disease and externally it is used to treat wounds.
- In Egypt fresh leaf juice administered intravaginally to use as a contraceptive before and after coitus.
- In Mexico taken orally for diabetes.

Therapeutic uses of Aloe barbadensis

Topical : Wound and burn healing; psoriasis, sunburn.

Aloe vera is reported to have antibacterial, antifungal and anti-inflammatory properties. Utilized in cosmetic products as a moisturizing emollient and widely used for radiation and thermal burns. Aloe is also used as skin healer for cuts, insect bites, bruises, acne, poison ivy, welts, skin ulcers, eczema and for varicose veins, skin cancer, arthritis and AIDS.

Products of Aloe vera

These are derived from the mucilage located in the parenchymatous cells of the *Aloe vera* leaf and should not be confused with aloes. The mucilaginous gel has been used from early times for the treatment of numerous conditions but in recent years its use in the herbal and cosmetic industries has become very big business in USA, Europe and Elsevier.

Aloe vera gel

Herbal's superior quality *Aloe vera* gel is prepared from freshly picked organically grown leaves and does not contain any added water or extender. No artificial fertilizer or pesticides are used. The plants are irrigated with natural spring water and individual leaves are harvested from only the ripest plant.

When used internally, it has antiviral, antibacterial, antifungal, anti-inflammatory and potent stimulant laxative properties.

Aloe gel has action on dead epithelial cells on the skin surface, which cause ageing of skin due to cellular build up on the outer layer. Aloe gel softens these dead cells and their removal from the surface leaving the skin smoother.

Aloe gel has an astringent action besides; it has shown remarkable results on sun-damaged skin with its moisturizing, softening and healing action.

Aloe vera gel is also used for variety of purposes such as in the preparation of balms, different skin creams, suntan preparation, body lotions, shampoos, bath salts, soaps, talc, body powder and detergents.

Friar's balsam : (Compound tincture of benzoin)

Aloe constitutes an important ingredient of the Friar's balsam.

IPECAC

Ipecac consists of dried roots and rhizomes of *Cephaelis ipecacuanha* or Brazilian ipecac (Rubiaceae) indigenous to Brazil, from where most of the present supplies originate. The plant is a small shrubby about a foot high found growing in clumps or patches in moist shady woods. It is also cultivated to a limited extent in India and Malaysia. *C. acuminata* referred to as Cartagena or Nicaragua or Panama ipecac is indigenous to Colombia, Panama and Nicaragua.

Production of the Drug

In the Mattto Grosso district of Brazil the drug is collected from wild plants. The roots are dried in the sun or by fires and transported down river to

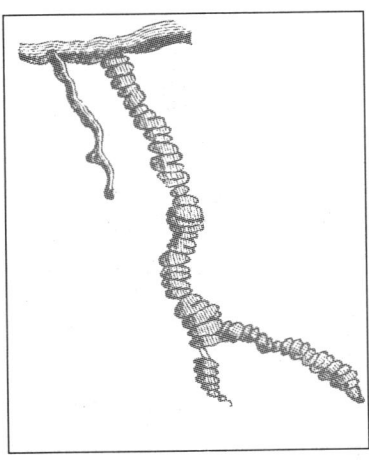

IPECAC ROOT *(Cephaelis ipecacuanha)*
(for colour, see Plate 2, Fig. 6)

port such as Rio de Janeiro, Bahia and Pernambuco from where it is exported in bales.

In India cultivation of Rio-ipecac is being done in West Bengal, which is known by the name of **Johore ipecac** but the lower foot hills of Eastern Himalayas is the best area for the better yield, **cultivation is done by seed propagation**. The seeds are sown in the month of Jan. to Feb. Two months old seedling are transplanted at spacing of 10 × 15 cm. For the yield of alkaloid, nitrogen fertilizer along with humid atmosphere and the temperature within the range of 25-35°C are the best conditions. The harvesting of the roots is done after three years.

The production and supply of Ipecac had been very erratic for many years and high price favours cultivation, hence, stimulated efforts to produce alkaloids by **cell culture**. The production of ipecacuanha alkaloids was increased by **artificial culture** obtained by the induction of hairy root culture in contrast to whole roots. It has been reported that cell culture, produces more yield of cephaeline than emetine, and **immobilized cell systems** give higher amounts of **cephaeline** compared with **static cell culture** mainly used for domestic manufacture of emetine.

It is also reported that by co-cultivation of three plantlets of *Eclipta alba* associated with one *C. ipecacuanha* produced higher emetine content (1, 29 mg) and a three-fold biomass increase of ipecac.

The principal producer of *C. ipecacuanha* are **Brazil** (Matto Grosso) and **India**. Small quantities are produced in **Malaysia**. *C. acuminata* is produced chiefly in Costa Rica and Nicaragua and smaller quantities are obtained from Columbia and Panama. Production data from India indicate that production has fallen from 25-30 tonnes to 9-10 tonnes of dry roots annually from cultivation.

Production of Phytoconstituent of Ipecac

The main phytochemical constituent is emetine for which laid down procedure is shown in schematic diagram given in Fig. 4.12.

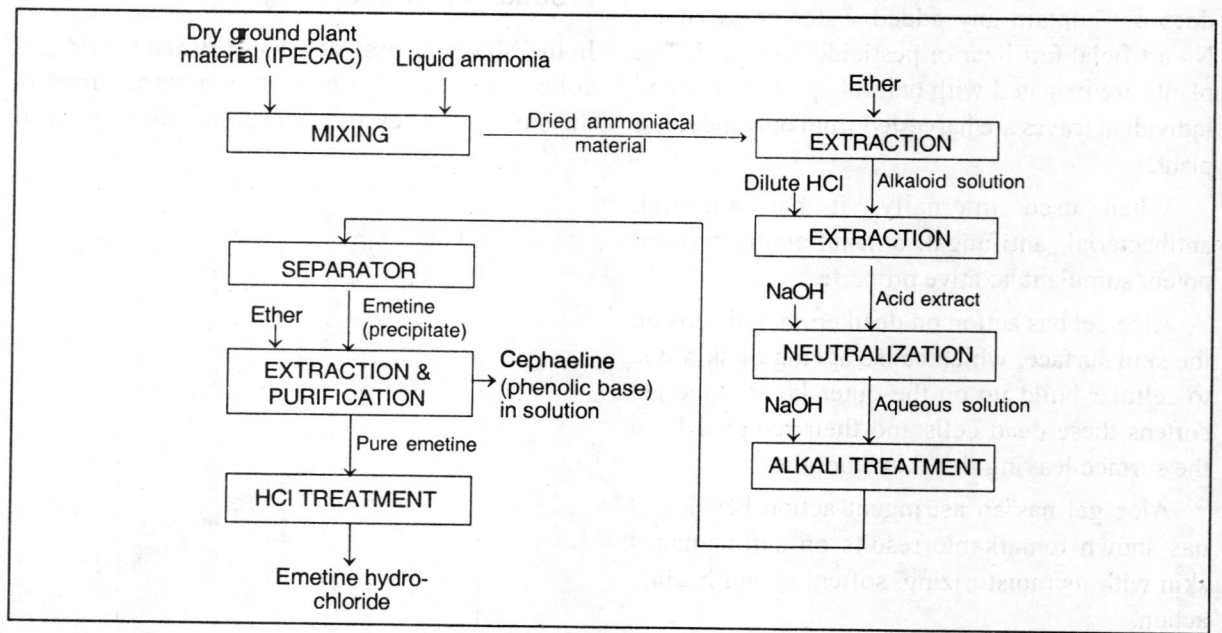

Fig. 4.12. Schematic diagram for Emetine hydro-chloride.

Utilization of Ipecac

The drug ipecac is used in the form of crude extract as **emetic and expectorant**. It is also used as a **source of emetine**, which is used to treat **amoebic dysentery**.

Ipecac powder (1 part) along with 1 part opium (Dover's powder) used as **diaphoretic**.

Ipecac in small doses along with aconite or belladonna used in the treatment of **pneumonia** especially in children.

Five drops of ipecac syrup in a half glass of water and a teaspoonful every hour is useful in the treatment of acute bronchitis. It is an excellent remedy in amoebic hepatitis and hepatic abscess.

In smaller doses ipecac is used as bitter tonic to improve the digestion.

SENNA

Senna leaves are the dried leaflets of *Cassia senna* (*C. acutifolia* (leguminosae) known in commerce as **Alexandrian or Khartoum senna** and *C. angustifolia* known in commerce as **Tinnevelly senna** or a mixture of both species, containing not less than 2.5% of anthraquinone glycosides calculated as sennoside B.

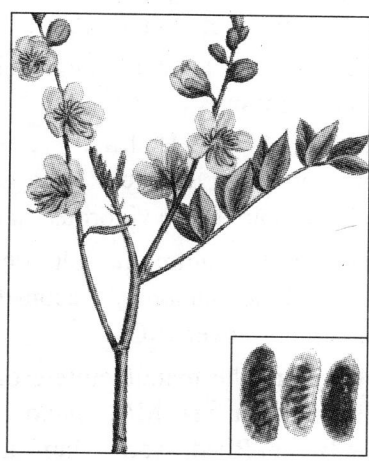

SENNA *(Cassia angustifolia)*
(for colour, see Plate 2, Fig. 7)

Senna pods are the dried or nearly ripe pods of *Cassia senna* (*C. acutifolia* Family leguminosae), known in commerce, as **Alexandrian senna** and of *C. angustifolia* known in commerce, as **Tinnevelly senna**, the principal active constituents of senna pods are also Sennoside A and Sennoside B. Alexandrian pods contain about 2.5–4.5% of these glycosides and Tinnevelly pods about 1.2-2.5%. European Pharmacopoeia specifies not less than 4% of hydroxyanthracene derivatives calculated as Sennoside B for alexandrian pods and not less than 2.5% for Tinnevelly pods. Indian senna leaflet contains 2.5%; and pods 3.5-4% sennosides.

Alexandrian senna is cultivated extensively in Sudan.

Tinnevelly senna is cultivated in India; the important states where cultivation is being done are Tamil Nadu, Maharashtra, Gujarat and Rajasthan.

Cultivation in India

Senna is an annual crop, sometimes, but rarely cultivated as a perennial. In India its cultivation is mainly concentrated in the Tinnevelly, Maudrai and Ramanathapuram district of Tamil Nadu and on small scale in other states mentioned above. The plant is also found to grow wild in Kutch, a district of Gujarat.

In Tamil Nadu the crop is cultivated under dry conditions (purely rain-fed) or under irrigated (garden land) conditions, but by far the larger area is being covered under rain fed conditions only. The crop is cultivated on red soil as well as on black soil. There are two main seasons for sowing the crop, one is March-April and other is November-December. Propagation method is by seed propagation followed by irrigation at sowing and thinning stage. Fertilizer required is 80 kg N: 40 kg P_2O_5 and 20 kg K_2 quantity per hectare. Nitrogen in 4 equal splits (sowing 30 days thinning stage, after first and second harvest) the crop remains in the field for 8-9 months. Senna is cultivated mostly as a pure crop but on a small scale as a mixed crop along with chillies and coriander.

The branches bearing leaves and pods are dried in the sun (shade). The pods and large stalks are separated by means of sieves. After separation from leaves they are hand picked into various qualities, the finer quality being sold in cartons and the inferior ones used for making galenicals.

Production

Total area under production in India is approximately 25000 hac. and the total production is about 22500 tonnes of leaves and is about 7500 tonnes of pods.

Preparation for the Market

For drying, the harvested leaves are spread in thin layers on a floor under the shade avoiding over lapping. In order to ensure uniform drying, the material is frequently stirred by means of rakes or with feet. The drying process takes from week to ten days time (leaves develop a yellowish green color). The pods are also dried in the similar way but when the leaves and pods are dried directly under sun, (this method of drying) give poor color and hence, lowers the quality.

During the drying process sticks, stems, stalks, sand, stones etc. are removed by means of sieving.

Production of Phytochemical Constituents

The principal active constituent of the senna leaves and pods is sennoside for which it is cultivated. Both leaves and fruits are used for the production of sennosides in the form of calcium sennoside. The technology for the production of calcium sennoside supplied by:

Amsar Pvt. Ltd. Indore; Mehta Pharmaceutical

Pvt. Ltd. Amritsar and by Chemiloids Vijayawada is given below.

Sennoside

Method A :

Extracted the senna leaves with 70% methanol at room temperature by shaking for 4 hours, filtered and concentrated to 1/8th volume under Vaccu, then acidified with hydrochloric acid [pH 3], followed by filtration and extraction of the aqueous solution with chloroform to remove the soluble aglycone if any, then neutralised with ammonia and centrifuged to separate the sennoside.

Method B

1. Extraction with benzene at room temperature by shaking for 2-3 hours, filter and recover the benzene under vacuum distillation.
2. Dry the marc left after the benzene extraction, at room temperature or in hot air oven temperature not exceeding 40°C.
3. Dry marc extracted with 70% methanol at room temperature on shaker for 4-6 hours.
4. Repeat extraction with methanol for two hours.
5. Mix both the methanol extracts.
6. Concentrate to 1/8th of the volume under reduced pressure.
7. Adjust pH 3 with HCl and set aside for 3 hours and filter, to the filtrate add $CaCl_2$ (28/25 ml spirit) with vigorous shaking.

Adjust pH to 8 by ammonia solution, set aside for 2 hours, filter the solution by vacuum distillation, dry the precipitate over P_2O_5.

Following are the manufacturers of calcium sennosides in India, viz. M/s. Glaxo Labs Ltd., (Dr. Annie Besant Road, Worli, Mumbai 400 018) M/s. Sandoz India Ltd. (Sandoz House, Dr. Annie Besant Road, Mumbai 400018) and M/s. Chemical

Industrial and Pharmaceutical Laboratories Ltd. (Mumbai), M/s. CIPLA, M/s. Alembic Chemical Works (Baroda), M/s. Kothari Phytochemical International, Madurai and M/s. Bengal Immunity Co. Ltd. (Calcutta).

Utilization

The leaves and fruits (pods) of senna have been used from time immemorial in India and abroad as cathartic. Sennosides, the main constituent of senna, are useful purgative for either habitual constipation or for occasional use. It lacks astringent after effect of rhubarb. Despite the availability of a number of synthetic preparations, sennoside preparations remain among the most important pharmaceutical laxatives.

TROPANE ALKALOIDS

The major tropane alkaloids of pharmacological or therapeutical importance are:

(i) Those occurring in a number of species of the plant belonging to Family **Solanaceae**.

(ii) Those occurring in certain Erythroxylon species (**Erythroxylaceae**).

A number of species of the genera Atropa, Datura, Hyoscyamus, Duboisia and Scopolia, all belonging to family Solanaceae, produce varying quantities of **tropane alkaloids**, hyoscyamine (of which racemic form is atropine), scopolamine (also called hyoscine), meteloidine, belladonine and several other alkaloids chemically related to these, hyoscyamine and scopolamine are the major ones both in the terms of quantity and therapeutically.

All these alkaloids are often collectively referred to as **Solanaceous alkaloids**. These "Solanaceous alkaloids" sometimes are also referred to as the **"Belladonna alkaloids"**, although they occur in great many plant species other than *Atropa belladonna*. For the production of commercial atropine, USP, NF and BPC recognize only *Atropa belladonna*, *Datura Stramonium* and *Hyoscyamus niger* as crude drug (dried plant material).

Belladonna Herb
(Deadly night shade plant)

Belladonna consists of fresh or dried leaves and flowering tops of *Atropa belladonna* Linn (Known as European belladonna) or *Atropa acuminata* Royle Ex (known as Indian belladonna).

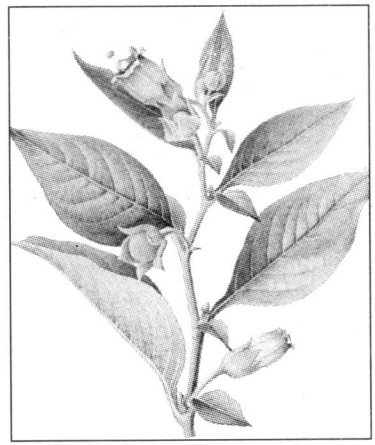

ATROPA *(A. belladonna)*
(for colour, see Plate 2, Fig. 8)

It is indigenous to and cultivated in England and other European countries.

In India, it is found in Western Himalayas from Shimla to Kashmir.

The plant is a tall perennial herb producing dull-purple bell-shaped flowers followed by conspicuous shiny black cherry fruits. The plant is propagated from seeds. The leaves are said to be richest in alkaloid at the end of June or in July. Plants about 3 years old are sufficiently large to give good yield of leaves. The tops of the plant are harvested 2-3 times per year and dried immediately after collection and stored carefully (Belladonna herb).

To obtain good colored leaves, drying is done in thin layers starting with a moderate heat, which is gradually increased to about 60°C and then gradually decreased. Roots from 3-4 years old plants are collected for the isolation of alkaloids but generally the roots contain small quantities of alkaloids.

In India cultivation is being extensively done in Kashmir and Tamil Nadu. Over the years and centuries it has been procured only from wild sources.

Atropa acuminata has been entitled as an endangered medicinal plant.

Stramonium leaves (Thorn apple leaves). It consists of dried leaves or dried leaves and flowering tops of *Datura stramonium* and its species (Solanaceae). The drug is required to contain not less than 0.25% of alkaloid calculated as **hyoscyamine**.

The generic name Datura is derived from "Dhat", an Indian poison used by Thugs. The narcotic properties of Datura species, especially *D. metel*, have been known and valued in India for centuries.

The plant is cultivated in Europe and South America. In India plant is grown **wildly**. The leaves and tops are harvested when the plant is in flower. The plant can be harvested several times a year.

Commercial Datura leaf consists of the dried leaf/ leaves and flowering tops of *D. innoxia* and *D. metel*, which is obtained principally from India. Leaves contain about 0.5% alkaloids.

Utilization

Tropane alkaloids are reported to possess antispasmodic mydriatic and anticholinergic properties. Atropine, hyoscyamine and hyoscine are strongly mydriatic.

Belladonna extracts and total alkaloids are commonly used in ophthalmology to measure refractive error. Belladonna preparations are used as local soothing, pain relieving drug and as counter irritants for treating intercostal pains, rheumatism, lumbago, neuralgia and pleurisy.

Belladonna used in the form of plasters, and liniments for local applications and belladonna suppositories for the relief of spasm of anal fistula.

Belladonna herb and extract containing total alkaloids is used internally in various diseases like parkinsonism (paralysis agitans) and encephalitis. The natural drug and total alkaloids are employed as sedative, tranquilizers and are useful in labour, delirium tremins, toxic psychoses and in maniacal state. The leaves extracts are also used in the preparation of proprietary pharmaceutical for the treatment of various diseases like gastro-intestinal hypermotility, hypersecretion, peptic ulcer, spastic constipations, spastic dysmenorrhea, nocturnal enuresis, bronchial asthma and whooping cough.

The belladonna berries are used as specific antidote to opium and muscarine poisoning although its berries are highly poisonous.

Atropine alkaloid is CNS stimulant and has depressant action on nerve ending of the secretory glands and plain muscle.

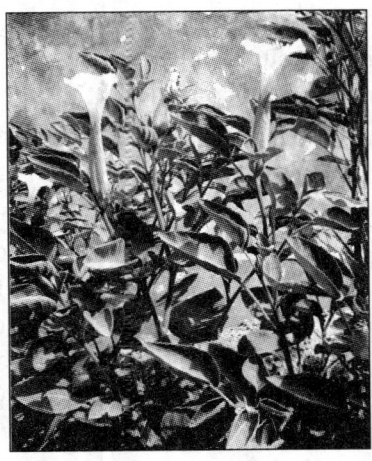

DATURA *(D. stramonium)*
(for colour, see Plate 2, Fig. 9)

Hyoscine lacks the CNS stimulant action of atropine but it is used in motion sickness (sedative properties) atropine and hyoscine are used to a large extent in ophthalmic practice to dilate the pupil of the eye.

Marketed preparations are:

(i) Atropine eye drops

(ii) Ateonex injection

(iii) Atropine eye ointment

(iv) Atropine injection 0.6 mg

(v) Atrogen eye drops

Production of Phytochemical Constituent

Regional Research Laboratory, Jammu has developed technique for production of total phytochemical constituent Fig. 4.13.

Based on this process total alkaloids are being extracted from the Belladonna leaves at the Drug factory of CIMAP, Jammu. Total production in the year 1979-80 was 25 kg of total alkaloids, valued at Rs. 375,000.

Trade

About (*Atropa acuminata*) 2304.566 tonnes belladonna roots were exported from India costing about Rs. 331.184 lakhs in the year 2000-2001; whereas about 16.532 tonnes of leaves costing about Rs. 84.640 lakhs were exported.

HYOSCYAMUS LEAF

Hyoscyamus leaf (Henbane) consists of dried leaves and flowering tops of *Hyoscyamus niger* (Solanaceae). It is required to contain not less than 0.05% of total alkaloids calculated as **hyoscyamine**.

Henbane is a **biennial** or annual plant. It generally grows wildly, chiefly near old building, both in U.K. and in the rest of Europe.

Hyoscyamus muticus is indigenous to India and Upper Egypt. It has been introduced into Algiers.

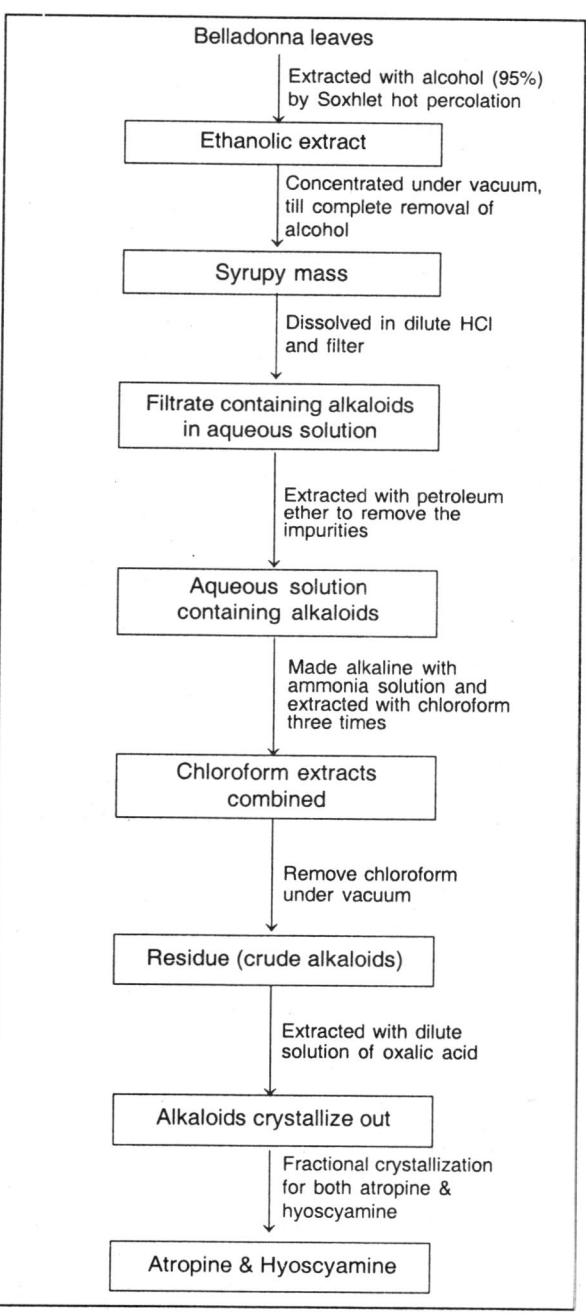

Fig. 4.13. Isolation of Tropane alkaloids (atropine/hyoscyamine).

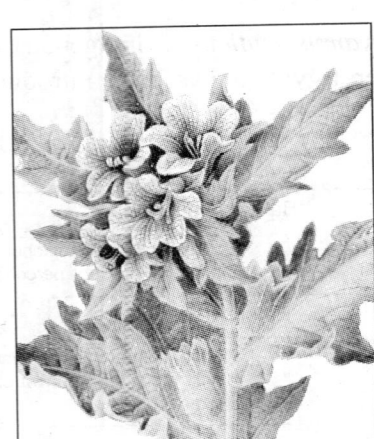

HYOSCYAMUS *(H. niger)*
(for colour, see Plate 3, Fig. 1)

Indian Henbane

It is dried leaves and flowering tops of *Hyoscyamus niger* and its closely related species *Hyoscyamus reticulatus* (Solanaceae) that grow wildly and cultivated in India and Pakistan.

Under this name considerable quantities of drug were imported into Britain during Second World War.

Egyptian Henbane

It consists of the dried leaves and flowering tops of *Hyoscyamus muticus* (Solanaceae). It is indigenous to desert regions in Egypt, Arabia, Iran, Baluchistan, Sind, Western Punjab and has been introduced into Algiers and is cultivated in Southern California. In Egypt it is collected from wild plant by Arab Shepherds.

Duboisia Leaves

The genus **Duboisia** (Solanaceae) is represented by three species *D. myoporoides* R. Brown; *D. leichhardtii* F. Muell. and *D. hopwoodii* F. Muell.

Three species of duboisia indigenous to Australia and two of these *D. myoporoides* and *D. leichhardtii* have been a major world source of

tropane alkaloids for the last 50 years. Third species *D. hopwoodii* contain principally nicotine and related alkaloids and was used by Australian aborigines for the preparation of "Pituri" held in the check pouch.

Duboisia species have considerable prospectus for replacing or at least supplementing Atropa. Datura and Hyoscyamus are source of hyoscine and hyoscyamine, which are used extensively in medicine throughout the world because of their mydriatic, antispasmodic and anticholinergic properties. The homoeopaths use the tincture and the alkaloid in paralysis and eye infections.

Leaves of *D. myoporoides* contain 2-4% of total alkaloids (about 60% hyoscine and 30% hyoscyamine) and are the main source of **tropane alkaloids** in the world. Commercial cultivation of duboisia is done only in Australia mainly in the Queensland area, from where it is exported to European countries for further processing. Cultivation of Duboisia species has also been successfully carried out in Japan.

Production in India

Duboisia myoporoides is a larger bushy tree and may grow as 14 m high. It flowers in spring; flowers are small, white and bell shaped. The fruits are small black globular berry about 5 mm in diameter. The plant is propagated through **root cuttings and seeds**.

Usually three harvests are obtained in early two years, but number of harvests depends mainly on season. When conditions are favourable, first harvest is obtained from new plantation after 7-10 months. Succeeding harvests are obtained at about 7-8 months intervals, yield vary considerably where 740 to 980 trees are planted per hectare, the average yield of leaf is about 450 kg per hectare. The average yield of dry leaf from plant cultivated at Bangalore is about three times higher than the plants cultivated at Lucknow. The climatic conditions at Bangalore are found to be very much favourable. The plantation of more than 200 trees have been established at Kodimanchanahalli in Bangalore.

Trade

Most of the Australian crop (Approx. 1200 tonnes) is exported to West Germany, Switzerland and Japan. Plantation has also been established in Ecuador.

Scopolia

All the available species of scopolia contain **tropane alkaloids**, similar to those found in belladonna. This plant is not much used in Western Europe but these plants constitute a useful source of hyoscyamine and galenicals in the area where the plant is available locally. Source of the drug is *Scopolia carniolica* indigenous to Eastern Europe. In shape and size it resembles those of belladonna.

The following are the other species of Scopolia, which are used as source of hyoscyamine. *S. japonica*, *S. caucasia*, *S. lurida* and *S. tangutica*. The last two species are source of hydroxy-hyoscyamine alkaloid named **Daturamine** (anisodine) and hyoscyamine on commercial scale in China.

COCA LEAF AND COCAINE

Coca leaves are derived from shrubs of the Erythroxylaceae (Bolivian or Huanuco) namely *Erythroxylum coca* (Bolivian) and *E. truxillense* (Peruvian or Truxillo) cultivated in Peru, Bolivia, Colombia and Indonesia.

They were formerly reserved for the sole use of native chief and Incas. It was introduced in Europe in about 1688 and **cocaine** was isolated in 1860. It was introduced into medicine sometime in the latter half of 19th Century.

Cocaine and its salts were the earliest of the modern local anaesthetic but because of their toxic

and addictive properties their use is now almost entirely confined to ophthalmic ear, nose and throat surgery. Its trade has been banned.

Production of Raw Material (leaves)

Coca leaves contains the **tropane alkaloids**, mainly **Cocaine**. Though it has local anesthetics effects, it has hallucinogenic actions, leading to addiction. Because of this property, the plant is strictly governed by Narcotic Drugs and Psychotropic Substances Act 1985 in India and by relevant acts in other countries.

Propagation is done by seeds in nursery beds. The seedlings on attaining a height of about 15-20 cm are transplanted to open fields at 2 m distance in each plant.

The drug is collected over a period of three years, at one year interval. The leaves are collected in dry weather and dried in the shed or by artificial means. Coca is native to South American countries like Peru and Bolivia. Commercially, it is cultivated in Java, Peru, Bolivia, Columbia, Sri Lanka and India. Since ancient time, the coca leaves have been used by South Americans as a masticatory and were reserved for only native chiefs. It was considered as "Divine plant".

Phytochemical constituents

The drug contains 0.7-1.5% of total alkaloids. The majority of alkaloids are tropane esters (ecgonine derivatives):

Production of Cocaine : The crude alkaloids may be extracted with dilute sulphuric acid or by treatment with lime and petroleum ether or other organic solvents. Non-alkaloidal matter is roughly separated by transferring the alkaloid from one solvent to another. The crude alkaloid is obtained in solid form either as free base by precipitation with alkali or as hydrochloride by concentrating an acidified solution.

Pure cocaine is prepared from the leaves, the

crude bases or crude hydrochloride. The process depends on the fact that cocaine, cinnamyl-cocaine and α-truxilline are closely related derivatives of ecgonine, which is produced by hydrolysing them with dilute hydrochloric acid.

Cocaine → ecgonine + methyl alcohol + benozic acid

Cinnamyl-cocaine ⟶ ecgonine + methyl alcohol + cinnamic acids.

α-Truxilline ⟶ ecgonine + methyl alcohol + (α-Isoatrophyl-cocaine) α Truxillic acid

R	R¹	Name of the Tropane alkaloid
H	H	Ecgonine
CH_3	C_6H_5CO	Cocaine
H	CH_3	Methyl Ecgonine
H	$C_6H_5CH=CHCO$	Cinnamoyl Ecgonine
H	C_6H_5CO	Benzoyl Ecgonine

The Ecgonine hydrochloride is purified and converted into the free base. This is benzoylated by interaction with benzoic anhydride and the benzoyl ecgonine purified. The benzoyl ecgonine is methylated with methyl iodide and sodium methoxide in methyl alcohol solution to give **methylbenzoyl ecgonine or cocaine**. The latter is converted into the hydrochloride and purified by recrystallization.

Utilization

Cocaine and its salts were the earliest of the modern local anesthetics but because of their toxic and addictive properties their use is now entirely confined to ophthalmic, ear, nose and throat surgery.

Food

Coca extract after the removal of cocaine is used together with extracts of kola, cinnamon, ginger, lime, orange peel and other as a flavour component in cola drinks (0.02%). Other food products in which it is used are alcoholic beverages, frozen dairy desserts, and candy (maximum level 0.055%).

What is Cocaine?

Cocaine is a powerfully addictive stimulant that directly affects the brain. Cocaine has been labeled the drug of the 1980s and 90s because of its extensive popularity and use during this period. However, cocaine is not a new drug. In fact it is one of the oldest known drugs. The pure chemical cocaine hydrochloride, has been an abused substance for more than 100 years and coca leaves (source of cocaine) have been ingested for thousands of years.

Pure cocaine was first extracted from the leaf of *Erythroxylum coca* Bush which grows primarily in Peru and Bolivia, in the mid-19th century. In the early 1990s, it became the main stimulant drug used in most of the tonics/elixirs that were developed to treat a wide variety of illness. Today, cocaine is a **Schedule two** drug, meaning that it has high potential for abuse but can be administered by a doctor for legitimate medical uses such as a local anesthetic for some eye, ear, and throat surgeries.

There are basically two chemical forms of cocaine: the **hydrochloride salt** and the **"freebase"**. The **hydrochloride salt** is powdered form of cocaine, dissolves in water and, when abused, can be taken intravenously (I/V) or intranasal (in the nose). **Freebase refers** to a compound that has not been neutralized by an acid to make the hydrocholride salt. The freebase form of cocaine is smokable.

Cocaine is generally sold on the street as a

fine, white, crystalline powder, known as "coke", "C", "snow", "flake", or "blow". Street dealers generally dilute it with such inert substances as cornstarch, talcum powder and/or sugar, or with such active drugs as procaine (a chemically-related local anesthetic) or with such other stimulants as amphetamines.

Cocaine Abuse and Addiction

Cocaine dosage form

The principal routes of cocaine administration are oral, intranasal, intravenous, and inhalation. The slang terms for these routes are, respectively, "chewing", "snorting", "mainlining", "injecting", and "smoking" (including freebase and crack cocaine).

Snorting is the process of inhaling cocaine powder through the nostrils, where it is absorbed into the bloodstream through the nasal mucosa.

Injecting releases the drug directly into the bloodstream and heightens the intensity of its effects.

Smoking involves the inhalation of cocaine vapour or smoke into the lungs, where absorption into the bloodstream is as rapid as by injection.

The drug can also be rubbed onto mucous tissues. Some users combine cocaine powder or crack with heroin in a "speedball".

Cocaine use ranges from occasional use to repeated or compulsive use with a variety of patterns between these extremes. There is no safe way to use cocaine. Any route of administration can lead to absorption of toxic amounts of cocaine, leading to acute cardiovascular or cerebrovascular emergencies that could result in sudden death. Repeated cocaine use by any route of administration can produce addiction and other adverse health consequences.

Aspects of Trade

Coca, opium and hemp, though excellent drugs but are habit forming substances and as such their use is restricted i.e. import and export is a danger from the social point of view. Natives of Peru, Bolivia and other Latin American countries were known to indulge in chewing coca leaves as early as 15th century. It is now known that its active constituent, cocaine has a very powerful effect on the brain and its continued use leads to very serious problems.

After the World War 1 and the formation of the League of Nations, a meeting of some nations was held to consider ways and means of suppressing the contraband traffic in and abuse of the dangerous drugs, especially derived from coca leaves. The various laws which came into force about this drug are as follows:

1. Opium Act, 1857
2. Opium Act, 1878
3. Dangerous Drugs Act, 1930
4. Narcotic Drugs and Psychotropic Substances Act, 1985

List of Manufacturers

1. Govt. Opium Factory, Ghazipur (M.P.)
2. Govt. Opium Factory, Neemuch (M.P.)

SOLANUM KHASIANUM

The genus Solanum comprise of about 2000 species distributed in the warmer region of the world. On the basis of presence of tubers the genus is divided into two main groups.

(a) *Tuberous group :* Represented about 100 species including potato.

(b) *Non-Tuberous Group :* Include the rest of the species and have been reported to contain glyco-alkaloid **solasodine**.

Solasodine is an alkaloid analogue of diosgenin with nitrogen atom in ring 'F'. It occurs in the form of a glycoside in *S. laciniatum*; *S. aviculare* G. and in spine-free mutant of *S. khasianum*.

Solanum khasianum consists of dried berries of *Solanum khasianum* C.B. Clarke (Solanaceae) grown in Central India and also in Myanmar and China. It is a stout much branched under shrub varying in height between 0.75–1.5 m with about straight prickles. Sometimes mixed with few curved spines on the stem, leaves are ovate, lobed, lobes are triangular hirsute (hairy) and prickly on both the surface. Flowers white in lateral 1-4 flowered recemes, brown-yellowish or greenish globcse, seeds smooth.

It is widely distributed in subcontinent extending from sea level to 2000 m and is reported from Khasia, Jaintia, and Naga hills, Assam, Bengal, Orissa and Upper gingetic plain in Nilgiris.

Production of Raw Material

Seed propagation

The seeds are sown in nursery beds. When the seedling sufficiently grown they are transplanted into open fields at the distance of 50 × 50 cm distance. Urea, potash and super-phosphate is used as fertilizer. After six month plants are harvested for collections of berries. They are immediately dried in shade or artificially at low tempt to reduce large content of moisture.

The berries are greenish to brownish in color with compressed smooth brown seeds.

The berries contain about 3% steroidal glycoalkaloid called **solasodine**. The berries also contain 8-10% of greenish-yellow fixed oil.

Isolation of the Constituents

For the isolation of solasodine, the berries are dried, powdered and the oil is removed by defatting. The defatted material is extracted with ethanol. The extract is concentrated, treated with concentrated hydrochloric (HCl) and refluxed for 6 hours. After this ammonia is added to basify the extract and again refluxed for one hour, it is filtered and the residue is washed, dried and dissolved in chloroform. This mixture is filtered and solasodine in the form of residue is obtained by evaporating the solvents.

Utilization

Solasodine is used as a precursor for steroid synthesis. Like diosgenin, it is first converted into 16-dehydro-pregnenelone acetate. The latter is precursor for steroids like corticosteroids, pregnane, androstanes and 19 NOR steroids. All of these are useful as sex hormones and oral contraceptive etc.

The large genus (over 1000 spp.) is noted for the production of C_{27} steroidal alkaloids in many species.

Some of these alkaloids are nitrogen analogues of C_{27} sapogenins (e.g. solasodine and diosgenin).

Another series of C_{27} compounds contain a tertiary nitrogen in a condensed ring system e.g. **Solanidine**. These compounds can also employed in the partial synthesis of steroidal drugs for commercial production.

(–) Solasodine (Steroidal alkaloid)

Solanidine

ANNEXURE I
LIST OF GOVERNMENT INSTITUTIONS INVOLVED IN THE DEVELOPMENT OF PLANT BASED INDUSTRIAL TECHNOLOGY

1. Regional Research Laboratory
   BHUWANESWAR - 751 013

2. Central Drug Research Institute
   LUCKNOW

3. Regional Botanical Research Institute
   LUCKNOW - 226 001

4. Regional Research Laboratory
   JORHAT - 785 001

5. Regional Research Laboratory
   TRIVANDRUM - 695 019

6. Central Institute of Medicinal &
   Aromatic Plants,
   Post Bag No. 1, P.O. Ram Sagar Misra, Nagar
   LUCKNOW

7. Regional Research Laboratory, Mungpoo
   DARJEELING

8. National Chemical Laboratory
   PUNE - 411 018

9. Regional Research Laboratory
   JAMMU TAWI (J&K) - 18 0 001

10. West Bengal Pharmaceutical and Phytochemical
    Development Corporation Ltd.,
    CALCUTTA

11. Regional Research Laboratory
    HYDERABAD

12. National Research Development Corporation
    Zamroodpur Community Centre,
    NEW DELHI - 110 048

13. Centre for Advance Research on
    Standardization, Quality Control and
    Formulation of Traditional
    Remedies/Natural Products
    (Established under Indian Council of Medical
    Research with effect from 1st April 1990)

14. Govt. Opium & Alkaloid Works
    GHAZIPUR - 233 001

15. Govt. Quinine Factory,
    MUNGPOO - 734 313

16. Drug Research Laboratory
    (Farms and Factories J&K)
    JAMMU TAWI - 18001

17. Indian Institute of Chemical Technology
    HYDERABAD - 500 007

18. National Bureau of Plant Genetic Sources
    Pusa, NEW DELHI - 110 012

19. Indian Agriculture Research Institute
    Pusa, NEW DELHI - 110 012

A. MANUFACTURERS OF HERBAL COSMETICS

1. Combii Organochem Pvt. Ltd.
   1205, New Delhi House,
   Barakhamba Road, NEW DELHI - 110 001

2. Herba Indica
   351, Industrial Area II,
   CHANDIGARH - 160 018

3. Balsara Hygienic Products Ltd.
   A-2/11, G.I.D.C., VAPI - 396 195

4. Shehnaz Herbals
   Okhla Industrial Area Phase I,
   NEW DELHI - 110 020

5. Ayurved Sewasharm Ltd.,
   Station Road, UDAIPUR

6. Ayurved Sewashram Ltd.
   Saidabad, HYDERABAD

7. Dabur India Ltd.,
   Sahibabad, GHAZIABAD

8. M.G. Shahni (Delhi) Pvt. Ltd.
   Delhi Faridabad Road, FARIDABAD

9. My Fair Lady Limited
   Z-37, Okhla Phase-II, NEW DELHI - 110 020

B. PRODUCERS OF EUCALYPTUS OIL

1. Blue Hills Eucalyptus Oil Distillery,
   13/295, Observatory, KODAIKANAL

cont'd...

2. Chordia Eucalyptus Oil Company
   25, Mount Road, COONOOR

3. Ganesh Eucalyptus Oil Distillery,
   Ganesh Hall, 101 Walshama Road,
   OOTACAMUND - 643 001

4. Geranco Aromatics Pvt. Ltd.,
   103, N.M.M. Road, Aninjskarai,
   MADRAS - 600 029

5. Highland Eucalyptus Oil Refinery,
   37, Main Bazar, OOTY

6. Jain Eucalyptus Oil Factory,
   IX/64, Mount Road,
   COONOOR - 643 102

7. Jos Eucalyptus Oil Distillery,
   17/39, Salmpur Kett Post, Dist. NILGIRIS

8. Jupiter Eucalyptus Oil Refinery,
   Mount Pleasant, COONOOR

9. Kaleeswari Ecalyptus Oil Co.
   8, Rathinaswarny Cottage,
   Govt. Hospital Road, KODAIKANAL

10. Kishore Eycalyptus Oil Col.
    75, Upper Bazar, OOTACAMUND

11. Mahavir Eucalyptus Oil Co.,
    5, Rolston club Road,
    OOTACAMUND

12. Mini Eucalyptus Oil Refineries,
    116, Gulshan Bunglow,
    Devi Road, OOTACAMUND

13. Nilgiris Eucalyptus Oil distilleries,
    D-404, Madan Chand Building,
    Main Bazar, OOTACAMUND

14. Nilgiris Green land Eucalyptus Oil Col.
    17/246, N.H. Road, COIMBATORE

15. Ootacamund Eucalyptus Oil Refinery,
    II/107, Wrem Benett Bledg.,
    Charin Cross, OOTACAMUND

16. Prabha Eucalyptus Oil Distilleries,
    31-26, Bazar Road, Kotagiri,
    Dist. NILGIRIS

17. Reliance Eucalyptus Oil Co.,
    IX/1361, Mount Road,
    COONOOR

18. Royal Eucalyptus Oil Co.,
    18-A, Garden Road, OOTACAMUND

ANNEXURE II
MANUFACTURERS OF HERBAL FORMULATIONS

1. Ansar Drugs Laboratories
   Salabatpura, Moti Begumwade
   SURAT - 359 002

2. Acis Laboratories
   118/177, Kaushalpuri
   KANPUR - 208 012

3. Aimil Pharmaceuticals (India) Pvt. Ltd.,
   2699, Main Patel Road, Patel Nagar (W)
   NEW DELHI - 110 008

4. Alrasin Marketing Pvt. Ltd.
   Plot No. 2, A-32, Road No. 3, MIDC,
   P. Box No. 9416, Opp ESIS Hospital
   Andheri (E), BOMBAY — 400 093

5. Allen Laboratories Pvt. Ltd.
   224/H, Maniktala Main Road,
   CALCUTTA - 700 054

6. Bharati Rasyanagar
   26, Nakuleswar Bhattacharjee lane
   CALCUTTA - 700 026

7. Dabur India Ltd.,
   22, Site IV, Sahibabad,
   GHAZIABAD - 201 005

8. Dattatraya Krishan Sandu Bros
   (Chembur) Pvt. Ltd.
   Sanduwadi, D.K. Sandu marg
   Chembur, BOMBAY - 400 071

9. Herbals (APS) Private Ltd.,
   B.M. Das Road, PATNA - 800 004

10. Herbo - Med (P) Ltd.,
    68, Hemchandra Naskar Road,
    CALCUTTA - 700 010

11. The Himalaya Drug Co.,
    Shivsagar 'E', Dr. Annie Besant Road,
    BOMBAY - 400 018

12. Indian Herba Research & Supply Co.,
    Post Box No. 5, Sharda Nagar,
    SAHARANPUR - 400 018

13. J & J Dechane Laboratories Pvt. Ltd.,
    4-1-324, Residency Road,
    HYDERABAD - 500 001

14. Madona Pharmaceutical Research Pvt. Ltd.,
    208/7, Rishi Bankim Chandra Road,
    CALCUTTA - 700 028

15. Kruzer Herbals
    B-20/2, Okhla Phase II
    NEW DELHI - 110 020

16. Shilpachem
    47-D, Industrial Estate,
    Fort, INDORE - 452 006

17. Hamdard (Wakf) Laboratores
    Hamdard Marg, DELHI - 110 006

18. Zandu Pharmaceutical Works Ltd.,
    Gokhdle Road (South)
    Dadar, BOMBAY - 400 025

19. Shri Baidyanath Ayurved Bhavan (P.) Ltd.,
    Baidyanath Baven Road, PATNA - 1

20. Ayurved Sewashram Ltd.
    Station Road, UDAIPUR

21. Charak Pharmaceuticals
    501/A, Poonam Chambers,
    Dr. Annie Besant Road,
    Worli, BOMBAY - 400 015

ANNEXURE III
MANUFACTURERS OF STANDARDIZED HERBAL EXTRACTS, PHYTOCHEMICALS AND ESSENTIAL OILS

Name & Address	Main Products	Name & Address	Main Products
1. Amsar Private Limited, 47, Laxmibai Nagar, Indl. Estate Fort INDORE	Extracts Phytochemicals Essential Oils	12. Bombay Extractions Pvt. Ltd. Daya Mandir, 1st Floor 123-25, Mumbadevi Road, BOMBAY - 400 003	Castor Oil
2. Ansar Drugs Laboratories Salabbatpura, Moti Begumwadi SURAT - 395 002	Extracts	13. Chemical, Industries & Pharmaceuticals Laboratories Ltd. Vikhroli, BOMBAY - 400 079	Phytochemicals
3. Alchem International Pvt. Ltd., 240, Jhanhewalan Extension, NEW DELHI - 110 055	Phytochemicals	14. CIPLA Research Centre & Factory, Virgonagar P&T Office, BANGALORE	Phytochemicals
4. Alembic Chemical Works BARODA	Extracts	15. CIBA - Giegy of India Ltd., Bhandup, BOMBAY - 400 078	Phytochemicals
5. Alkaloids Corpn, 8, Bentick Street, CALCUTTA - 700 001	Phytochemicals	16. Central Institute of Medicinal and Aromatic Plants Post Beg No. 1, Ram Sagar Misra Nagar, LUCKNOW - 226 016	Essential Oils
6. Auro Impex Pvt. Ltd., 8, Camac Street, 2nd Floor CALCUTTA - 700 017	Phytochemicals	17. Chemiloids 40-45, 10 B, Brindavan Colony, Labbipet VIJAYAWADA - 510 010	Extracts Phytochemicals Essential Oils
7. Bengal Immunity Co. Ltd., 153, Dharamtala Street, CALCUTTA - 700 013	Extracts	18. Drug Research Laboratory (Farm and Factories J&K) JAMMU-TAWI - 180 001	Extracts Phytochemicals
8. Biological Evans Ltd., C-1-4936, Dehgam Road, Industries Towrship, VAPI - 396 195	Phytochemicals	19. Enzo Chem Laboratories Pvt. Ltd. YBOLA - 423 401 MAHARASHTRA	Papain
9. Bengal Chemicals and Pharmaceuticals Ltd. 164, Maniktala Main Road, CALCUTTA - 700 054	Extracts	20. Govt. Opium and Alkaloid Works, GHAZIPUR (U.P.)	Opium Alkaloids
10. Bhavnagar Oil & Chemicals Industries Pvt. Ltd., 1411, Dalamal Tower, Nariman Point, BOMBAY - 400 021	Castor Oil	21. Govt. Quinine Factory, MUNGPOO	Quinine Salts
11. Bicon India Pvt. Ltd. 20th K.M. Hosur Road, Hebbagodi - 562 158 BANGALORE Dst.	Papain	22. Govt. Quinine Factory, Anamallais, TAMIL NADU	Quinine Salts
		23. Glaxo Laboratories (I) Ltd. Dr. Annie Besant Road, Worli, BOMBAY - 400 018	Phytochemicals

cont'd...

Name & Address	Main Products	Name & Address	Main Products
24. Herbochem 38, Technocrats Industrial Estate, Balanagar, HYDERABAD - 500 037	Extracts	34. Polybond Chemicals, 4, Bhaktinagar Station Plot, RAJKOT - 360 002	Papain
25. Indo German Alkaloids, Mahakali Caves Road, Andheri (East), BOMBAY - 400 093	Phytochemicals	35. Rathi Papains Pvt. Ltd., 75-76-A, Mittal Court, Nariman Point, BOMBAY - 400 021	Papain
26. Jayant Oil Mills, 13, Sitalwadi, Mazgaon, BOMBAY	Castor Oil	36. Regional Research Laboratory JAMMU TAWI	Phytochemicals Essential Oils
27. Kothari Phytochemicals, International, 766, Anna Nagar, MADURAI - 625 020	Phytochemicals	37. Scopa Pvt. Ltd., JAMMU TAWI	Phytochemicals
28. Kisalaya Pharmaceuticals Pvt. Ltd., Plot No. 548, Sector - III, Industrial Area, Pitampur Dist., DHAR (M.P.)	Tannic Acid	38. Sandoz India Ltd., Sandoz House, Dr. Annie Besant Road, Worli, BOMBAY - 400 018	Phytochemicals
29. Kumaon Chemcial Products, Village Shivalalpur, P.O. Kamnagar - 244 715 NAINITAL	Phytochemicals Ginger Oil	39. Smith Stanistreet Pharmaceuticals Limited, 18, Convent Road, CALCUTTA - 700 014	Phytochemicals
30. Liberty Oil Mills Pvt. Ltd., 302, Dalamal House, 206, Nariman Point, BOMBAY - 400 021	Castor Oil	40. Shashi Phytochemical Industry, 1, Old Industrial Area, ALWAR	Phytochemicals
31. Mehta Pharmaceuticals Pvt. Ltd., G.T. Road, Chheharta, AMRITSAR - 143 105	Phytochemicals	41. Sheeba Laboratories Pvt. Ltd., B-151, Avas Vikas Colony, Delhi Road, SAHARANPUR - 247 001	Phytochemicals
32. New India Agro Chemcial Industries, 4013, Yawai Road. BHUSAWAL	Phytochemicals	42. Standard Essential Oil Distillers 84/113, Carvalongar, KANPUR - 208 003	Essential Oils
33. Organokem Laboratories, Near Janata Vidyala, Yeola Dist. NASIK	Phytochemicals	43. True Food Corporation 17, Kamer Building, 38, Cawaji Patel Street, BOMBAY - 400 023	Papain

Chapter 5

Utilization of Aromatic Plants and Derived Products

INTRODUCTION

The natural essential oils and their perfumes had played vital role directly or indirectly in human life, since the beginning of civilization. The art of perfume making was first conceived and employed in the east, specially in India, Egypt, Persia and China. Rose flavours had been available in India since 1000 B.C. and during Mughal period, oriental type of perfumes like 'Attars' were produced and exported to other countries as a traditional produce of essential oils.

India is an emporium of aromatic and medicinal plants and has one of the oldest, richest and most diverse cultural customs associated with the uses of aromatic medicinal plants e.g., fragrance, flavour curative, antiseptic, antioxidant, antibacterial, food technology, industry insecticides, preservatives and alternative medicine (Fig. 5.1, Table 5.1).

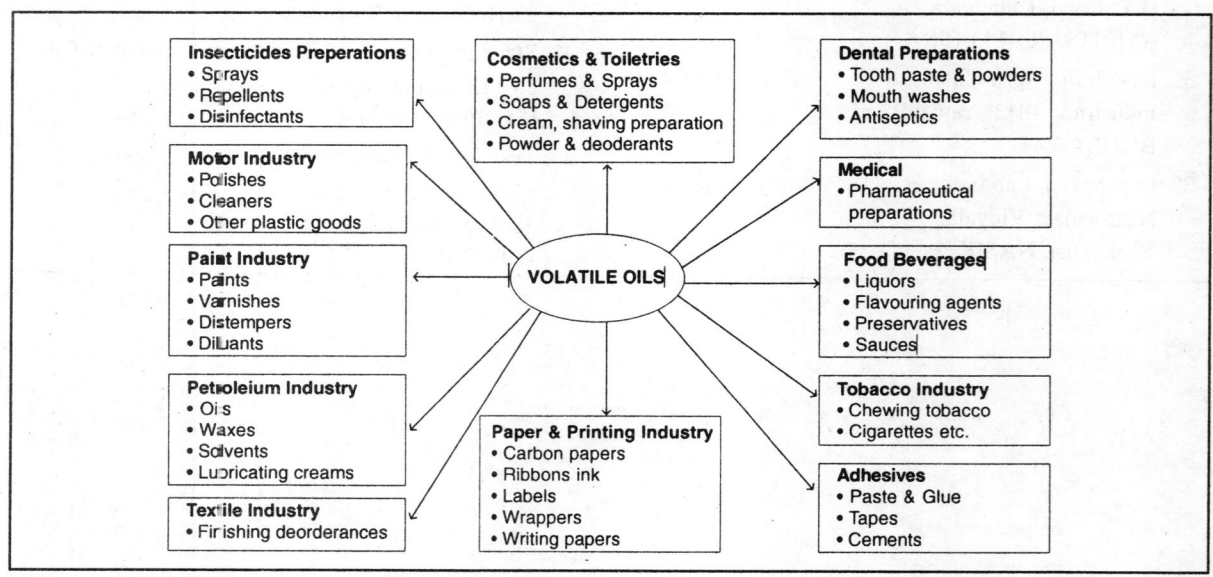

Fig. 5.1. Utilization of volatile oils.

Table 5.1. Pharmacological and therapeutical uses of volatile oils

Therapeutic Properties		Aromatic medicinal plants
Antiseptic	To kill the pathogenic bacteria and remove the infections	Anise, bergamot, cedar wood, Cyperus, *Eucalyptus*, geranium, lavender, lemon, peppermint, pine, rose and turpentine oil
Sedative	Calming, soothing, toning, relaxing	Benzoin, chamomile, cedarwood, jasmine, lemongrass, marjoram, patchouli, rose, rosemary, sandalwood, valeriana
Stomachic	Digestives	Anise, basil, bergamot, chamomile, cinnamon, clove, coriander, cumin, cyperus, dill, *Eucalyptus*, fennel, geranium, hyssop, juniper, lemongrass, marigold, mint and nutmeg
Cardiac	Heart toners	Anise, cinnamon, cumin, cyperus
Hypnotic	Sleeping agents	Basil, chamomile, juniper, lavender, orange, rose and sandalwood
Diuretic	Bladder and kidney remedies	Anise, cedar wood, cumin, *Eucalyptus*, geranium, lavender, lemon, pine, rosemary, sage and sandalwood
Anthelmintic	Against parasites-worms	Bergamot, chamomile, cinnamon, clove, cumin, *Eucalyptus*, lemon, mint, thyme, turpentine and chenopodium
Analgesic	Pain killers	Chamomile, cinnamon, clove, *Eucalyptus*, geranium, jasmine, juniper, lavender, lemon, marigold, marjoram, mint, nutmeg, pepper, rosemary, sage and turpentine
Anti-rheumatic	Rheumatic cure	Benzoin, chamomile, camphor, Cyperus, juniper, lemon, marjoram, mint, rosemary, sage and turpentine
Antigripe	Cold remedies	Basil, camphor, cedar wood, cinnamon, cyperus, *Eucalyptus*, juniper, lavender, pepper, pine and rosemary
Bronchodilator	Cough and bronchitis treatment	Anise, basil, bergamot, camphor, cedar wood, cyperus, *Eucalyptus*, jasmine, lemon, lavender, mint, myrrh, pine, sage, sandalwood and thyme
Bio-stimulant	Stimulating life processes and improving resistance to infections, cancer protection	Bergamot, chamomile, cinnamon, cyperus, *Eucalyptus*, geranium, hyssop, juniper, lavender, peppermint, rosemary, sage and thyme
Carminative		Anise, chamomile, cumin, fennel
Stimulant	Stimulating, energizing	Basil, bergamot, camphor, geranium, ginger, jasmine, juniper, lemon, melissa, patchouli, pepper, peppermint, rosemary, sage, sandalwood, verbena and ylang-ylang

Fragrance

The essential oils have been known for their fragrance and curative effects on the body, mind and spirit. These aroma molecules of the oil contain numerous and very potent organic plant chemicals, which are natural and highly potent medicine, benefiting in numerous ways the health of our body, mind and spirits e.g. geraniol of palmarosa oil (Cymbopogon martinii); (+) and (–) Linalool, (+) citronellal, eugenol and safrole, these are starting materials for the synthesis of the active principle of medicine, vitamins and fragrance. One example of the use of safrole (extracted from Brazilian ocotea or from cinnamomum species from China) is to synthesize heliotropin, used in perfumery or piperonyl butoxide, a pyrethrinoid synergist. They can be antibacterial, antiviral, anti-inflammatory, support the immune system and other systems of the body – hormonal, glandular, emotional, circulatory nervous system, calming or heightening the body awareness including memory enhancement and alertness and tranquillizing effect. Aroma signals causes release of a certain neurochemical, which bring the desired change and feeling of relief. The aroma of calming oils would cause release of **serotonin**. Similarly, euphoric oil cause release of **endorphin** and stimulating oil will cause release of **noradrenalin**, thus bringing the desired effect on the mind and the body. This is because of "Psychodynamic" action of fragrance (aromatherapy and effects of scents) on "**hedonic**" mechanism (influence on behaviour of the pleasure or displeasure linked to an odour) and a "**semantic**" mechanism (memory linked between odour and an exceptionally emotional situation). Till the end of 19th century natural essential oils were the main components of fragrance and flavours. However, the availability of number of aroma chemicals and the use of natural oils as fragrances has been reduced considerably with times.

Antiseptic

The essential oil obtained from thyme, cinnamon, clove, lavender and eucalyptus, have antiseptic activity against various pathogenic bacteria; even for those, which are reported to be resistant against certain antibiotics and fungi which are responsible for mycosis and also against yeast (candida). The plant components like citral, geraniol, linalool and thymol have antiseptic activities many times more than phenol. There are reports that thymol is 20 times stronger than phenol.

Product such as turpentine when applied locally on painful area, increases the blood circulation in the blood capillary (substantial rubefacient), causes heat sensation and in some cases causes local anaesthetic activity and similar action in the case of severe gum pain as observed for clove oil. These days many ointments, creams or gels based on essential oil are formulated to relieve sprains, soreness, strains or other joint and muscular pains.

When used topically/externally, like while taking bath or a massage (aromatherapy), the oils are absorbed through skin and carried by body fluids to the main body systems (nervous and muscular

system) because most essential oil constituents are lipophilic, therefore they are rapidly absorbed by the pulmonary, cutaneous or digestive route. The essential oils are to be applied to skin only after dilution in a vegetable oil (aromatherapic massage). It is always important not to use prior dilution in an appropriate solvent (because some are harsh on mucous membrane or on the skin) or they should be used in dosage form (Table 5.2).

Table 5.2. Marketed menthol dosage forms

Dosage form	Market products
Oral products	Tooth paste, mouth washes, oral sprays
Pharmaceutical products	Cough drops, cough lozenges, analgesic balms and inhalers
Confectionary items and beverages	Chewing gums, hard candies, (chocolates), aerated drinks and liquors
Tobacco goods	Cigarettes, pipe tobacco, chewing tobacco
Perfumed products for cooling effects	Lotions, after shave lotion, foot sprays, shampoos, refreshing towels, cooling gels

Antibacterial

Antibacterial, antifungal properties of essential oil play important role in their topical application on cuts, burn & wound and joint pains & sprains.

Oral hygiene

Main functions of the dental preparation and mouthwashes are that of oral hygiene. Since cleanliness is associated with the removal of bacteria, slight antiseptic properties are usually sought often in these gargling preparations.

The essential oils generally used in oral hygiene preparations are peppermint, cassia, anise, thyme, caraway, clove, myrrh spearmint, geranium, otto of rose, menthol, salol and eucalyptol etc. (Table 5.3).

Table 5.3. Major commercial essential oils of India

Product	Price (Rs./kg)	Product	Price (Rs./kg)
Ajowan oil	500	Galangal alpine oil	9000
Anise oil	550	Galangal kaempferia oil	10000
Basil oil	225	Ginger oil	3500
Betle leaf oil	16000	Ginger grass oil	400
Black pepper oil	6000	Geranium South Indian oil	4500
Cajuput oil	600	*Hedychium* (kapoor kachri) oil	1300
Calamus oil	1300	Jamarosa oil	400
Chamomile blue oil	14000	Lemon grass oil	545
Camphor oil	70	*Mentha arvensis* (shivalik) oil	350
Caraway oil	4000	*Mentha citrata* (bergamot mint)	700
Cardamom oil	14000	*Mentha spicata* (spearmint) oil	500
Carrot seed oil	3000	Marjoram oil	7000
Cassia oil	9000	Mandarain oil	1000
Cedarwood himalayan oil	180	Nutmeg oil	2500
Celery seed oil	1500	Orange oil	80
Cinnamon leaf oil	1200	Palmarosa oil	500
Citronella oil	350	Pine oil	40
Clove bud oil	1500	Sandalwood oil	15000
Coriander seed oil	14000	Sugandh kokila oil	2000
Costus root oil	15000	Thuja oil	1300
Cumin seed oil	3500	Tomar seed (*Zanthoxylum*) oil	1500
Curry leaf oil	5000	*Tagetes* oil	3000
Dill seed (anethi) oil	1800	Turmeric (*Curcuma aromatica*) oil	1500
Davana oil	8000	Turmeric (*Curcuma longa*) oil	1600
Elemi oil	1500	Tulsi (*Ocimum sanctum*) oil	3200
Eucalyptus globulus oil	300	Vetiver (khus) oil	13000
Eucalyptus citriodora oil	400	Valerian root (sugandh bala) oil	15000
Fennel seed oil	1500		

Antioxidant

Due to their proven anti-aging and anti-oxidant properties, essential oils find use in rejuvenating and restorative preparations having cosmetic and curative value. The aroma therapy has now assumed an important position in the holistic approach towards better health and cure (stresses, depressions and psychosomatic disorder).

Pharmaceutical Industry

With the advancement in analytical methods like GC, GLC, GC+MS it is possible to know most of the constituents of essential oils and their substitutes developed for many of the essential oils, but natural products still occupy a formidable position in industry. Infact there has been an increasing demand for aromatic raw material for industrial formulations. Natural products obtained as plant isolate may be useful directly or may serve as starting material for the synthesis of an active agent e.g. Limonene content of the orange oil is used for the production of synthetic carvone. Citral content of the lemon-grass oil is for the synthesis of Vit. A and the lemon oil is used for making substitute of bergamot oil.

Food Technology

Few herbs containing essential oils are used in dried powder form as spices e.g. cardamom, caraway, cumin, coriander, turmeric, cinnamon bark, clove etc. These drugs have power to stimulate gastric secretion, affecting digestion, stomachic and other metabolism.

In the food technology sector – alcoholic, non alcoholic beverage, confectionary, dairy products, meat product, sauce, soups, snacks, bakery products all are enriched with natural flavour to make food tasty and have psychodynamic influence on the consumers.

Alternative Medicine

Many essential oils of aromatic plants like sweet basil, chamomile. clove, balm, mint, thyme and angelica have showed marked spasmolytic activity on isolated guinea pig ileum and thus proved to be efficacious in decreasing or suppressing gastrointestinal spasms. They stimulate the gastric secretion and hence play role in the improvement of certain insomnias, miscellaneous psychosomatic disorders, decrease in "nervousness" and sea-sickness. This establishes their extensive use in folk medicine as well as in alternative medicine.

Few essential oil have decongestant and bronchodilating properties (e.g. eucalyptus and tulsi oil), advocating their use as alternative medicine in cold and cough (Table 5.1).

Essential Oil Industry Waste

The waste of essential oil Industry (Ligno-cellulosic residues) are economically utilized in paper and board industry for the manufacture of straw boards, fibre boards and paper pulp.

The **world trade** in essential oils and its products is vast and the oils of major importance are aniseed, citronella, clove, geranium, lemon grass, pepper-mint patchouli, sandalwood and vetiver. The sandalwood, mint oil, zinger oil, lemon grass oil, palmarosa occupies a prominent position in the world market of medicinal and aromatic plants serving as raw materials to pharmaceutical and other plant industry.

TOXICITY OF ESSENTIAL OILS

With the latest therapeutic trend towards aromatherapy and excessive use of essential oil under the labels of natural products, the knowledge of toxicity of essential oil has become important to avoid their abusive use.

As a general rule, the acute toxicity of essential oils by the oral route is low or very low; e.g. many of the oils used have an LD-50 between 2 and 5g/kg body weight (e.g. anise, eucalyptus & clove) and for most of them greater than 5g/kg body weight (e.g. chamomile, citronella, lavender, marjoram and vetiver). Other oils have further low LD50 between 1 and 2 g/kg for sweet basil, taragon, hyssop (1.5 g/kg), savory (1.37g/kg), sassafras (1.9g/kg), winter green (0.9–1.25g/kg), chenopodium (0.25g/kg), thuja (0.83g/kg), pennyroyl (0.4g/kg) and mustard oil (0.34g/kg).

A review of the available literature shows that serious accident involves the young children, due to the ingestion of oils such as clove (eugenol) eucalyptus, pennyroyl (Pulegone), winter green (methyl salicylate deadly) and Parsley (apiole)in large quantity.

The chronic toxicity of essential oil is also not well known at least for uses, such as aromatherapy as well as for any other route of administration; because the doses in which they are used are too low for chronic toxicity.

At present in India about 30% of the fine chemicals used annually in perfumes and flavour are obtained from essential oils. The total consumption of perfumery and flavouring materials in India is about 4800 metric tonnes/annum. The food technology, oral hygiene and pharmaceutical flavour share around 900 metric tonnes and rest represents perfumery.

> **UTILIZATION OF SPECIFIC OIL AND DERIVED PRODUCTS (As Per AICTE Syllabus)**

MENTHOL

Menthol is a colorless crystalline compound, having peppermint like odour. It is derived either from peppermint oil or other species of mint (*Mentha arvensis, Mentha spicata,* or *Mentha piperita*) or is synthetically produced from limonene, thymol, myrcene and citronellal.

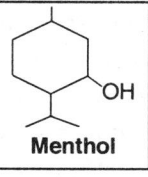

Menthol

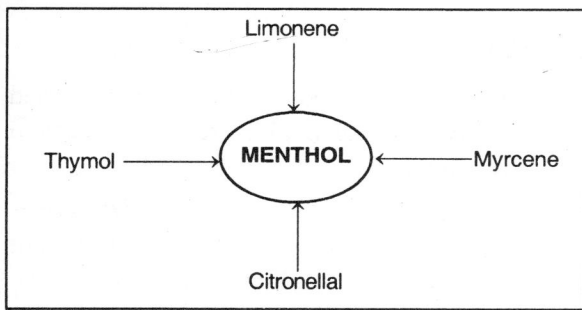

India has become the world's largest producer of *Mentha arvensis* oil, which is mainly used for production of menthol.

Utilization

Menthol is used in various dosage form for its following properties:

- Cooling sensation.
- Flavouring property
- Antipruritic
- Anti spasmodic and
- Carminative

Cooling Sensation

For over a century menthol has been used as a decongestant, this reflects a purely subjective sensation, linked to the cooling sensation, which

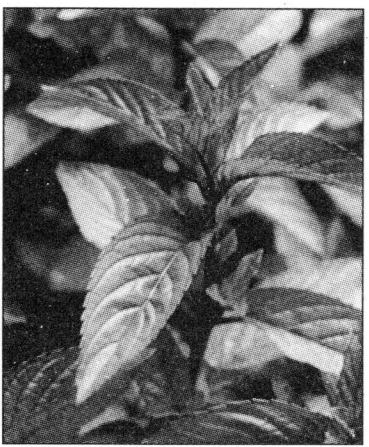

MENTHA (PEPPERMINT)
(M. Piperita)
(for colour, see Plate 3, Fig. 2)

may be due to the stimulation of thermoreceptors of the nasal cavity. Traditionally it is topically used to relieve nasal congestion in the common cold and as a analgesic for mouth and pharynx infection (collutoria, lozeges). It is also used in mouth wash formulation for oral hygiene and cooling sensation.

Flavouring Property

Menthol is used as flavour in medicine as well as in other pharmaceutical and hygiene preparations.

For food technologies, it is used in liquors, soda, concentrated syrups, confectionary (candy, chewing gum and chocolates) and also in tobacco industry.

Antipruritis

Topically it is used as an adjunctive, emollient and itch relieving treatment for skin diseases as well as topic protective agent for cracks, bruises, frost bite and insect bites.

Antispasmodic and Carminative

Orally menthol is used for symptomatic treatment of functional dyspepsia, including epigastric bloating, impaired digestion, eructation and flatulence.

In France it is being used as an antispasmodic during colonscopy or rectal barium sulfate administration for X-ray visualisation as it decreases the frequency of spasm and decrease the need of additional administration of intravenous spasmolytic drugs.

It is also used traditionally as oral component in combinational therapy for the painful relieve of functional dyspepsia and to enhance urinary and digestive elimination and in functional dyspepsia of hepatic region.

In Pharmacy

It is an ingredient of itch-reliving creams and preparations designed to decongest the upper respiratory tract in rhinitis. It is also incorporated in shaving cream and other shaving products (deodorant, after shaves) along with ester of a pyrolidinic acid.

It is a component of non-prescription products for short-term relief of minor *sore throat* and minor mouth or throat irritation. Menthol is also an ingredient in combination products used for the relief of muscle aches, *sprains* and similar conditions.

Following is list of dosage form and the marketed products, in which menthol is used (Table 5.3).

Laevo or Racemic forms are only therapeutically active. Menthol obtained from natural or synthetic source has melting point between 41–44°C.

CITRAL

Citral is a mixture of two geometric isomers : Geranial (citral A) and Neral (citral B). It is a aliphatic terpene aldehyde obtained from volatile oil of Lemon verbena (*Aloysia triphylla*)

(Verbenaceae), lemon grass, **citrus limon**, lemon balm, orange, Limetta and Pimento. It is also derived from wild plant *Backhousia citriodora* growing wildly in eastern and

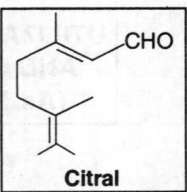

Citral

southern Australia and *Litsea cubeba*, small tree growing in Indo-China and now cultivated in Taiwan, Java and China. It is also known as Chinese lemon grass oil.

Citral is slightly yellowish oily liquid, with penetrating odour of lemons. Specific gravity 0.893–0.897. Boiling point 117°–119°C. It is optically inactive.

Utilizations

1. Citral has lemon odour, It is commonly used in flavours like apple, grape, orange and strawberry etc.

2. A large number of semisynthetic derivatives of citral are available with wide spectrum of odour of commercial importance.

3. Ionone, a derivative of citral, has powerful odour of violets and is extensively used in the preparation of artificial violet perfumes.

4. Citral is also employed in aromatherapy, having sedative properties. It also has antiseptic properties.

VETIVER OIL
(Khus-Khus)

Vetiver oil is obtained from *Vetiveria zizanioides* L. (Gramineae) a grass that can be found in both tropical and subtropical parts of the world. This oil is steam distilled from cleaned and washed rootlets of the herb.

Vetiver is native to south India, Indonesia and Sri Lanka.

Vetiver oil is one of the essential oils which has no synthetic substitute.

Constituents

The main constituents of vetiver oil are vetiverone, vetiverol, vitivene and cadinene.

Pharmacological Properties

Antiseptic : Skin care of acne, cuts and dry skin.

Antispasmodic : Muscle pain and spasm

Rubefacient : Increases blood flow to sore muscle

Circulatory stimulant : It revitalizes by fortifying red blood cells

Fixative : Soaps, cosmetics and perfumes

Above all vetiver is an excellent oil for maintaining the emotional equilibrium – It is an effective oil in the midst trauma condition, when a patient have severe anxiety and flashbacks. It is also used in aromatherapy for muscular rheumatism, arthritis, anxiety, insomnia and depression.

Indigenous uses of Vetiver Oil

Vetiver oil has played an important part in indigenous medicine since antiquity. The most important use is as a refrigerant. During hot summer month the oil bath or local application help to beat the external heat. It is also used to treat flatulence, colic and obstinate vomiting. The **hydrosal** is widely used in preparing a delicious sharbat, a favourite summer drink and a great variety of regional dishes (especially sweets).

It is also used in the production of eugenol, isoeugenol and their esters and ethers. At one stage it was used as a raw material for producing vanillin.

It is used in fine fragrances as stimulant. It is also used in burns, sores and as diaphoretic.

GERANIUM OIL

Geranium oil of commercial use is obtained by the steam distillation of the tender parts of the plants of various species of the genus *Pelargonium* (Geraniaceae). True oil of geranium is obtained from *Macrorrhizum* Linn, which grow wild in Bulgaria. The cultivated species are:

P. graveolens, L. Herit, *P. capitatum*, L. Ant, *P. odoratissium* Linn and *Radulata* var. *Roseum*, L. Herit.

The principal growing areas in the world are Reunion Islands, Algeria, Morocco, Belgium, Congo, Grecce, Spain, Corsica and East Africa.

Indian plant *P. graveolens* was introduced in the plantations of Tamil Nadu, Government Cinchona Department in 1993. At present Department is cultivating on the Shevroy hills (altitude 1400–1500 m), Nilgiri hills (altitude 1400–2100 m) and Kodai Kanal hills (Altitude 1800–2000 m).

P. graveolens is the main commercial variety cultivated for its oil. Three cultivators of *Pelargonium graveolens* called Algerian, Bourbon and Kelkar were introduced in Northern Indian plains at Lucknow.

Essential oil is obtained by steam distillation from leaves, stalks and flowers. An absolute and concentrate are also produced in Morocco.

Geranium oil possesses strong somewhat rose like odour, which is reported to improve with age when properly stored.

The oil is non-toxic, non-irritant, generally non-sensitising; possible contact dermatitis in hypersensitive individuals, especially with **Bourbon** type oil.

The chief constituents of the oil are geraniol and citronellal in various proportions depending upon the source of the oil. The esters of these alcohols as formate are also present; other components are linalol, menthone, isomenthone, phellandrene and limonene.

Properties

The reported medicinal properties of the oil are of extensive range such as antidepressant, antibacterial, antifungal, **nematicide and insectcidal**. It is mild analgesic and sedative and may be used for neuralgia. As an antiseptic it is an excellent remedy for burns.

Utilization

The oil is used in the treatment of inflammation, with its mild soothing effect. It is a stimulant of the adrenal cortex and can be used to balance the production of androgens or octoroons, which occurs during the menopause.

Geranium oil is a good **insecticide** due to its **terpene** content making it effective as a mosquito repellant. It is also used in the treatment of lice and ringworm. It has great value in skin care hence it is used on almost any type of skin disease such as eczema and psoriasis and can assist the healing of burns and abrasions.

Aromatherapy : In aromatherapy it is used as a fragrance in all kinds of cosmetic products and oil massage; soaps, creams, perfumes etc. Its aroma is reputedly beneficial for menstrual and hormonal problems.

It is also employed as flavouring agent in most food products, alcoholic and soft drinks.

Geranium oil blends well with lavender, patchouli, clove, rose, sandalwood, jasmine, juniper, bergamot and other citrus oils.

Besides rose like odour, oil of *Pelargonium graveolens* is one of the most important essential oil, employed for the isolation of rhodinol and its esters which form a part of most high grade perfumes.

EUCALYPTUS OIL

The British Pharmacopoeia (BP) describes Eucalyptus oil as the oil distilled from the fresh leaves of *E. globulus* and other species (Myrtaceae).

The essential oil of Eucalyptus used in medicine is obtained by aqueous distillation of the fresh leaves. It is a colourless or straw-coloured fluid when freshly prepared, with characteristic odour and taste, soluble in its own weight of alcohol. The most important constituent is

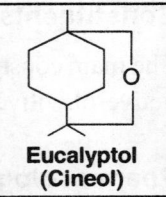
Eucalyptol (Cineol)

eucalyptol (cineol) present in *E. globulus* up to 70% of its volume. It consists chiefly of a terpene (cymene).

Utilization

The oil may be roughly divided into three classes of commercial importance.

(i) *Medicinal oils :* The medicinal oils are distilled from *E. globulus* (small amounts of eucalyptol); and

E. polybractea (contains 85% of eucalyptol)

(ii) *The Industrial oils :* The industrial oils contain terpenes, used for flotation purpose in mining operation.

(iii) *The Aromatic oils :* The oil obtained from *E. citriodora*, which is characterized by aroma.

E. smithii

E. australiana + E. bakeri (contains about 70–77% of eucalyptol and other aromatic substance identical with those of found in *E. polybractea*).

Medicinal action and uses – stimulant, antiseptic, aromatic.

Stimulant and Antiseptic Properties

Antiseptic power of the oil is increased especially when it is old, due to the ozone formation on exposure to air.

Eucalyptus oil is used as a stimulant and antiseptic gargle, locally it impairs sensibility because of tannins; the drug exert an astringent effect on the inflamed mucous membranes of the throat. It is also recommended to swallow the infusion slowly for better result. In Germany the use of eucalyptus is recommended for catarrh of the upper respiratory tract and for bronchitis.

It increases cardiac action.

It is also used for parasitic skin infections.

Internally the oil in the form of emulsion is used as a urethral injection for urethral infection and orally in drachm doses used in pulmonary tuberculosis and other microbial diseases of lungs and bronchitis.

The oil is one of ingredient of catheter oil, used for sterilizing and lubricating urethral catheters but in large doses, it is irritant to the kidneys and has marked nervous depression leading to failure of respiratory systems.

In veterinary practice, eucalyptus oil is used internally for horses in the treatment of influenza, to dogs in distemper and to all animals in septicaemia.

The cineol content of the oil is responsible for its powerful antiseptic, anti-viral and expectorant effect, especially when used as steam inhalation because of their antiseptic and "decongestant" activity, syrup, lozenges, nasal drops, preparation for inhalation (These are proposed to relieve the symptoms of ordinary respiratory disorders, such as non-productive, hacking coughs).

Chest massage with eucalyptus oil can ease congestion and relax the chest because of cineol, which facilitate the transcutaneous absorption of other substance.

It also stimulates immune system. When used as a vaporiser, the essential oil reduces air-borne microbes.

Formulation/Dosage Form

The oil 1/2–3 minims, to be used for the purpose of **inhalation**, for asthma, diphtheria, sore throat etc.

For local application in the **treatment of ulcer and sores**, 1 ounce of the oil is added into 1 pint of lukewarm water.

For the purpose of irrigation 1/2 ounce is added to 1/2 pint lukewarm water.

The fluid extract in the doses of 1/2–1 drachm, is taken for the treatment of scarlet fever, typhoid and for intermittent fever.

Formulation

I. Eucalyptol, USP dose 5 drops.

II. Ointment (BP)

Commercial Utilization

The oil obtained from *E. amygdalina* and *E. dives.* contain little eucalyptol, having sp. gravity from 0.866–0.885 and optical rotation −59 to −79 degree, the chief constituent is phellandrene irritating to be inhaled. This oil is used for flotation purposes in the extraction of ores. It is used in mining industry in the separation of metalic sulphide from ores.

The oil is in demand in new Sothwales for the cheap *phellandrene*.

For Aroma Purpose

Eucalyptus oil obtained from *E. citriodora* has lemon scent, contains citronellal (up to 98%); and is much used in perfumery.

Oil obtained from *E. odorata*, is odorous oil used by soap-maker in Australia. The oil obtained from *E. macarthurii* contains up to 75 per cent of **geranyl acetate** and is in demand as a **source of geraniol**.

The Eucalyptus oils obtained from *E. piperita*, *E. dives* (peppermint gum) and *E. radiata* (white top peppermint) yield oils with strong peppermint flavour and these oils can be used in the synthesis of menthol.

Market Preparations

I. Compound Resin Ointment BPC

Resin	–	20 gm
Oil of Eucalyptus	–	1.5 ml
Hard paraffin	–	10 gm
Soft paraffin	–	55 gm

II. Eucalyptus Ointment

Elder oil	–	12 ounces
White wax	–	2 ounces
Spermaceti	–	1/2–1 ounces
Eucalyptus oil	–	2 drachm
Wintergreen oil	–	20 drops

These ointments are used for skin, containing antiseptic and healing properties. It produces very satisfactory results in scruf, chapped hands, chafes, dandruff, tender feet, enlargement of glands, spot on the chest, arms, back and legs, pain in joint and muscles.

SANDALWOOD OIL

The term "sandalwood" in the world market is, however, a general term, which is used for a variety of woods that yields oil somewhat similar in smell to the east **Sandal oil**. Today, almost all the sandalwood oil traded internationally is called East Indian sandal wood oil distilled from the heartwood and roots of *Santalum album* (Santalaceae). Australian sandalwood oil are obtained from *S. spicatum* and West Indian and African "Sandalwood" oils are no longer produced.

Sandalwood oil has a characteristic sweet, woody odour, which is widely employed in the fragrance industry, but more particularly in the higher priced perfumes. It has excellent blending properties and the presence of high boiling point constituents of (almost 90%) the oil Santalols makes it a valuable fixative for other fragrance.

Sandalwood oil is used to calm and cool the body and to ease sunstroke. It is sedative and used in massage blend or burnt in vaporizer to treat anxiety and depression. In India, it is used for the manufacture of traditional attars such as rose attar, the delicate floral oils are distilled directly into Sandalwood oil.

It is very gentle antiseptic and diuretic and is useful in urinary problem like cystitis. Because of its soothing and anti-inflammatory nature the oil is beneficial for acne.

Plant Tissue Culture

INTRODUCTION

Tissue culture is *in vitro* cultivation of plant cell or tissue under aseptic and controlled environmental conditions, in liquid or on semisolid well – defined nutrient medium for the production of primary and secondary metabolites or to regenerate plant. This technique affords alternative solution to problems arising due to current rate of extinction and decimation of flora and ecosystem.

The whole process requires a well-equipped culture laboratory and nutrient medium. This process involves various steps viz. preparation of nutrient medium containing inorganic and organic salts, supplemented with vitamins, plant growth hormone(s) and amino acids. Sterilization of explant (source of plant tissue), glassware and other accessories; inoculation and incubation.

ADVANTAGES OF TISSUE CULTURE TECHNIQUE OVER THE CONVENTIONAL CULTIVATION TECHNIQUES

1. **Availability of raw material :** Some plants are difficult to cultivate and are also not available in abundance. In such a case, the biochemicals/bioproducts from these plants cannot be obtained economically in sufficient quantity. Unlimited cutting of plants also leads to deforestation, natural imbalance and sometimes may lead to extinction of a particular species. Hence, tissue culture is considered a better source for regular and uniform supply of raw material, manageable under regulated and reproducible conditions in the medicinal plants industry for the production of phytopharmaceuticals.

2. **Fluctuation in supplies and quality :** The production of crude drugs is subject to variation in quality due to changes in climate, crop diseases and seasons. The method of collection, drying and storing also influence the quality of crude drug. All these problems can be overcome by tissue culture techniques.

3. **Patent rights :** Naturally occurring plants or their metabolites cannot be patented as such. Only a novel method of isolation can be patented. For R&D purpose, the industry has to spend a lot of money and time to launch a new natural product but can't have patent right. Hence, industries prefer tissue culture for production of biochemical compounds. By this method, it is possible to obtain a constant supply and new methods can be developed for isolation and improvement of yield, which can be patented.

4. **Political reasons :** If a natural drug is successfully marketed in a particular country of its origin, the government may prohibit its export to up-value its own exports by supplying its phytochemical product, e.g. *Rauwolfia serpentina* and *Dioscorea* spp. from India. Similarly the production of opium in the world is governed as such by political consideration. In such case, if work is going on the same drug, it will be either hindered or stopped. Here also, plant tissue culture is the solution.

5. **Easy purification of the compound :** The natural products from plant tissue culture may be easily purified, because of the absence of significant amounts of pigments and other unwanted impurities. With the advancement of modern technology in plant tissue culture it is also possible to biosynthesise those chemical compounds which are difficult or impossible to synthesise.

6. **Modifications in chemical structure :** Some specific compounds can be achieved more easily in cultured plant cells rather than by chemical synthesis or by micro-organism.

7. **Disease free and desired propagule :** Plant tissue culture is advantageous over conventional method of propagation in large scale production of disease free and desired propagules in limited space and also the germplasm could be stored and maintained without any damage during transportation for subsequent plantation.

8. **Crop improvement :** Plant tissue culture is advantageous over the conventional cultivation technique in crop improvement by somatic hybridization or by production of hybrids.

9. **Biosynthetic pathway :** Tissue culture can be used for tracing the biosynthetic pathways of secondary metabolites using labeled precursor in the culture medium.

10. **Immobilization of cells :** Tissue culture can also be used for plants preservation by immobilization of cell further facilitating transportation and biotransformation.

HISTORICAL DEVELOPMENT OF PLANT TISSUE CULTURE

Although the feasibility of aseptic culture of **cells, tissues and organs** on defined nutrient medium had been recognized at the beginning of the century. But it is only some few decades ago that modern developments in the cultivation of plants cell as a callus or as a suspension liquid culture actually came into existence. It is only in the last **two decades** its implication have been realized and in particular pharmaceutical importance of this modern technique was appreciated. The principles of tissue culture were involved as early as 1838–1839 in cell theory advanced by **Schleiden and Schwann**. But according to noted biologist **Gautheret** (1985), the discovery of tissue culture could be considered with the **Henri-Louis Duhamel du Monceau's** (1756) pioneering experiment on wound healing in plants, demonstrated spontaneous callus formation on the decorticated region of the Elm plant. Further contribution to plant tissue culture could be attributed with the **Haberblandt's** hypothesis (1902) that a cell is capable of autonomy and have potential for totipotency (the potential of cell to develop into an organism by regeneration is termed as **totipotency** by Morgan) hence the isolated plant cell should be capable of cultivation on artificial medium.

The development of multicellular or multiorganed body of a higher organism from a single cell (zygote) support the totipotent behaviour of a cell. But **Haberblandt and co-worker** have tried to demonstrate the hypothesis but could not succeed. In 1904 another physiologist **Hannig** started research work, by taking embryogenic tissue instead of single cells, for *in vitro* cultivation in an artificial medium consisting of mineral salts and sugar solution. He excised nearly matured embryos of some crucifers (*Raphanus sativus, R. landra, R. caudatus* and *Cochlearia donica*) and successfully cultivated them up to maturity. Thus it became an important area of investigation, using an in vitro technique.

Simon (1908) obtained more promising results as he achieved success in the regeneration of bulky callus, buds and roots from Popular stem segments and thus he succeeded in establishing the basis for **callus culture** and to some extent also micropropagation.

In vitro, technique of culture was carried out further by many biologists. In 1922, **Kotte** (Germany) and **Robbin** (USA) simultaneously conceived a new approach to tissue culture and reported that true in vitro culture could be made easier by using meristematic cells (**root tips or buds**). **Kotte** carried out number of experiments and successfully cultivated, small excised root tips of pea and grew the culture for two weeks by using a variety of nutrients containing salts of Knop's solution, glucose and several nitrogenous compounds (such as asparagine, alanine and yeast extract). **Robbin** working independently maintained maize root tip culture for longer period, by subculturing, but growth gradually diminished and ultimately culture was lost.

White (1934–39) carried out the in vitro technique of tissue culture by changing the nature of media. He replaced the yeast extract in a medium containing inorganic salts and sucrose, with three vitamins (pyridoxine, thiamine and nicotinic acid) and was able to maintain the root tip culture, hence **White's** synthetic media later proved to be one of the basic media for cell and tissue culture.

The number of workers continued efforts to develop a complete media, this will be discussed latter on under the media composition.

Gautheret (1934) successfully cultured cam-

bium cells of some tree species (*Acer pseudoplatanus, Ulmus campestre, Robinia pseudoacacia* and *Salix caprea*) on the surface of the media (Knop's solution containing glucose and cysteine hydrochloride) solidified with agar and observed that after six month, proliferation of callus was ceased but on addition of auxin enhanced the proliferation of cambial culture and making it possible to prepare subculture.

Van Overbeek et al (1941) used coconut milk (embryo sac fluid) for **embryo development** and callus formation in *Datura*, which proved to be turning point in the development of **embryo culture**, which latter on proved to be helpful in the development of several **hybrids**.

Loo (1945) got success in developing whole plant from **stem tip culture**. He obtained excellent cultures from stem tips of Dodder and Asparagus, subsequently **Ball** (1946) able to identify the exact part of the shoot meristem, which give rise to whole plant. This method is now being used in plant propagation at industrial scale throughout the world.

Muir (1953) demonstrated that on transferring the callus tissues of these two plants in to liquid medium and on subsequent **agitating on a shaking machine** it is possible to break down the callus tissue into single cell and small cell aggregates, which on subculturing into fresh liquid medium can multiply while remaining in the medium under constant shaking. **Muir and associates** (1954) reported that the pieces of callus of *Tagetes erecta* and *Nicotiana tabacum* can be cultured in the form of cell suspension.

Van Overbeek et al (1941) had suggested earlier that liquid endosperm (coconut milk) is a good medium for embryo culture. Latter in 1955 **Skoog** and collaborator finally isolated adenine derivative from the embryo sac known as **kinetin**, which helps in the proliferation of embryo.

Skoog & Miller (1957) proposed the concept of hormonal control of organ formation. They demonstrated that root and bud initiation were conditioned by balance between auxin and kinetin in addition to other ingredients of the define medium. High proportions of auxin promoted rooting, whereas proportionately more kinetin initiated bud or shoot formation.

Bergmann (1960), developed **plating technique** for cloning a large number of isolated single cells. He demonstrated the technique by using **callus culture** of *Nicotiana tabacum* and *Phaseolus vulgaris* and reported population of nearly 90% of free cells. In the same year, i.e. 1960 **Jones et al** used hanging drops of free cells for the **microculture propagation**, this technique proved useful to have continuous observation of cell growth in the culture.

In 1960, **Cocking** introduced **protoplasmic plant tissue culture**. He succeeded in isolating the protoplasts of plant tissue by using cell wall enzymes like cellulase, hemicellulase, pectinase and protease. The enzyme was extracted from fungus *Trichoderma viride*. Earlier **Michel** (1939) had demonstrated the role of sodium nitrate in fusion of protoplasts. In the same year, **Steward and co-worker** had successfully raised a large number of plantlets from carrot root suspension culture. In year 1960, **Moral** initiated **micropropagation technique** and produced virus free orchid, *Cymbidium*.

Steward & Co-worker in 1966 raised large number of plantlets from carrot root suspension culture via **somatic embryogenesis**. Actually **Rienert** (1968) introduced somatic embryogenesis in callus, cultured on a semisolid medium. This phenomenon of somatic embryogenesis for the production of plantlets was later reported in many species. All these discoveries contributed to the establishment of totipotency power of the cells under suitable environment thereby accomplishing the theory introduced by **Haberblandt**.

In 1970, **Power et al** demonstrated the intra- and interspecific fusion between the protoplasts of different plant roots; subsequently in 1972 **Carlson et al**, succeeded in obtaining the first interspecific **somatic hybrid** by protoplasts fusion of *Nicotiana* species (*N. glauca* and *N. longsdorfi*). In 1981, **Vilnken**, brought new approach of electrical fusion of protoplasts. Later **Gamborg and Neabors** (1987) described a number of variations in protoplasts fusion.

During last two decades, procedures for culture of **somatic cells, pollens and protoplasts** have been refined and many new developments in regenerating plants from such cultured cells have been made. Protoplast fusion has been used to obtain novel somatic hybrid plants among several sexually incompatible species and to produce hybrids, difficult to obtain through conventional methods. Defined tissue culture procedures have made it possible to introduce foreign DNA and cloned genes into cultured cells, protoplasts and plant organs from diverse biological systems and to regenerate transgenic plants (Table 6.1).

BASIC REQUIREMENTS FOR A TISSUE CULTURE LABORATORY

For the successful achievement of any type of tissue culture technique, a tissue culture laboratory should have the following general basic facilities.

- Equipment and apparatus
- Washing and storage facilities
- Media preparation room
- Sterilization room
- Aseptic chamber for culture
- Culture rooms or incubators fully equipped with temperature, light and humidity control devices.
- Observation or recording area well equipped with computer for data processing.

Table 6.1. Brief review of historical developments in plant tissue culture technology

Year	Authors	Results	Species
1892	Klercker	First attempts to isolate protoplasts mechanically	
1902	Haberblandt	First cultivation experiments with isolated plant cells; cell growth, but no cell division obtained	*Tradescantia*
1904	Hannig	Establishment of embryo culture for the first time	*Cochleria Raphanus*
1909	Kuster	First observation of fusing cells	
1922	Kotte, Robins	*In vitro* cultivation of root tips, no permanent cultures obtained	*Zea, Pisum*
1924	Dieterich	Embryo rescue - "artificial premature birth"	*Linum*
1925	Laibach		
1934	White	First permanent root cultures beginning in 1934 - terminated in 1968!	*Lycopersicum*
1934	Gautheret	First permanent callus culture using B-vitamins and auxins	*Daucus*, Nicotiana
1934	Nobecourt		glauca × *N. langsdorffi*
1942	Gautheret	Observation of secondary metabolites in plant callus culture	
1946	Ball	Micropropagation: First development of stem tips and subadjaent regions: plantsfree of viruses	*Tropaeolum*
1952	Morel and Martin		*Lupinus, Dahlia*
1954	Muir et al	First suspension cultures of single cells or cell aggregates: nurse culture	*Tagetes, Nicotiana, Daucus, Picea, Phaseolus*
1955	Mothes and Kala	First reports of secanary metabolite production **in liquid media**	
1956	Routien and Nickell	US patent No. 2747334 for the production of substances from plant tissue culture	*Phaseolus*
1958	Wickson & Thimann Reinert Steward et al	Establishment of axillary branching Somatic embryogenesis in tissue cultures	*Daucus*
1959	Tulecke and Nickell	First report of large-scale (1341) culture of plantcells: carboy system	*Ginkgo, Lolium, Rosa, Ilex*
1960	Bergmann	**Cell clones obtained from single cultures cells plated in** an agar medium	*Nicotiana Phaseolus*
1960	Jones et al	Hanging drop culture in conditioned medium	*Nicotiana*
1960	Cocking	Method for obtaining large numbers of protoplasts from plant tissue	*Lycopersicon*
1965	Morel	Clonal multiplication of horticulture plants (orchids) through tissue culture: protocorm formation	*Cymbidium*
1965	Vasil & Hilderbrandt	Regeneration of a plant from one single cell cultivated in a hanging droplet	*Nicotiana*
1966	Kohlenbach	First cell division and culture of differentiated mesophyll cells	*Macleaya*
1967	Kaul and Staba	Reports of the yields of certain products in cell culture equal to those in intact plants	*Ammi*
1967	Bourgin & Nitsch; Guha & Maheshwari	*In vitro* production of haploid plants from immature pollen within cultured anthers	*Nicotiana Datura*
1970	Carlson	Isolation of auxotrophic mutants from cultured cells	*Nicotiana*
1971	Nagata and Takebe	Regeneration of plants from cultured protoplasts	*Nicotiana*
1972	Carlson et al	First interspecific somatic hybrid plant from fusd protoplasts	*Nicotiana*
1977	Noguchi et al	Cultivation of tobacco cells in 20 000 1 reactors	*Nicotiana*
1978	Melchers et al	First intergenetic somatic hybrid plant from fused protoplasts	
1978	Zenk	Manifold increase in product yields by selection over parent plant documented for a variety of plant metabolites	
1979	Brodlius et al	Alginate beads used to immobilize plant cells for biotransformation and secondary mtabolite production	
1981	Shuler	Use of hollow fiber reactor for secondary metabolite production	
1983	Mitsui Petrochemical Ind. Ltd	First industrial production of secondary plant products by suspension cultures	*Lithospermum*

Equipment and Apparatus

Culture vessels and glassware

Many different kinds of vessels may be used for growing cultures. Callus culture can be grown successfully in large test tubes (25 × 150 mm) or wide mouth conical flasks (Erlenmeyer flask). In addition to the culture vessels, glassware such as graduated pipettes, measuring cylinders, beakers, filters, funnel and petri dishes are also required for making preparations. All the glasswares should be of pyrex or corning.

Equipment

- Scissors, scalpels and forceps for explant preparation from excised plant parts and for their transfer.
- A spirit burner or gas micro burner for flame sterilization of instruments.
- An autoclave to sterilize the media.
- Hot air oven for the sterilization of glassware etc.
- A pH meter for adjusting the pH of the medium.
- A shaker to maintain cell suspension culture.
- A balance to weigh various nutrients for the preparation of the medium.
- Incubating chamber or laminar airflow with UV light fitting for aseptic transfer of explants to the medium and for subculturing.
- A BOD incubator for maintaining constant temperature to facilitate the culture of callus and its subsequent maintenance.

Washing and Storage Facilities

First and foremost requirement of the tissue culture laboratory is provision for fresh water supply and disposal of the waste water. Space for distillation unit for the supply of distilled and double distilled water and de-ionized water. Acid and alkali resistant sink or wash basin for apparatus/ equipment washing. The working table should also be acid and alkali resistant.

Sufficient space is required for placing hot air oven, washing machine, pipette washers and the plastic bucket or steel tray for soaking or drainage of the detergent bath or extra water.

For the storage of dried glassware separate dust proof cupboards or cabinet should be provided. It is mandatory to maintain cleanliness in the area of washing, drying and storage.

Media Preparation Room

Media preparation room should have sufficient space to accommodate chemicals, lab ware, culture vessels and equipments required for weighing and mixing, hot plate, pH meter, water baths, bunsen burners with gas supply, microwave oven, autoclave or domestic pressure cooker, refrigerator and freezer for storage of prepared media and stock solutions.

Sterilization Room

For the sterilization of culture media, a good quality ISI mark autoclave is required and for small amount domestic pressure cookers, can also serve the purpose. For the sterilization of glassware and metallic equipments hot air oven with adjustable tray is required.

Aseptic Chamber/Area for Transfer of Culture

For the transfer of culture into sterilized media, contaminant free environment is mandatory. The simplest type of transfer area requires an ordinary type of small wooden hood, having a glass or plastic door either sliding or hinged fitted with UV tube. This aseptic hood can be conveniently placed in a quiet corner of the laboratory.

These days, modern laboratory have laminar airflow cabinet having vertical or horizontal airflow, arrange over the working surface to make it free from dust particles/microcontaminants.

The air coming out of the fine filter (a 0.3 μm HEPA filter) is ultraclean (free from fungal or bacterial contaminant) and having adequate velocity (27±3 m/min) to prevent microcontamination of the working area by worker sitting in front of the cabinet.

Inside the cabinet, there is arrangement for bunsen burner and a UV tube fitted on the ceiling of the cabinet (to make area free from any live contamination).

The advantage of working in the laminar airflow cabinet is that the flow of air does not hamper the use of bunsen burner and moreover, the cabinet occupies relatively small space within the laboratory (Fig. 6.1).

Incubation Room or Incubator

Environmental factors have great effect on the growth and differentiation of cultured tissues. Therefore, it is very much essential to incubate all types of cultures in well-controlled environmental conditions, like temperature, humidity, illumination and air circulation. A typical incubation chamber or area should have both light and temperature controlled devices managed for 24 hours period. Air conditioners or room heaters are required to maintain the temperature at 25±2°C. Light is adjusted in the terms of photo-period duration (specified period for total darkness as well as for higher intensity light). Further the requirement for humidity range of 20–90% controllable to ±3% and uniform forced air circulation can be achieved.

The incubation chamber or room should have the provision for storing the culture vessels (flask, jars and petri dishes). Shelves should be designed in such a way so that the culture vessels can be placed in the shelf or trays in such a way, that there should not be any hindrance in the light, temperature and humidity maintenance. A label having full detail about date of inoculation, name of the explant, medium and any other special information should stuck on each tray and rack to ensure identity and for maintaining the data of experiment.

In the case of suspension culture arrangement for shaker should also be made.

These days BOD incubators (Fig. 6.2) with all the requisite environmental condition maintenance

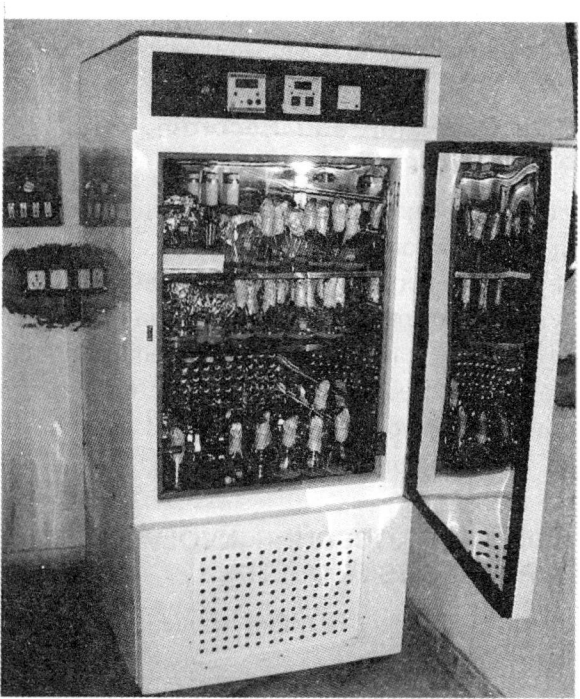

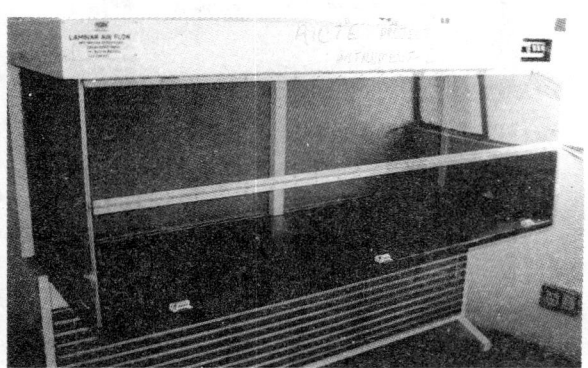

Fig. 6.1. Laminar air flow.

Fig. 6.2. BOD incubator.

are available in the market, they occupy less space and manageable with small generator or automatic invertor in the case of electricity failure to maintain the necessary light and temperature conditions. Failure of electricity may ruin important experiment and in the case of suspension culture the whole culture may get damaged due to stoppage of the shaker.

BOD Incubators required to maintain the culture conditions should have the following characteristics:
- Temperature range, 2–40°C
- Temperature control ±0.5°C
- Automatic digital temperature recorder
- Twenty four hours temperature and light programming.
- Adjustable fluorescent lighting up to 10,000 lux.
- Relative humidity range 20–98%.
- Relative humidity control ±3%.
- Uniform forced air circulation
- Shaker
- Capacity up to 0.7 m³ of 0.5 m² shelf space.

Data Collection and Recording of the Observation

The growth and maintenance of the tissue culture in the incubator should be observed and recorded at regular intervals. All the observations should be done in aseptic environment, i.e. in the laminar airflow. Whereas for microscopic examination separate dust free space should be marked for microscopic work. All the recorded data should be fed in computer.

GENERAL PROCEDURE INVOLVED IN PLANT TISSUE CULTURE

In vitro culturing of plant tissue involves the following steps:
- Sterilization of glassware tools/vessels
- Preparation and sterilization of explant.

- Production of callus from explant.
- Proliferation of cultured callus.
- Subculturing of callus.
- Suspension culture.

Sterilization of Glassware Tools/Vessels

Cleaning of glassware

All the glassware to be used in tissue culture laboratory should be of pyrex or corning. To make them free from any dirt, waxy material or bacteria, all the glassware should be kept overnight dipped in sodium dichromate-sulphuric acid solution. Next morning, glassware should be washed with fresh running tap water, followed by distilled water and placed in inverted position in plastic bucket or trays to remove the extra water. For drying the glassware, it is placed in hot air oven at high temperature about 120°C for **1/2–1 hour** (Fig. 6.3).

In the case of plastic labware, washing should be carried out with a mild non-abrasive detergent followed by washing under tap water or the plasticware after general washing with dilute sodium bicarbonate and water followed by drainage of extra water, rinsed with an organic solvent such as alcohol, acetone and chloroform.

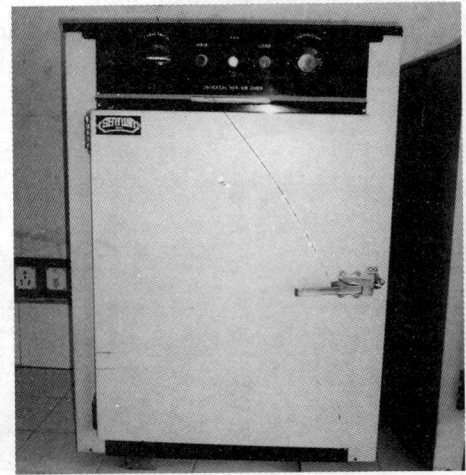

Fig. 6.3. Hot Air Oven.

Washed and dried glassware or plasticware should be stored in dust proof cupboards.

To prevent reinfection following sterilization, empty containers are wrapped with aluminium foil. Stainless steel, metals tools (knives, scalpels, forceps etc.) are also wrapped with the aluminium foil and pads of cotton wool are stuffed into the opening of the pipettes, which are either also wrapped in aluminium or placed in an aluminium or stainless steel box.

The period of sterilization usually ranges between 1–4 hours.

Note : The object with different thermal expansion coefficients may not be mixed together during the treatment period of at least 30 min. The accuracy of calibrated instruments is often reduced.

Preparation of Explant

Explant can be defined as a portion of plant body, which has been taken from the plant to establish a culture. Explant can be obtained from plants, which are grown in controlled environmental conditions. Such plants will be usually free from pathogens and are homozygous in nature. **Explant may be taken from any part of the plant like root, stem, leaf, or meristematic tissue like cambium, floral parts like anthers, stamens etc.**

Age of the explant is also an important factor in callus production. Young tissues are more suitable than mature tissues. A suitable portion from the plant is removed with the help of sharp knife and the dried and mature portions are separated from young tissue. When seeds and grains are used for explant preparation, they are directly sterilized and put in nutrient medium. After germination, the obtained seedlings are to be used for explant preparation.

Surface Sterilization of Explant

For the surface sterilization of the explant, **chromic acid, mercuric chloride (0.11%), calcium hypochlorite, sodium hypochlorite (1–2%) and alcohol (70%)** are used. Usually the tissue is immersed in the solution of sterilizing agent for 10 seconds to 15 minutes and then they are washed with distilled water. Repeat the treatment with sodium **hypochlorite for 20 minutes** and the tissue is finally washed with sterile water to remove sodium hypochlorite. Such tissue is used for inoculation.

The explants are sterilized by exposing to aqueous sterilized solution of different concentration as shown in Table 6.2. In the case of leaf or green fresh stem the explant needs pretreatment with wetting agent (70–90% ethyl alcohol, Tween 20), 5–20 drops in 100 ml of purified water or some other mild detergent to be added directly into the sterilization solution to reduce the water repulsion (due to waxy secretion).

Procedure to be followed for respective explant is as follow:

Seeds

1st Step : Dip the seeds into absolute ethyl alcohol for 10 second and rinse with purified water.

2nd Step : Expose seeds for 20–30 minutes to 10% w/v. aqueous calcium hypochlorite or for 5 minutes in a 1% solution of bromine water.

Table 6.2. Surface sterilizing agent

Name of Chemical	Concentration (%)	Exposure (min.)
Bromine water	1-2	2-10
Benzalkonium chloride	0.01-0.1	5-20
Sodium hypochlorite	0.5-51	5-30
Calcium hypochlorite	9-10	5-30
Mercuric chloride	1-2	2-10
Hydrogen peroxide	3-10	5-15
Silver nitrate	1-2	5-20

3rd Step : Wash the treated seeds with sterile water (three to five times) followed by germination on damp sterile filter paper.

Fruits

1st Step : Rinse the fruit with absolute alcohol.

2nd Step : Submerge into 2% (w/v) solution of sodium hypochlorite for 10 minutes.

3rd Step : Washing repeated with sterile water and remove seeds of interior tissue.

Stem

Clean the explant with running tap water followed by rinsing with pure alcohol.

Submerge in 2% (w/v) sodium hypochlorite solution for 15–30 minutes.

Wash three times with sterile water.

Leaves

Clean the leaf explant with purified water to make it free from dirt and rub the surface with absolute ethyl alcohol.

Dip the explant in 0.1% (w/v) mercuric chloride solution, wash with sterile water to make it free from chloride and then dry the surface with sterile tissue paper.

Production of Callus from Explant

The sterilized explant is transferred aseptically onto defined medium contained in flasks. The flasks are transferred to BOD incubator for maintenance of culture. Temperature is adjusted to 25±2°C. Some amount of light is necessary for callus (undifferentiated amorphous cell mass) production. Usually sufficient amount of callus is produced within 3–8 days of incubation.

Proliferation of Callus

If callus is well developed, it should be cut into small pieces and transferred to another fresh medium containing an altered composition of hormones, which supports growth. The medium used for production of more amount of callus is called proliferation medium.

Subculturing of Callus

After sufficient growth of callus, it should be periodically transferred to fresh medium to maintain the viability of cells. This subculturing will be done at an interval of 4–6 weeks.

Suspension Culture

Suspension culture contains a uniform suspension of separate cells in liquid medium. For the preparation of suspension culture, callus is transferred to liquid medium, which is agitated continuously to keep the cells separate. Agitation can be achieved by rotary shaker system attached within the incubator at a rate of 50–150 rpm. After the production of sufficient number of cells sub-culturing can be done.

CULTURE MEDIA

Nutritional requirements for optimal growth of a tissue culture may vary with the species. Even tissues from **different parts of a plant may** have different requirements for proper satisfactory growth. As such no single medium can be suggested as being entirely sufficient for the satisfactory growth of all types of plant tissues and organs, hence with **every new system** it is essential to work out a medium by hit and trial that would fulfill the specific requirements of that particular tissue. List of several culture media developed by scientists to culture diverse tissues and organs are Gautheret (1942), White (1943), Haberblandt et al (1946), Haller (1953), Nitsch and Nitsch (1956), Murashige and Skoog (1962), Eriksson (1965) and B5 (Gamberg et al 1968) (Table 6.3).

Table 6.3. Composition of some plant tissue culture media

Comnstituents	Media (amount in mg l^{-1})						
	White (1963)	Heller's (1953)	MS (1962)	ER	B (1968)	Nitsch (1951)	NT
Micronutrients							
$MnSO_4 \cdot 4H_2O$	5	0.1	22.3	2.23	–	25	22.3
$MnSO_4 \cdot H_2O$	–	–	–	–	10	–	–
$ZnSO_4 \cdot 7H_2O$	3	1	8.6	–	2	10	–
$ZnSO_4 \cdot 4H_2O$	–	–	–	–	–	–	8.6
$CuSO_4 \cdot 5H_2O$	0.01	0.03	0.00025	–	0.025	0.025	0.025
$CoSO_4 \cdot 7H_2O$	–	–	–	–	–	–	0.03
$Fe_2(SO_4)_3$	2.5	–	–	–	–	–	–
$FeSO_4 \cdot 7H_2O$	–	–	27.8	27.8	–	27.8	27.8
KCl	65	750	–	–	–	–	–
KI	0.75	0.01	0.83	–	0.75	–	0.83
H_3BO_3	1.5	1	6.2	0.63	3	10	6.2
$Na_2MoO_4 \cdot 2H_2O$	–	–	0.25	0.025	0.25	0.25	0.25
MoO_3	0.001	–	–	–	–	–	–
$CoCl_2 \cdot 6H_2O$	–	–	0.025	0.0025	0.025	–	–
$AlCl_3$	–	0.03	–	–	–	–	–
$NiCl_2 \cdot 6H_2O$	–	0.03	–	–	–	–	–
$FeCl_3 \cdot 6H_2O$	–	1.00	–	–	–	–	–
EDTA							
$Zn \cdot Na_2EDTA$	–	–	–	15	–	–	–
$Na_2EDTA \cdot 2H_2O$	–	–	37.3	37.3	–	37.3	37.3
Vitamins							
Nicotinic acid	0.05	–	0.5	0.5	1	5	–
Pyridoxine HCl	0.01	–	0.5	0.5	1	0.5	1
Thiamine HCl	0.01	–	0.10	0.5	10	0.5	1
Glycine	3.0	–	2.0	2.0	–	2	–
Folic acid	–	–	–	–	–	0.5	–
Macronutrients							
NH_4NO_3	–	–	1650	1200	–	720	825
HNO_3	80	–	1900	1900	2527.5	950	950
$NaNO_3$	–	600	–	–	–	–	–
$Ca(NO_3)4H_2O$	300	–	–	–	–	–	–
$CaCl_2 \cdot 2HO$	–	75	440	440	150	–	220
$CaCl_2$	–	–	–	–	–	166	–
$MgSO_4 \cdot 6H_2O$	750	250	370	370	246.5	185	1233
$(NH_4)_2SO_4$	–	–	–	–	–	–	–
KH_2PO_4	–	–	170	340	–	68.0	68.0
$NaH_2PO_3 \cdot H_2O$	19	125	–	–	150	–	–
Growth regulators							
Inositol	–	–	100	–	100	100	100
2,4-D	–	–	0.1	1.0	–	–	–
IAA	–	–	1.0	30.0	–	–	–
Kinetin	–	–	0.04	10.0	0.02	0.1	–
NAA	–	–	–	1.0	–	–	–
Myo-inositol	–	–	100.0	–	100.0	–	–
pH	–	–	5.7	5.8	5.5	–	–
Sucrose	2%	–	3%	4%	2%	2%	1%

MS – Murashige and Skoog (1962), ER – Eriksson, B – Gamberg et al (1968), NT – Nagata and Takebe (1971).

Note: Growth regulators and complex nutrient mixtures described by various authors are not included.

Media Composition

To maintain the vital functions of a culture, the basic medium consisting of inorganic nutrients (macronutrients and micronutrients) adapted to the requirements of the object in question, must be supplemented with organic components (amino acids, vitamins), growth regulators (phytohormones) and utilizable carbon (sugar) source and a gelling agent (agar/phytogel).

Inorganic Nutrients

Mineral elements play very important role in the growth of a plant. For example magnesium is a part of chlorophyll molecule, calcium is a component of cell wall and nitrogen is an important element of amino acids, vitamins, proteins and nucleic acids. Iron, zinc and molybdenum are parts of certain enzymes.

Essentially about **15 elements** found important for whole plant growth have also been proved necessary for the growth of tissue(s) in culture. Elements required in the life of a plant greater than 0.5 mmol l^{-1} are referred as **macronutrients** and those less than 0.5 mmol l^{-1} as **micronutrients**.

Macronutrients : The macronutrients include six major elements: nitrogen (N), phosphorus (P), potassium (K), calcium (Ca), magnesium (Mg), and sulphur (S) present as salts that constitute the various above mentioned defined media. The concentration of the major elements like calcium, phosphorus, sulphur and magnesium should be in the range of 1–3 mmol l^{-1} where as the nitrogen in the media (contributed by both nitrate and ammonia) should be 2–20 mmol l^{-1}.

Micronutrients : The inorganic elements required in small quantities but essential for proper growth of plant cells or tissues are: boron (B), copper (Cu), iron (Fe), manganese (Mn), zinc (Zn) and molybdenum (Mo). Out of these, iron seems more critical as it is used in chelated forms of

iron and zinc in preparing the culture media, as iron tartrate and citrate are difficult to dissolve. The concentration generally prescribed for all these elements are in traces:

Cu	0.1 μmol l^{-1},
Fe	1 μmol l^{-1},
Mo	5 μmol l^{-1},
Zn	1.5-30 μmol l^{-1},
Mn	20-90 μmol l^{-1} and
B	2-5100 μmol l^{-1}

These are added to culture media depending upon the requirement of the objective.

In addition to these elements certain media are also enriched with cobalt (Co), iodine (I) and sodium (Na) but exact cell growth requirement is not well established.

The composition of some plant tissue culture media reveal that the chief difference in the composition of various commonly used tissue culture media lies in the quantity of various salts and ions. Qualitatively, the inorganic nutrients required for various culture media appear to be fairly constant.

The active factor in the medium is the ions of different types rather than the salt (mineral salts on dissolving in water undergo dissociation and ionization). A single ion may be contributed by more than one salt. For example, in **Murashige and Skoog's** medium NO_3^- ions are contributed by NH_4NO_3 as well as KNO_3 and K^+ ions are contributed by KNO_3 and KH_2PO_4.

White's medium, one of the earliest plant tissue culture media includes all the necessary nutrients and was widely used for root culture. The experience of various investigators has however revealed that quantitatively the inorganic nutrients are inadequate for good callus growth (**Murashige and Skoog's** 1962), hence most plant tissue culture media, that are **now being widely** used (Table 6.3) are richer in mineral salts (ions) **as compared to White's medium. Aluminium and nickel used by Heller's** (1953) could not be proved to be essential and therefore, were dropped by subsequent workers, but **sodium, chloride and iodide** are indispensable.

In **Heller medium**, special emphasis was given to iron and nitrogen. In the **original White's medium** iron was used in the form of $Fe_2(SO_4)_3$ but **Street and co-workers** replaced it by $FeCl_3$ for root culture because of the impurities due to Mn and some other metallic ions. However, $FeCl_3$ also did not prove to be an entirely satisfactory source of iron. In this form iron is available to the tissue culture at or around pH 5.2 and within a week of inoculation the pH of the medium drift from 4.9–5.0 to 5.8–6.0 and the root culture started showing the iron deficiency symptoms. To overcome this difficulty, in most medium, iron is now used as FeEDTA, in this form iron remains available up to a pH of 7.6–8.0. However, unlike root, callus cultures can utilize $FeCl_3$ to pH 6.0 by secreting natural chelates. FeEDTA may be prepared by using $Fe_2(SO_4)_3 7H_2O$ and $Na_2EDTA \cdot 2H_2O$.

Inorganic nitrogen is supplied in the medium in the forms as nitrates and ammonium compounds, when nitrate is used alone the pH of the medium shifted toward alkalinity, to check this drift small amount of ammonium compound is added along with nitrate.

Following are the deficiency symptoms of the some of the elements shown by callus tissues:

- **Nitrogen :** Spectacular appearance of anthocyanins; vessels are not formed.
- **Nitrogen phosphorus and potassium :** Cell hypertrophy and a reduction of cambium tissue.
- **Sulphur :** Very apparent chlorosis
- **Iron :** Cessation of cell division

- **Boron :** Retardation of cell division and cell elongation.
- **Manganese or molybdenum :** Effect cell elongation.

Organic nutrients

Nitrogenous substances : Most cultured plant cells are capable of synthesising essential vitamins but not in sufficient amount. To achieve best growth it is essential to supplement the tissue culture medium with one or more vitamins and amino acid. Among the **essential vitamins thiamine** (vitamin B_1) has been proved to be essential ingredient. Other vitamins, especially pyridoxine (vitamin B_6), nicotinic acid (vitamin B_3) and calcium pentothenate (vitamin B_5) and ionositol are also known to improve growth of the tissue culture material. As shown in Table 6.3 there is variation in the quantities of essential vitamins used by various standard media.

Numerous **complex nutritive mixtures** of undefined composition, like **casein hydrolystate, coconut milk, corn-milk, malt extract, tomato juice and yeast extract** have also been used to promote growth of the tissue culture but these substances specifically fruit extracts may affect the reproducibility of results because of variation in the quality and quantity of growth promoting constituent in these extracts.

Carbon Source : It is essential to supplement the tissue culture media with a utilizable source of carbon to the culture media. **Haberblandt** (1902) attempted to culture green mesophyll cells, probably with the idea that green cells would have simple nutritive requirement, but this did not prove to be true. In fact even fully organized green shoot in cultures also did not show proper growth and proliferation without the addition of suitable carbon source in the medium.

The most commonly used carbon source is **sucrose** at a concentration of 2–5%. **Glucose**

and fructose also known to be used for good growth of some tissues. **Ball** (1953, 1955) demonstrated that autoclaved surcose was better than filtered sterilized sucrose. Autoclaving may do the hydrolysis of the sucrose thereby converting it into more efficiently utilizable sugar such as **fructose**. In general excised **dicotyledonous roots** grow better with sucrose where as monocots do best with **dextrose** (glucose). Some other forms of carbon that plant tissues are known to utilize include **maltose, galactose, mannose, lactose and sorbitol**. It has been reported that some tissues can even **metabolise starch** as the **sole carbon source** e.g. tissue cultures of Sequoia and maize endosperm.

Growth regulators (Hormones)

In addition to the nutrients, it is generally necessary to add one or more growth hormones e.g. **auxin, cytokinins and gibberellins** to support better growth of tissues and organs. However, the requirement of these hormones varies considerably with their endogenous levels.

(i) *Auxins :* Hormones of this group involved with elongation of stem and internodes, apical dominance, tropism, abscission, and rooting etc. In tissue culture auxin induces **cell division** and also **stimulate root formation/ differentiation**. Both natural IAA (Indole-3-acetic acid) and synthetic IBA (Indole-3-butyric acid) NAA (Naphthalene acetic acid) NOA (Naphthoxyacetic acid), 2, 4-D (2, 4 dichlorophenoxy acetic acid) and 2,4,5 T (triclorophenoxyacetic acid) are used.

Among auxins, IBA and NAA are widely used for rooting. In interaction with cytokinin, the auxins are used for shoot proliferation. 2,4-D and 2,4,5 T are very effective for the induction and growth of callus. IAA inhibits the bud formation and also play role in embryogenesis.

Auxins are generally dissolved in either ethanol or dilute NaOH.

Although the synthetic forms are relatively stable IAA is considered to be rapidly inactivated by certain environmental factors e.g. light.

(ii) *Cytokinin :* It is phytohormones occurring naturally in plant, which have a more specific effect on cell division (cytokinesis). Chemically cytokinins are **adenine derivatives** and have been employed in **tissue culture** work to promote the formation of adventitious buds and shoots from undifferentiated cells. In **cell cultures** they have been shown to promote the biosynthesis of berberine (*Thalictrum minus*), condensed tannins (*Onobrychis viccifolia*) and rhodoxanthin (*Ricinus*).

Cytokinin (adenine or kinetin) in the medium leads to the promotion of bud differentiation and development. **Kinetin** is 30,000 times more potent than adenine. **Kinetin** is originally detected as an artificial rearrangement product of the autoclaving process of herring sperm DNA (6-furfuryl aminopurine), while **kinetin** is only rarely used for callus induction aside from specific experimental purposes.

Other cytokinins which influence the induction of shoot buds include 6-benzylaminopurine (BAP) or 6-benzyladenine (BA), 6-γ-γ-dimethylamino-purine (2-iP), 6-tetrahydropyrane-adenine and zeatin. **Zeatin and 2-iP** are naturally occurring cytokinins while BA and kinetin are synthetically derived. **6 BAP** (6-benzyl-amino-purine) and **zeatin** are very commonly used to induce and maintain growth of callus and cell suspension cultures.

Cytokinins are generally dissolve in dilute HCl or NaOH.

Zeatin isolated from maize embryos at the milky stage. It is 6-substituted adenine derivative, 6-(4-hydroxy-3-methylbut-2-enyl)-amino-purine obtained from maize associated with zeatin riboside (1β-D-ribofuranose) and with phosphate ester of this compound.

(iii) **Gibberellins** : There are over 20 known gibberellins, of these, GA_3 is usually used to increase the **shoot elongation** in tissue culture. As compared to auxins and cytokinin, **gibberellins are used very rarely**. It is reported to stimulate normal development of plantlets from *in vitro* formed adventive embryos. GA is readily soluble in cold water up to 1000 mg^{-1}.

Solidifying Agents for Solidification of the Media

Due to improved oxygen supply and support to the culture growth, solid media are often preferred to liquid cultures. For this purpose, substance with strong gelling capacity is added into the liquid media. These reversibly bind water and thus ensure the humidity of the medium desired for culturing depending on the concentration.

GELLING AGENT USED TO SOLIDIFY LIQUID MEDIA

• Agar	• Hydroxyethylcellulose
• Alginate	• Polyacrylamide
• Carrageenan	• Starch
• Gelatin	• Silica gel

The most commonly used substance for this purpose is the phycocolloid agar-agar obtained from red algae (*Gelidium gracilaria*). It is generally used at a concentration of 0.8-1.0%, with higher concentration medium become hard and does not allow the diffusion of nutrients into the tissues medium. However, agar is not an essential component of the nutrient medium. Single cell and cell aggregates can be grown as suspension cultures in liquid medium containing inorganic, organic nutrients and other growth factors. Such culture should however be regularly aerated either by bubbling sterile air or gentle agitation. In nutritional studies, the use of agar should be avoided because of the impurities present in all the commercially available agar-agar especially of Ca, Mg, K, Na and trace elements.

Agar (Agarose) is extraordinary **resistant to enzymatic hydrolysis** at incubation temperature and only a few bacteria exist which are capable of producing degrading enzyme, agarase. This resistance to hydrolysis is the fundamental importance to the use of agar-agar in cell culture medium. It is also neutral to media constituents and thus do not react with them.

pH

pH of the medium is generally adjusted between 5.0 and 6.0 before sterilization. In general pH higher than 6.0 give fairly hard medium and pH below 5.0 does not allow satisfactory gelling of the Agar.

Media Preparation

For media preparation, there are two possible methods i.e.:

(i) To weigh the required quantity of nutrient, dissolved them separately and mixed at the time of medium preparation.

(ii) To prepare the stock solution separately for macronutrients, micronutrients, iron solution and organic components, store them in the refrigerator till not used. e.g., **Murashinge & Skoog's** media stock solution is prepared as under.

Procedure

All the ingredients may be grouped into following four groups:

Stock Solution Ingredients	Amount (mg/L)
Group I	
• NH_4NO_3	1650
• KNO_3	1900
• $CaCl_2 \cdot 2H_2O$	440
• $MgSO_4 \cdot 7H_2O$	370
• KH_2PO_4	170
Group II	
• KI	0.83
• H_3BO_3	6.2
• $MnSO_4 \cdot 4H_2O$	22.3
• $ZnSO_4 \cdot 7H_2O$	8.6
• $Na_2MoO_4 \cdot 2H_2O$	0.25
• $CuSO_4 \cdot 5H_2O$	0.025
• $CoCl_2 \cdot 6H_2O$	0.025
Group III	
• $FeSO_4 \cdot 7H_2O$	27.8
• $Na_2EDTA \cdot 2H_2O$	37.3
Group IV	
• Inositol	100
• Nicotinic acid	0.5
• Pyridoxine HCl	0.5
• Thiamine HCl	0.1
• Glycine	2

Concentration of the ingredients : For the preparation of stock solution the **Group I** ingredient are prepared 20 × concentrated solution. **Group II** 200 × concentrated, **Group III** Iron salts (200 × concentrated) and **Group IV** organic ingredient except sucrose (200 × concentrated).

Solution preparation : For the preparation of stock solution each component (analar grade) should be weighed and dissolved separately in glass distilled or demineralized water and then mix them together.

Stock solution may be prepared at the strength of 1 mmol l^{-1} or 10 mmol l^{-1}. All the stock solutions are stored in refrigerator till used.

For iron solution dissolve $FeSO_4 \cdot 7H_2O$ and $Na_2EDTA \cdot 2H_2O$ separately in about 450 ml distilled water by heating and constant stirring. Mix the two solutions, adjust pH of the medium

to 5.5 and final volume adjusted 1 L with distilled water.

Semisolid media preparation : Required quantities of agar and sucrose are weighed and dissolved in water by 3/4th volume of medium, by heating them on water bath.

Adequate quantities of stock solution (for 1L medium 50 ml of stock solution of Group I, 5 ml of stock solution II, III and IV group) and other special supplements are added and final volume is made up with double distilled water. After mixing well, pH of the medium is adjusted to 5.8 using 0.1 N NaOH and 0.1 N HCl.

Note : These days dry powdered media are available in the market. The available powder is to be dissolved in 3/4th volume of distilled water and after adding sugar, agar and other desired supplements the final volume is made up with distilled water pH is adjusted and the medium autoclaved.

Sterilization of Culture Media

Culture media packed in glass containers or vessels are sealed with cotton plugs and covered with aluminium foils and are autoclaved at pressure of 2–2.2 atm at 121°C for 15–40 minutes (time to be fixed from the time when temperature reaches the required temperature). The exposure time depends on the volume of the liquid to be sterilised as given below.

MINIMUM AUTOCLAVING TIME FOR PLANT TISSUE CULTURE MEDIA

Volume of the media per vessel (ml)	Minimum autoclaving time (min)
25	20
50	25
100	28
250	31
500	35
1000	40
2000	48
4000	63

Minimum autoclaving time include the time required for the liquid volume to reach the sterilising temperature (121°C) and 15 minutes at this temperature. Time may vary due to difference in autoclaves.

Moreover the actual success of sterilization can be tested using a **bioindicator**, commonly spores of the bacterium Bacillus stearothermophillus are used as such as a test organism. Together with culture medium and a pH indicator in ampoules sealed by melting, both autoclaved material and non-autoclaved controls are incubated for 24–48 hours at 60°C. If the spores are dead, the color of the pH indicator in the solution remains unchanged indicating no change in pH (Fig. 6.4).

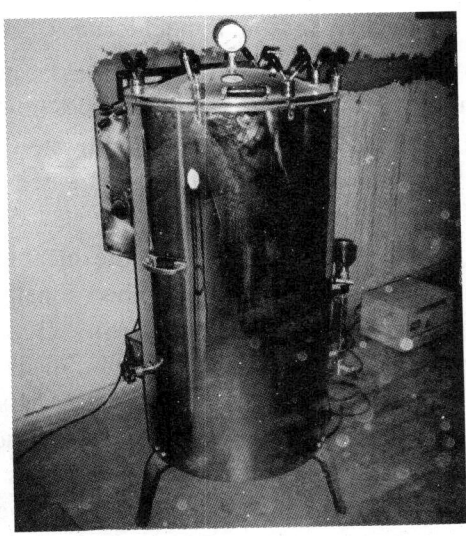

Fig. 6.4. Autoclave.

TYPES OF PLANT TISSUE CULTURES; THEIR ESTABLISHMENT AND MAINTENANCE

Plant tissue culture is a general term to culture the **isolated plant organs** (particularly of isolated roots but, to a lesser extent of stem tips, immature embryo, leaf primordia, flower structures and even the cells and the protoplasts) under aseptic environment.

Types of Cultures

Root tip culture : Tips of the lateral roots are sterilised, **excised** and **transferred** to fresh medium. The lateral roots continue to grow and provide several roots, which after **seven days**, are used to initiate stock or experimental cultures. Thus the root material derived from a **single radicle** could be multiplied and maintained in continuous culture, such genetically uniform root cultures are referred to as a **clone of isolated roots**.

Leaves or leaf primordia culture : Leaves (800 μm) may be detached from shoots, **surface sterilized** and placed on a solidified medium where they will remains in a **healthy conditions** for a long periods. Growth rate in culture depends on their stage of maturity at excision. **Young leaves have more growth potential** than the nearly mature ones.

Shoot tip culture : The excised shoot tips (100–1000 μm long) of many plant species can be cultured on relatively simple nutrient media containing growth hormones and will often **form roots and develop into whole plants**.

Complete flower culture : **Nitsch** in 1951 reported the successful culture of the flowers of several dicotyledonous species, the flowers remain healthy and develop normally to produce mature fruits. Flowers (2 days after pollination) are excised, sterilized by immersion in 5% calcium hypochlorite, washed with sterilized water and transferred to culture tubes containing an agar medium. Often fruits, which develop are smaller than their natural counterpart; but the size can be increased by supplementing the medium with an appropriate combination of growth hormones.

Anther and pollens culture : Young **flower buds** are removed from the plant and surface sterilized. The anthers are then carefully excised and transferred to an appropriate nutrient medium. Immature stage usually grow abnormally and there is **no development of pollen grains from pollen mother cells**. Anther at a very young stage (containing microspore mother cells, or tetrads) and late stage (containing binucleate starch filled pollen) of development are generally ineffective and hence for better response always select mature anther or pollen.

Mature anther or pollen grains (microspora) of several species of gymnosperms can be induced to form callus by spreading them out on the surface of a suitable agar media.

Mature pollen grains of angiosperms do not usually form callus, although there are one or two exceptions.

Ovule and embryo culture : Embryo is dissected from the ovule and put into culture media.

Very small globular embryos require a delicate balance of the hormones. Hence mature embryos are excised from ripened seeds and cultured mainly to avoid inhibition in the seed for germination. This type of culture is relatively easy as the embryos require a simple nutrient medium containing mineral salts, sugar and agar for growth and development.

The seeds are treated with 70% alcohol for about **two minutes**, washed with sterile distilled water, treated with surface sterilizing agent for specific period (Table 6.2), once again rinsed with sterilized distilled water and kept for germination by placing them on double layers of pre-sterilized filter paper, placed in petridish moistened with sterilized distilled water or placed on moistened cotton swab in petridish. The seeds are germinated in dark at 25–28°C and small part of the seedling is utilised for the initiation of callus.

Apart from above mentioned cultures, there are two more methods for culturing of plant tissues/cells:

- Protoplast culture,
- Hairy roots culture.

Protoplast Culture

Protoplasts are the naked cells of varied origin without cell walls, which are cultivated in liquid as well as on solid media. Protoplasts can be isolated by mechanical or enzymatic method from almost all parts of the plant : roots, tubers, root nodules, leaves, fruits, endosperms, crown gall tissues, pollen mother cells and the cells of the callus tissue but the most appropriate is the leaves of the plant.

Fully expanded young leaves from the healthy plant are collected, washed with running tap water and sterilized by dipping in 70% ethanol for about a minute and then treating with 2% solution of sodium hypochlorite for 20–30 minutes and then washed with sterile distilled water to make it free from the trace of sodium hypochlorite.

The lower surface of the sterilized leaf is peeled off and stripped leaves are cut into pieces (midrib).

The peeled leaf segments are treated with enzymes (**macerozyme** and then treated with cellulase) to isolate the protoplasts.

The protoplasts so obtained are cleaned by centrifugation and decantation method. Finally, the protoplast solution of known density (1×10^5 protoplast/ml) is poured on sterile and cooled down molten nutrient medium in petridishes. Mix the two gently but quickly by rotating each petridish. Allow the medium to set and seal petridishes with paraffin film. Incubate the petridishes in inverted position in BOD incubator. The protoplasts, which are capable of dividing undergo cell divisions and form callus within 2–3 weeks. The callus is then subcultured on fresh medium. **Embryogenesis** begins from callus when it is transferred to a medium containing proper proportion of auxin and cytokinin, the embryos develop into plantlets which may be transferred to pots (Fig. 6.5).

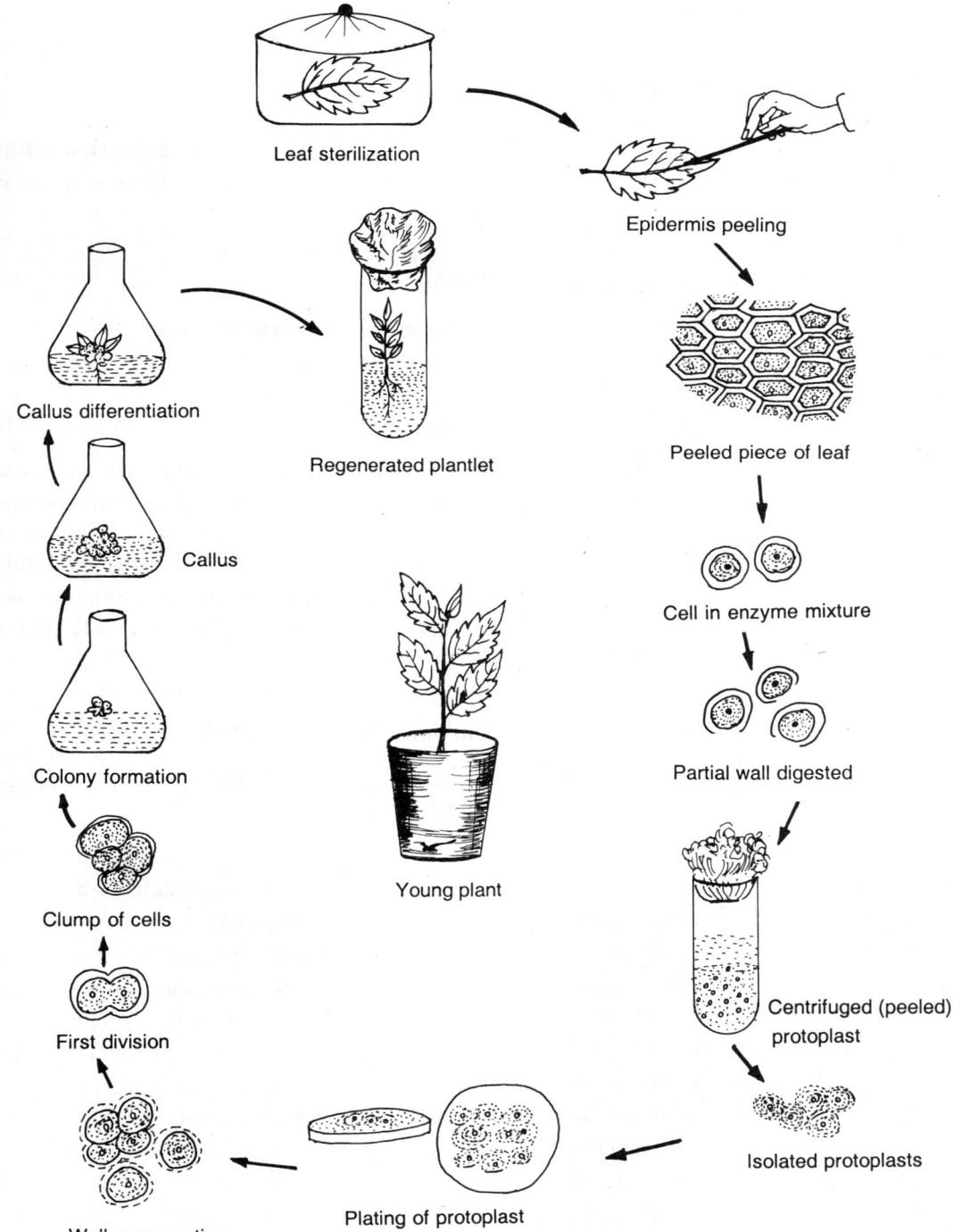

Leaf sterilization

Epidermis peeling

Peeled piece of leaf

Cell in enzyme mixture

Partial wall digested

Centrifuged (peeled) protoplast

Isolated protoplasts

Callus differentiation

Regenerated plantlet

Callus

Colony formation

Clump of cells

First division

Young plant

Wall regeneration

Plating of protoplast

Fig. 6.5. Schematic diagram showing the isolation, culture and regeneration of young plant from leaf protoplast.

Hairy Root Culture

The name "hairy root" was mentioned in the literature by **Steward** et al (1900). A large number of small fine hairy roots covered with root hairs originate directly from the explant in response to *Agrobacterium rhizogenes* infection are termed "hairy roots". These are fast growing, highly branched adventitious roots at the site of infection and can grow even on a hormone-free culture medium

Many plant cell culture systems, which did not produce adequate amount of desired compounds is being reinvestigated using hairy root culture methods. A diversified range of plant species has been transformed using various bacterial strains. One of the most important characteristics of the transformed roots is their capability to synthesize secondary metabolites specific to that plant species from which they have been developed. Growth kinetics and secondary metabolite production by hairy roots is highly stable and are of equal level and even they are higher to those of field grown plants (Fig. 6.6).

Establishment and Maintenance of Various Cultures

For the growth establishment and maintenance of various types of plant tissue cultures, there are three main **culture systems**, selected on the basis of the objective.

(i) Growth of **callus** masses on solidified media (**callus culture** also known as **static culture**).

(ii) Growth in liquid media (**suspension culture**) consists of mixture of single cells or cell aggregates.

(iii) **Protoplast culture.**

The protoplast culture can be grown as:

• Callus culture (static tissue culture); or

• Suspension culture.

Callus Culture

Callus is an amorphous aggregate of loosely arranged parenchyma cells, which proliferate from mother cells. Cultivation of callus usually on a solidified nutrient medium under aseptic conditions is known as **callus culture**, unlike tumor tissue, the cell division take place periclinally (Fig. 6.7 (a) & (b)).

Initiation of callus culture

(a) Selection and preparation of explant (also See at p.105)

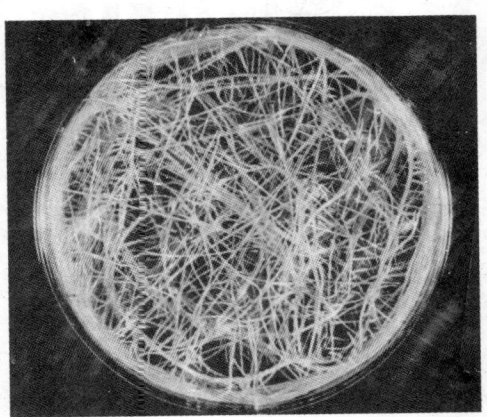

Fig. 6.6. Hairy roots

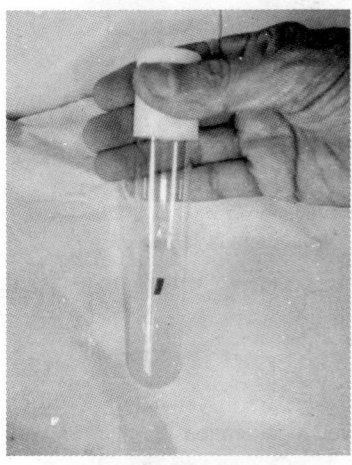

Fig. 6.7(a). Initiation of callus culture.

Selection : For the preparation of callus culture, organ or culture is selected such as segments of root or stem, leaf primordia, flower structure or fruit etc.

Preparation :

- **(i)** Excised parts of the plant organ are first washed with tap water, then sterilised with 0.1% of mercuric chloride (HgCl$_2$) or 2% w/v, sodium hypochlorite (NaOCl) solution for 15 minutes.

  In the case of plant organ containing waxy layer, the material is either pretreated with wetting agents [ethanol 70–90%; tween 20 (polyoxyethylene-sorbitan-monolaurate); 1–20 drops into 100 ml distilled water]; or other detergents are added to the sterilization solution to reduce the water repulsion.

- **(ii)** Washed the sterilised explants with sterile glass distilled water and cut aseptically into small segments (2–5 mm).

(b) Selection of culture medium

The organ is to be cultured in well-defined nutrient medium containing inorganic & organic nutrients and vitamins. The culture of the medium depends on the species of the plant and the objective of the experiment. The MS medium is quite suitable for **dicot tissues** because of relatively high concentration of nitrate, potassium and ammonium ions in comparison to other media (Table 6.3).

Growth hormones (auxin, cytokinin) are adjusted in the medium according to the objective of the culture. For example **auxins, IBA and NAA** are widely used in medium for rooting and in combination with cytokinin for shoot proliferation. 2, 4-D and 2, 4, 5-T are effective for good growth of the callus culture. This is also quite favourable for monocot tissues or explant.

The selected semi-solid nutrient is prepared. The pH of the medium is adjusted (5.0–6.0) and poured into culture vessels (15 ml for 25 × 150 mm culture tubes or 50 for 150 ml flasks) plugged and sterilised by autoclaving.

(c) Transfer of explant

Surface sterilised organs (explant) from stem, root or tuber or leaf etc. is transferred aseptically into the vessel containing semisoild culture medium.

(d) Incubation of culture

The inoculated vessels are transferred into BOD incubator with autocontrolled device. Incubate at 25–28°C using light and dark cycles of each 12 hours duration. Nutrient medium is supplemented with auxin to induce cell division. After 3–4 week callus should be about 5 times, the size of the explant. Many tissue explants possess some degree of polarity with the result that the callus is formed most early at one surface. In stem segment, callus is formed particularly from that surface which in vivo is directed towards the root.

The unique feature of callus is its ability to develop normal root and shoot, ultimately forming a plant. Commercially important secondary metabolites can also be obtained from static culture by manipulating the composition of media and growth regulators (physiological and biochemical conditions) but on the whole it is a good source for the establishment of suspension culture.

Callus is formed through three stages of development. They are:

- Induction,
- Cell division, and
- Cell differentiation.

Induction : During this stage metabolic activities of the cell will increase; with the result, the cell accumulates organic contents and finally divide into a number of cells. The length of this phase depends upon the functional potential of the explant and the environmental conditions of the cell division stage.

Cell division : This is the phase of active cell division as the explant cells revert to meristematic state.

Cell differentiation : This is the phase of cellular differentiation i.e. morphological and physiological differentiation occur leading to the formation of secondary metabolites.

Maintenance

After sufficient time of callus growth on the same medium following change will occur, i.e.–

• Depletion of nutrients in the medium,

• Gradual loss of water,

• Accumulation of metabolic toxins.

Hence for the maintenance of growth in callus culture it becomes necessary to **subculture the callus** into a fresh medium. Healthy callus tissue of sufficient size (5–10 mm in diameter) and weight 20–100 mg) is transferred under aseptic conditions to fresh medium. Subculturing should be repeated after every 4–5 weeks (Fig. 6.7(b)).

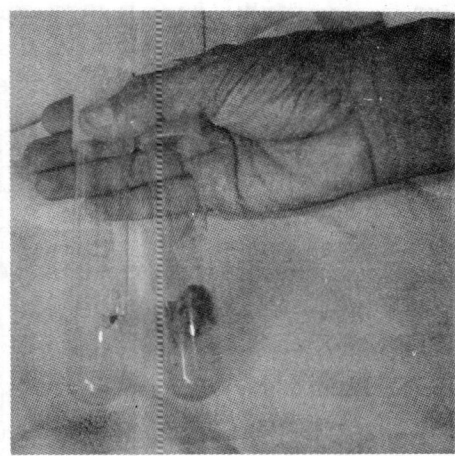

Fig. 6.7(b). Development of callus culture.

Many callus cultures, however remain healthy and continue to grow at slow rate for much longer period without subculturing, if the incubation is to be carried out at low temperature 5–10°C below the normal temperature (16–18°C). Normally total depletion takes about 28 days.

Callus tissue may appear of the following different colours:

• **White :** If grown in dark due to the absence of chlorophyll.

• **Green :** If grown in light.

• **Yellow :** due to development of carotenoid pigments in greater amounts.

• **Purple :** due to the accumulation of anthocyanins in vacuole.

• **Brown :** due to excretion of phenolic substance and formation of quinones.

Callus culture may vary widely in texture appearance and rate of growth. Some callus growth are heavily lignified and hard in texture while others are fragile.

The cells in callus tissue vary in shape from spherical to elongated.

Suspension Culture

Suspension culture contains a uniform suspension of separate cells in liquid medium. For the preparation of suspension culture, callus fragments is transferred to liquid medium (without agar), which is agitated continuously to keep the cells separate. Agitation can be achieved by rotary shaker system attached within the BOD incubator at a rate of 50–150 rpm. After sufficient number of cells are produced, subculturing can be done in fresh liquid medium.

Single cells can also be obtained from fresh plant organ (leaf).

Initiation of suspension culture

Isolation of single cell

(a) **From callus culture :** Healthy callus tissue is selected and placed in a petridish on a sterile filter paper and cut into small pieces with the help of sterile scalpel.

Selected small piece of callus fragment about 300–500 mg and transferred into flask containing about 60 ml of liquid nutrient media (i.e. defined nutrient medium without gelling agent), the flasks is agitated at 50–150 rpm to make the separation of the cells in the medium. Decant the medium and resuspend residue by gently rotating the flask, and finally transfer 1/4th of the entire residue to fresh medium, followed by sieving the medium to obtain the degree of uniformity of cells.

(b) From plant organ : From the plant organ (leaf tissue) single cell can be isolated by any of the following methods:

• Mechanical method

• Enzymatic method

Mechanical Method : The surface sterilised fresh leaves are grinded in (1:4) grinding medium (20 µmol sucrose; 10 µmol $MgCl_2$, 20 µmol tris-HCl buffer, pH 7.8) in glass pestle mortar. The homogenate is passed through muslins (two layers) cloth. Then washed with sterile distilled water, centrifuge with culture medium, sieved and placed on culture dish for inoculation.

Enzymatic Method : Leaves are taken from 60 to 80 days old plant and sterilised by immersing them in 70% ethanol solution followed by hypochlorite solution treatment. Then washed with sterile double distilled water, placed on sterile tile and peeled off the lower surface with sterile forceps.

Cut the peeled surface area of the leaves into small pieces (4 cm^2). Transfer them (2 g leaves) into an Erlenmeyer flask (100 ml) containing about 20 ml of filtered sterilised enzyme solution (macerozyme 0.5% solution, 0.8% mannitol and 1% potassium dextran sulphate).

Incubate the flask at 25°C for 2 hours, during incubation, change the enzyme solution with the fresh one at every 30 minutes.

Wash the cell twice with culture medium and place them in culture dish.

Growth pattern of suspension culture

Cell suspension culture is generally initiated by transferring an established (undifferentiated) callus tissue to a liquid nutrient medium, in flask culture vessel, which is agitated continuously during culture period. Agitation serves both, to aerate the cultures and to disperse the cell in medium. The composition of the medium for the establishment of suspension culture could be the same as for the callus culture except for the addition of agar. **After transferring the cells** into a suitable liquid medium they divide after **lag phase** and **linearly increase** their population. The soft callus generally forms a suspension culture without much difficulty. The release of cells and tissue fragments from less friable callus masses and the maintenance of good degree of cell separation may often be promoted by the presence of liquid medium of a high auxin concentration, an appropriate balance between yeast extract and auxin or between auxin and kinetin. After sometime depending upon the nutrient level and the rate of cell division, it comes to **stationary phase** (Fig. 6.8).

Stationary phase : The suspension culture are usually incubated at 25°C in darkness or low intensity fluorescent light at this stage, cell cultures are sub-cultured by dilution of stock culture 5–10 times (v/v) depending upon the growth of cells.

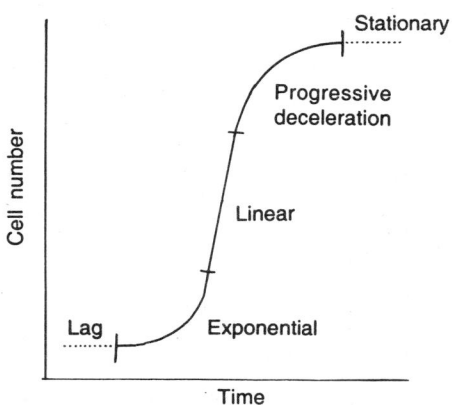

Fig. 6.8. Curve showing the growth pattern in the suspension culture.

The growth of suspension culture is higher than callus culture, and therefore it requires rapid sub culture (7–21 days) as compared to callus culture (4–8 weeks).

The incubation period from culture initiation to the stationary phase is determined primarily by:

(a) initial cell density,

(b) duration of lag phase, and

(c) growth rate of cell type.

The cell density used to subculture is critical and depend largely on the type of suspension culture to be maintained. The low initial cell density will prolong the lag phase and exponential phase of growth. At an initial cell density of $9–15 \times 10^3$ ml, the cell will generally undergo eight fold increase in cell number before entering the stationary phase. Normal incubation time of stock culture is 21–28 days, while for sub culture it is 14–21 days.

There are several **parameters** for measuring growth of cultured cells such as measurement of fresh and dry weights, cell mass, cell number, mitotic index or indirectly by the conductivity of the medium (King et al, 1973).

(i) **Fresh weight :** The value of callus cultures, frequently determined as total weight of callus medium layer and petridish. However in this method, there are variations due to evaporation via the medium's surface. Hence, more exact values are obtained by determining the weight after complete separation from the culture medium. This is possible when the material is cultured on separate layers of cellulose or nylon.

(ii) **Dry weight :** It requires repeated drying usually at 60°C to the point of constant weight, up to fresh weight of 500 mg, a Linear relationship between fresh and dry weight is assumed. This method excludes error due to varying endogenous water contents.

(iii) **Cell mass :** It may be determined by densification by centrifugation (Ca 2000 g, 5 min.) of a particular percentage of the volume (4–7 ml) in graduated conical centrifuge tubes. In order to avoid error, due to water absorption by the cells, the so-called packed cell volume (PCV) must be recorded immediately following the separation process.

(iv) **Cell number :** To determine the number of cell per unit volume, existing cell clumps or aggregates must be separated into isolated cell (callus culture and in most suspension cultures). This is commonly done using chrome-trioxide alone or in combination with hypochlorous acid. Possible alternative are EDTA and pectinase.

Procedure : Cell aggregates are treated with 5–15% chromic acid or pectinase. To 1 volume of cell suspension culture may be added 2 volumes of 8% chromic acid, trioxide solution and mixture is heated at 70°C for 2–15 min. The mixture is cooled and then agitated vigorously for 10 min. on a shaking machine.

The suspension is now centrifuged, the chromic acid is poured off and the pellet resuspended in 8% saline solution After 10–15 min. free cells are counted on a haemocytometer. Heating is avoided if an enzyme is used to disrupt the aggregates.

(v) **Conductivity :** The inverse relationship between the conductivity and fresh or dry weight of the medium allows the determination of growth without taking samples (which would affect the sterility of the culture). In fully synthetic media, conductivity is determined almost exclusively by salt concentration.

Coherence of salt concentration, especially KNO_3 and conductivity of a medium

Salt	Concentration (milligram equivalent/L)	Conductivity (ms/cm)
Usually used plant media	50–55	5.6
KNO_3 (0.5%)	50	5.5

As long as the pH of the medium remains above 3 (C^{H+}<10–3 ml/L) the concentration of hydrogen ions does not affect conductivity.

(vi) **Cellulose Concentration :** Calcofluor-white ST (0.1% aqueous) allow monitoring of changes in the concentration of cell wall polymers from β-glucoside bond glucose molecule such as cellulose or callose. The textile brightener specifically bonds to β-1, 4 glucans and intensely fluoresces following stimulation with short wave blue light. In this way even traces of these compound may be identified.

Maintenance of suspension culture

Maintenance of suspension culture can be done by following three ways (Fig. 6.9) :

(i) **Batch Suspension Culture :** In this technique, the cells are allowed to multiply in liquid medium, which is continuously agitated to break up cell aggregates. The system is **"closed"** with respect to additions or removal of culture, except for circulation of air. In this technique to commence the growth again on the stationary phase, more amount of nutrient medium is added to the original culture or the cells are to be transferred into fresh medium. Each fresh medium containing culture (suspension) constitutes a batch. Such cultures are grown again and again for the purpose of experiment to achieve certain specific objectives. In batch culture there is no steady state of growth, hence it is not ideal for commercial production of secondary metabolites.

(ii) **Semi Continuous Suspension Culture :** In this very type, the system is **open**. It is designed for periodic removal of culture and addition of fresh medium. Hence, the **growth** is continuously maintained.

(iii) **Continuous Suspension Culture :** Here, the volume of culture remains constant and fresh medium and culture are continuously added and withdrawn respectively. The important feature of the continuous culture is the proliferation of cell occurs under constant conditions. In this very suspension culture technique, a steady state is achieved by adding medium in which single nutrient has been adjusted so as to be growth limiting.

Continuous culture is **closed** and **open** type.

In the **Closed** type, addition of fresh medium is balanced by the outflow of spent medium. The cell passing through the outgoing medium are separated mechanically and reintroduced into the culture for the continuous growth of the cell biomass.

Open continuous system involves regulated new medium and balancing harvest of equal volume of culture. The open system is further of two type depending upon regulation technique: **chemostat and turbidostat.**

In chemostat the desired rate of growth is maintained by adjusting the level of concentration of nutrient by constant inflow of fresh medium.

In turbidostat, on the contrary, the input of medium is intermittent, and it is mainly required to maintain the cell density in the culture.

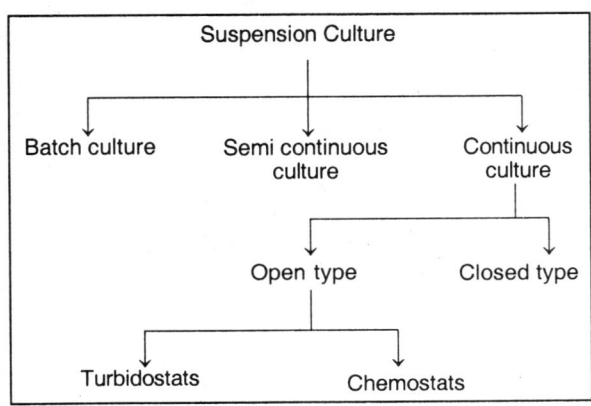

Fig. 6.9. Schematic Diagram Showing the Maintenance of Suspension Culture.

APPLICATIONS OF TISSUE CULTURE IN PHARMACOGNOSY

Plant tissue culture technology has been used in almost all the field of biosciences. The desirable products produced by plant tissue cultures are as diversified as is industry itself. Its applications include:

- Production of Phytopharmaceuticals,
- Biochemical Conversions,
- Clonal Propagation (Micropropagation), and
- Production of Immobilized Plant Cells.

Production of Phytopharmaceuticals

The use of plant tissue culture for the production of phytopharmaceuticals was started in 1959 when Wenstein et al, studied Agave, for the production of steroids using tissue culture method. Dioscorea was reported to contain industrially useful steroids by 1966 but it was 1969 when Kaul reported the production of 1.2% dry weight diosgenin by tissue culture of *D. sylvatica*.

During the last two decades advancement in tissue culture technology such as **development of hairy root cultures, immobilized plant cell systems, and technique to enhance the excretion of desired product into medium** has resulted in promising findings for a variety of medicinally important substance from several medicinal plants. Even the callus and suspension cultures are also capable of synthesising secondary metabolites and yields are comparable to the intact plant (Tables 6.4 & 6.5). There are report about few cell line producing secondary metabolites far in excess of that found in intact plants example:

Table 6.4. Phytopharmaceuticals of pharmaceutical significance

Compound	Plant Species	Culture type
Ajmalicine	*Catharanthus roseus*	S
Anisodamine (6-hydroxy-hyoscyamine)	*Anisodus tanguticus* (bioconversion)	S
Anthocyanins	*Euphorbia milli*	S
Anthraquinones	*Cassia angustifolia*	C
	Cassia obtusifolia	C
	Cassia tora	C
	Galium mollugo	S
	Morinda citrifolia	S
	Rubia species	S
Atropine	*Atropa belladonna*	Hairy root
Berberine	*Coptis japonica*	C&S
Betacyanins	*Chenopodium rubrum*	S
Caffeine	*Coffea arabica*	C
Carboline alkaloids	*Phaseolus vulgaris*	S
	Peganum harmala	S
Cardenolides	*Digitalis purpurea*	S&C
	Digitalis lanata	S (biotransformation)
Cinnamoyl putrescines	*Nicotiana tabacum*	S (reduction of phosphate)
Codeine	*Papaver somniferum*	S
Digoxin (Biotransformation)	*Digitalis lanata*	S
Diosgenin	*Dioscorea composita*	C
	Dioscorea deltoidea	S
	Solanum xanthocarpum	S
	Trigonella foenum-graecum	S

(Cont'd)

Compound	Plant Species	Culture type
L. dopa	Mucuna ruriens	S
Ginsenosides	Panax ginseng	S
Glycyrrhizin	Glycyrrhiza glabra	S
Harringtonine and homoharringtonine	Cephalotaxus sps	S
Hyoscyamine	Hyoscyamus niger Duboisia leichhardtii	S root culture
Indole alkaloids	Ipomoea violacea Rivea corymbosa	C & S
Isoprenoids (vol. oil)	Pelargonium fragrans	C & shoot proliferation
Morphine	Papaver sominiferum	S
Naphthoquinone	Lithospernum erythrorhizon	C & S
Nicotine	Nicotiana tobacum	S
Papain	Carcia papaya	C
Phenolics	Pinus resinosa	C
Protoberberines	Thalictrum species, Coptis japonica & Berberis species	S
Psoralen	Ruta Graveolens	S
Quinoline alkaloids	Chinchona ledgeriana	C & S
Quinine & quinidine	Chinchona ledgeriana	Root culture
Reserpine	Rauwolfia serpentina	S
	Alstonia constricta	C
Rosamarinic acid	Coleus blumei	C & S
Scopolamine	Duboisia leichhardtii	Root culture
Serpentine & other monomeric alkaloids	Catharanthus roseus	C & S
Shikonin	Lythospermum erythrorhizon	C & S
Steroidal glycoalkaloids	Solanum acculeatissimum	C
	Salanum khasianum (Organogenesis)	C
	Solanium xanthocarpum	C
Trigonelline	Trigonella foenum-graecum	S
Tropane alkaloids	Datura innoxia	S
	Datura innoxia (regeneration)	S
	Datura stramonium	C & S
	Hyoscyamus niger	S
	Scopolia parviflora	C
Ubiquinone 10	Nicotiana tabacum	S
Undecanone & other volatile components	Ruta gravealens	C
Vrbascoside	Syringa vulgaris	S
Vinblastine	Catharanthus roseus	C (differentiation)
Vindoline	Vatharanthus roseus	S
Visnagin	Ammi visnaga	S
Xanthotoxin	Ruta graveolens	S

C: callus; S: Suspension.

Table 6.5. Induced production of metabolites in cell cultures by various elicitors

Elicitor	Plant-cell suspension culture	Effect
High light intensity	*Coffea arabica*	Stimulation of caffeine production
Colchicine	*Valeriana wallichi*	Sixtyfold increase in valepotriates with six new compounds (not due to higher ploidy level)
Copper sulphate	*Lithospermum erythrorhizon*	Greatly increased shikonin production
	Various Solanaceae	Induced formation of sesquiterpene phytoalexins of lubimin type
Thiosemicarbazide	*Panax ginseng*	Promotes biosynthesis of saponins and inhibits phytosterol production
L-Tryptophan (a biosynthetic precursor of quinoline alkaloids)	*Cinchona pubescens, C. ledgeriana*	Enhanced alkaloid production
Phytophthora megasperma preparation	Tobacco plant	Accumulation of capsidiol
Non-viable conidia of the wilt-producing fungus *Vertiicillium dahliae*	*Gossypium arboreum*	One hundred fold increase in gossypol after 120 h incubation
Yeast carbohydrate preparation	*Thalictrum rugosum*	Up to four fold enhancement of berbrine
Yeasts (free and immobilized)	*Ruta graveolens*	Increased production of acridone epoxides but not rutacridone
Phytophthora cinnamomi and *Aspergillius niger* (sterilized mycelia)	*Cinchona ledgeriana*	Increase in anthraquinone production
Sterilized fungal mycelia (*Pythium, Phytophthora, Verticillium*), etc. or	*Pimpinella anisum Petroselinium crispus Ammi majus*	Stimulation of coumarin synthesis
	Catharanthus roseus	Production of catharanthine and other major indole alkaloids stimulated
	Cephalotaxus harringtonia	Dramatic increase in alkaloid content
	Cinchona ledgeriana	Increase in anthraquinone production
	Gossypium arboretum	One hundredfold increase in gossypol after 120 h incubation
Yeast, yeast extracts and alkaloid carbohydrate preparations	*Escholtzia california*	Large and rapid increase or benzophenanthridine
	Thalictrum rugosum	Upto fourfold enhancement of berberine
	Ruta graveolens	Increased production of acridone expoxides but not rutacridone
	Orthosiphon aristatus	Stimulation of rosmarinic acid production

Table 6.6. Important plant alkaloids and their pharmacological activities

Alkaloids	Plant source	Culture type	Pharmacological use
Ajmalicine	*Catharanthus roseus*	Cell suspension	hypotensive
Atropine	*Atropa belladonna*	–	anticholinergic
Berberine	*Berberis* spp., *Coptis japonica*	Cell suspension	antispasmodic, antiprotozoal
Codeine	*Papaver somniferum*	–	sedative, analgesic
Colchicine	*Colchicum autumnale*	Callus culture	antimitotic
Caffeine	*Coffea arabica, Camellia sinensis*	–	stimulant
Camptotecine	*Camptotheca acuminata*	Cell suspension	Antitumour
Emetine	*Cephaelis ipecacuanha*	Root culture	emetic
Ellipticine	*Ochrosia elliptica*	Cell suspension	antitumour
Ephedrine	*Ephedra gerardiana*	–	spasmolytic
Morphine	*Papaver somniferum*	Cell suspension	analgesic, sedative
Papaverine	*Papaver somniferum*	–	spasmolytic
Quinine	*Cinchona lederiana*	Cell suspension	antimalaria
Reserpine	*Rauwolfia serpentina*	Cell suspension	hypotensive
Vinblastine, vincristine	*Catharanthus roseus*	Shoot culture	anticancer

Berberis for jatrorrhizine, **lithospermum** for shikonin; **coleus** for rosamarinic acid production and **coptis** for berberine.

During the last few years, plant tissue culture of several medicinal plants has been initiated and in many cases interesting compound with high yields of secondary metabolites are produced. For example, ten times more production of anthra-quinone derivative from *Cassia tora* (6%) as compared to the crude drug. A twenty times more production of anthraquinone content in suspension culture of *Morinda citrifolia* and similar results were obtained from the suspension culture of *Galium* species. The suspension culture of *Dioscorea deltoidea* could produce up to 1.5% dry weight content of diosgenin. The cell culture of *Dioscorea deltoidea* yielded 26 mg/g dry weight of diosgenin where as the plant produce only 20mg/g of diosgenin. The *Catharanthus roseus* cell culture yielded four times more ajmalicene and serpentine than the whole plant. The production of ginsenoside (21% of dry weight) from the cell culture of *Panax ginseng* has also been reported. The selected cell lines of *Euphorbia*

millic produce seven times as much anthocyanin as the original calluses.

Nowadays, pharma industry is using plant tissue culture as source of variety of pharmaceuticals, which includes **alkaloids, terpenoids, glycosides and steroids** (Tables 6.6 & 6.7).

Table 6.7. Steroids and saponins produced through tissue cultures

Plant species	Product formation
Sponins	
• *Aesculus hippocastamum*	Aescin
• *Agave sisalana*	Hecogenin
• *Dioscorea deltoidea*	Diosgenin
• *Glycyrrhiza glabra*	Glycyrrhizin
• *Panax ginseng*	Ginseng saponins
Cardiac glycosides	
• *Digitalis lanata, D. purpurea*	Digoxin, Digitoxin
• *Strophanthus* sps.	Quabain
• *Ureginea maritima*	Proscilariddin
Other steroids	
• *Holarrhena antidysenterica*	Sitosterol, stigmasterol, cholesterol
• *Solanum xanthocarpum*	Solasodine
• *Withania somnifera*	Withanolides

Industrial Production of Secondary Metabolite

It has been possible to establish large-scale production of biomass containing useful secondary metabolites by defining nutritional requirements and ensuring proper environmental conditions for their growth.

Secondary metabolism products compete with primary metabolism for precursors and potential bottlenecks for the former may involve those enzymes linking the primary and secondary pathways, as tryptophan dicarboxylase converting tryptophan to tryptamine in the formation of Indole alkaloids and cyclase enzymes involved in the synthesis of cyclohexanoid monoterpenes from geranyl pyrophosphate.

With cell cultures, as distinct from whole plants, particular genes may be repressed and need to be activated by suitable elicitors (Table 6.5).

Elicitors are the compounds (phytoalexins) produced in normal plants in response to stress; induce the accumulation of secondary products. When cell cultures are subjected to such elicitors, some genes are derepressed, resulting, among other things in the formation of secondary metabolites, which are found in the entire plants.

For the production of secondary metabolites in large amounts, the plant cells should be grown in bioreactor, in the form of suspension culture (continuous), having proper effective aeration, optimum heat, light and pH adjustment necessary for optimum production and isolation of natural substances. Some times callus cultures are also used for secondary metabolite production.

As mentioned earlier, different classes of secondary metabolites are produced by plant cell cultures. Some suspension cultures were reported to produce product at a level, which is equal or higher than plant itself.

Factors affecting the production of secondary metabolites

Media Composition and Environmental Factors

Variations in the relative **hormonal contents** of the growth medium affect the metabolism, for example: **cytokinins** have been found to enhance secondary metabolites accumulation in a number of tissue cultures-Indole alkaloids (C. roseus) condensed tannins (Onobrychis species), Coumarins (Nicotiana species), Rhodozanthin (Ricinus species), Berberine (Thalictrum minus) **mixture of naphthalene, acetic acid** and **kinetin** has affected the concentration of ginkgolides in the cell culture of Ginkgo biloba in medium, as the production medium not only support the level of growth required to obtain an appropriate biomass but also the secondary metabolite. Addition of **IAA and zeatin riboside** has effected the concentration of alkaloid biosynthesis (five-fold increase in alkaloid contents of Cinchona ledgeriana have been reported, on transfering the cell from 2, 4-D, benzyl adenine medium, to a medium containing IAA and Zeatin riboside).

The presence or absence of **phosphate** in a medium, greatly affect the production and accumulation of some secondary products. About 50% increase in anthraquinone accumulation was reported in cell culture of Morinda citrifolia on increasing the phosphate concentration to 5g/l; paradoxically the overall accumulation of tryptamine and Indole alkaloids could occur only by shifting Catharanthus roseus cells to a medium devoid of phosphate concentration. Similar type of sensitivity has been reported in the cell culture of Nicotiana tabacum.

Source of carbon, nitrogen, vitamins and ions have all played significant role in altering the expression of secondary pathways. The addition of sucrose, NO^{3-}, Cu^{2+} or SO_4^{2-} in the culture media above the optimum level have a profound effect on shikonin biosynthesis. Ion concentration and sugar has been reported to have increased the production of Ubiquinone-10 in tabacco cell culture and anthraquinone in *Morinda* suspension cultures.

Precursors

Addition of precursors to the culture medium affect the growth and concentration of secondary metabolites – addition of conferrin (a phenyl propane) to cell suspension culture of Podophyllum hexandrum improved podophyllotoxin production by 128 fold. An increase in quinoline alkaloids has been reported, with the addition of L-tryptophan in the cultures of Cinchona ledgeriana. Cinnamic acid or α-phenylalanine precursors, affect the increase of flavonoids and tropic acid biosynthesis of tropane alkaloids.

Light intensity

The intensity of light and certain wave lengths of light have been reported to have a stimulating effect on the production of some secondary metabolites in various tissue cultures. It has been reported that **blue light** enhances whereas **red light** decreases diosgenin production in *Dioscorea deltoidea* callus cultures.

Selection of Cell-lines

To increase the yield of secondary metabolite a tissue culture should be started from an explant of high yielding variety of plant and capable of yielding high secondary metabolites and capable of accumulating higher levels of the desired metabolites is done. The yield can then be further improved by selection of cell lines originating from individual protoplast, taking advantage of the somaclonal variation. In the case of *Catharanthus roseus* cultures; the dimeric alkaloids vinblastine and vincristine (important anticancer drugs), are produced at the end of a complex biogenetic

pathway in which monomers are first produced. The latter, as corynanthe, strychnos and aspidosperma type alkaloids can all be produced (0.1–1.5%) in culture using Zeink's alkaloid production medium. Different cell cultures derived from any one species of plant may vary enormously in their synthetic capacities, so that in above cases, distinct ajmalicine producing and high serpentine producing stains are possible. Example of other plants for which somaclonal variation has been exploited are *Nicotiana tabacum* and *N. rustica* (Nicotine), *Coptis japonica* (berberine) *Lavandula vera* (biotin) and *Thalictrum minus* (berberine), a strain giving a 350 fold increase in alkaloid production has been reported.

Genotype of Mother Plant

A range of variability in the amount and type of secondary metabolite has been observed in cell cultures raised from different mother plants and sometimes even from the same mother plant. This is because of the difference between the genotype of mother plant and relative productivity of cell cultures.

Cell cultures are known to show gradual loss of productivity and very little is known about the factors that inhibits the secondary metabolite synthesis in tissue cultures or cause of its re-emergence upon re-differentiation.

High yielding lines are rather easily distinguished from low-yielding lines where cell synthesizes visible metabolites e.g. anthocyanins, quinones, betacyanins and carotenoids. For other compounds, quantitative analysis of cellular accumulation patterns of specific metabolites (rosemarinic acid and cinnamyl putrescines) may be determined by micro-spectrophotometry.

Age of Cell Culture

The accumulation of metabolites at any particular instant in the cell culture is the result of a dynamic balance between rate of its biosynthesis and biodegradation, in which a variety of metabolisms are involved. Hence, there is no strict particular time in the cell cycle for harvesting the cells in order to obtain the maximum yield of the secondary compounds. Most of the secondary metabolites accumulate during the late stages of growth in tobacco batch cultures although under same conditions certain metabolites in *Catharanthus cell* cultures accumulate even during the **lag phase**.

Instability of cell line : It is well known that changes in the genetic characteristic of cell occur within a culture so that callus selected for specific biochemical properties may need reselection after a period of time.

Isolation of secondary production : Secondary metabolites synthesis occurs intercellularly. For cultivation and production of active metabolite it is preferable, that the metabolite be excreted into the medium rather than retained within the cells. **For the better excretion, media should be of lower pH**. The biomass then can be separated from the nutrent liquid from which the active constituents are extracted. **Two phase culture system** have been described i.e. a **Silicone product** is added to the fermentation tank to extract the metabolites and in this way the development of culture is not disturbed.

Second method is the use of **media at low pH**, and application of **DMSO sonication** with continuous ultrasound and electrical treatment inducing permeabilisation of cell in culture.

To date over 30 classes of compounds have been produced in appreciable quantities by plant cell cultures, these include *Digitalis* **glycosides, diosgenin-derived steroid hormone precursors, shikonin, rosemarinic acid, opium alkaloids** (codeine and morphine), **ginsenosides, ajmalicine and other indole alkaloids, including vinblastine and vincristine,** and possibly complex mixtures such as rose and jasmine oil. Mitsui Petrochemical Industries of Japan have been producing shikonin, a red coloured phenolic naphthoquinone compound from cell cultures of *Lithospermum erythrorhizon*, which is used as a dye and as an astringent. A West-German Pharmaceutical company is in process of producing Digitalis glycosides by biotransformation in cell cultures. The worldwide research in commercial production of anti-cancer alkaloids of *Catharanthus* shall be soon a practical reality. The factors that limit the success of plant culture include slow growth of plant cells and low accumulation of metabolites. The desired secondary product is often retained within the cells.

List of phytopharmaceuticals of medicinal & industrial importance produced by plant tissue cultures is given in Tables 6.4, 6.8–6.10 (Fig. 6.10).

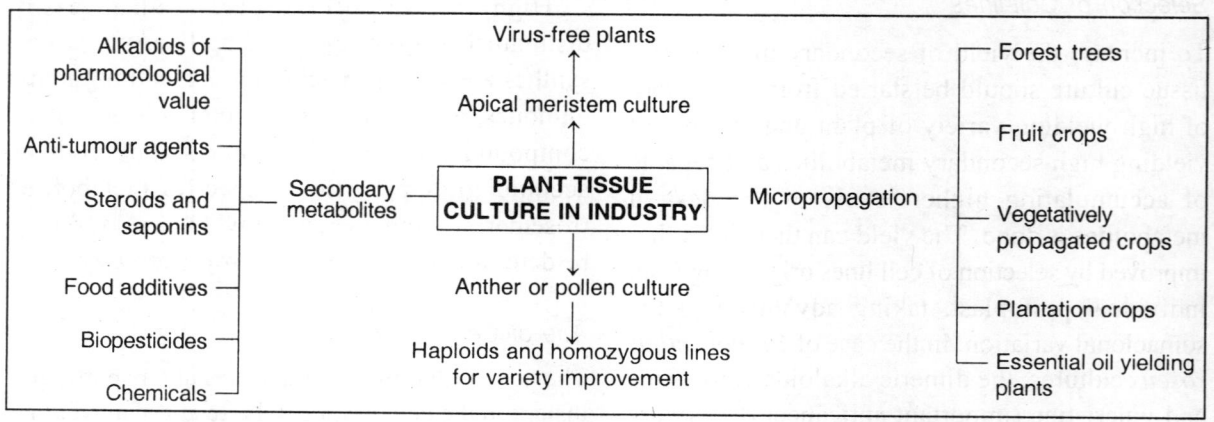

Fig. 6.10. A Schematic Presentation of Role of Plant Tissue Culture in Industry.

Table 6.8. Antitumour agents produced in culture

Plant species	Compound
Baccharis megapotamica	Baccharin
Brucea antidysenterica	Bruceantine
Camptotheca acuminata	Camptotaecine
Catharanthus roseus	Vincristine, vinblastine
Cephalotaxus harringtonia	Harringtonine, homo-harringtonine
Fagara zanthoxyloides	Fagaronine
Heliotropium indicum	Indicine=N-oxide
Maytenus bucchananii, Putterlickia verrucosa	Maytansine
Ochrosia elliptica	Ellipticine, 9-methoxy-E
Podophyllum peltatum, P. hexandrum	Podophyllotoxin
Taxus brevifolia, T. baccata	Taxol
Thalictrum dasycarpum	Thalicarpine
Tripterygium wilfordii	Tripdiolide, tryptolide
Withania somnifera	Withanolide-A, withaferine

Table 6.9. Production of food additives by plant tissue culture

Food activities	Plant species
Colours	
• Anthocyanin	*Dacus carota*
• Anthocyanin	*Euphorbia milli*
• Anthocyanin	*Vitis vinifera*
• Betalaines	*Beta vulgaris*
• Crocin, crocetin	*Crocus sativus*
Flavours	
• Onion flavour	*Allium cepa*
• Capsicum, capsaicin	*Capsicum annuum*
Frutescens	
• Safranal	*Crocus sativus*
• Vanilla, vanillin	*Vanilla planifolia*
Sweetner	
• Stevioside	*Stevia rebaudiana*
• Thaumatin	*Thaumatococcus danielli*

Table 6.10. Insecticides of plant origin

Plant species	Insecticides
Azadirachta indica	Azadirachtin
Derris elliptica, Tephrosis vogelii, Lonchocarpus utilis	Rotenoids
Chrysanthemum cinerariaefolium, Tagetes erecta	Pyrethrins
Nicotiana rustica, N. tabacum	Nicotine
Quassia amara	Quassin

Biochemical Conversion (Biotransformation)

The conversion of small part of a chemical molecule by means of biological systems is termed biotransformation. It is a process in which the substrate can be modified. For example, *Digitalis lanata* cell cultures have a ability to effect hydroxylation, acetylation, glycosylation etc. It is reported that *D. lanata* strain 291 can convert β-methyl digitoxin into β-methyl digoxin. Cell suspension culture of *Strophanthus gratus* affects various biochemical conversions of digitoxigenin.

Monoterpene bioconversions are reported with mentha cell culture. It can convert (–) menthone to (+) neomenthol and pulegone to isomenthone.

Podophyllum peltatum in semi-continuous culture can produce anticancer drugs by biotransformation of synthetic dibenzyl butanolides to lignans suitable for conversion to etoposide.

In some tissue culture stereospecific biotransformation is also reported, which is important for the isolation of optically active compound from racemic mixture. Example of cell culture of *Nicotiana tabacum* selectively hydrolyse R-configurational form of monoterpenes like bornyl acetate and isobornyl acetate.

Apart from the above mentioned biochemical conversions many other, like saponifications, esterification, epoxidation, oxidation, methylation and isomerization are also reported.

Clonal Propagation (Micropropagation)

Clonal propagation (micropropagation) is the technique to produce entire plant from single individual by asexual reproduction, constitute a clone. This fact can be commercially utilized to produce high yielding crops of the desirable characters in a short period of time, which otherwise show variation when grown using seeds. For example, *Foeniculum vulgare* (fennel) shows wide variations in the yield and composition of the volatile oil and by this technique it has been reported to have uniform clones of fennel with narrow variation in the volatile oil composition, in comparison to the normal cultivation.

Somaclonal Variation

In clonal propagation, clones are produced from tissue culture with uniform characters but few clones may show variations among the population of clones, which were not present in the parent cells. This formation of variant clones from cultured tissue is called as **Somaclonal variations**. Variants are of two types:

Desirable Variants & Undesirable Variants

Desirable variants can be used for the improvement of crops. The clone showing high productivity can be used for commercial purposes.

Immobilization of Plant Cells

The immobilization of plant cell or enzymes has increased the utility of plant cell biotechnology for production of **pharmaceuticals**. The plant cells can be immobilized by using matrices such as alginates, polyacrylamides, agarose and polyurethane fibres. The immobilized plant cells can be utilized in the same way as immobilized enzymes to effect different reactions.

Immobilized cell systems may be used for bioconversions such as (–)**codeinone to (–)codeinine and digitoxin** to **digoxin** or for synthesis from added precursors, e.g. production of ajmalicine from tryptamine and secologanin. The suspension cultures of *Anisodus tanguticus* have been reported to convert hyoscyamine to anisodamine in good quantity. Subsequently, the cultures convert anisodamine into scopolamine. The biotransformation reactions such as glycosylations, hydroxylation, acetylation, demethylation etc, have been successfully attempted in immobilized cell systems. The hydroxylation or glycosylation of cardiac glycosides in cultures of *Digitalis lanata* and *Daucus carota* have also been reported.

Immobilized plant cells can be used for tracing the biosynthetic pathways of secondary metabolites and also can be used for carrying out biotransformation or biochemical reactions.

Chapter 7

Chemotaxonomy of Medicinal Plants

INTRODUCTION

The subject of chemotaxonomy is concerned with the application of chemical characters in relation to taxonomy. This rapidly expanding discipline of plant taxonomy has been variously called as chemotaxonomy, chemosystematics, biochemical systematic or comparative phytochemistry.

TAXONOMY

It is a branch of science, which deals with the laws governing the classification of plants. It contributes to the orderly arrangement and study of plants and to systematisation of our knowledge about the plants.

The classification of plants may be tabulated as:

Division	(Thallophyta, Bryophyta, Pteridophyta or Embryophyta, as given by Engler and Prantl) (Table 7.1).
Subdivision	Gymnospermae and angiospermae
Class	Monocotyledonae and dicotyledonae.
Subclass	Archichlamydeae
Order	Rosales, generally ending - ales
Suborder	Rosineae, generally ending with - Ineae
Family	Rosaceae, generally ending - aceae (Compositae, Graminae and Labiatae exception).
Subfamily	Rosoideae, generally ending with - oideae
Tribe	Roseae generally ending with - eae
Sub-tribe	Rosinae generally ending with - inae
Genus	Rosa
Species	Rosa indica

Categories below the rank of species in descending order are as follow:

Sub-species, Varieties, Sub-varieties, Forma.

The major taxonomic categories used in taxonomy, in the ascending order are, species, genus, family, order, class and division.

The earlier systems of classification were of the following categories.

1. Artificial systems
2. Natural systems
3. Phylogenetic systems

Artificial Systems

These systems of classification were artificial and since very little information was available about the plants, these systems were based on one or a few characters and the system remained dominant from 300 BC to about 1830. The artificial systems propounded by early botanist were based on habit (trees, shrubs, herbs etc.) and the **Carolus Linnaeus's** (1707-1778) sexual system based on floral characters (particularly the number of stamens and pistils/carpels).

Natural Systems

The systems that followed were based on natural

Table 7.1. Plants can be arranged in six chief groups

I Algae (sea weeds)	Mostly photosynthetic aquatic plants; Thallus unicellular to multicellular; Include several taxonomic divisions such as cyanophyta, chlorophyta, rhodophyta and phaeophyta
II Fungi (slime molds, molds, mushrooms, toac-stools and lichens)	Mainly terrestial; non-photosynthetic (except in lichens in which an Ascomycete is combined with a blue or green algea); Thallus often a mycellium formed by so called hyphae. Include Myxophyta, Fungi (Phycomycetes. Ascomycetes, and Basidomycetes) and lichens.
III Bryophyta (mosses and moss allies)	Green non vascular terrestrial plants. Include the two classes Hepaticae (liverworts) and Musci (true mosses)
IV Pteridophyta (Ferns and fern allies or vascular cryptogams)	Green vascular land plants include lycopsida (club mosses), Psilotopsida, Articulatae (horsetails) and Filices (true ferns)
V Gymnospermae	Green, vascular, woody, terrestrial plants, dispersal by seeds. Include cyacadopsida, coniferopsida, taxopsida, and chlamydospermae (Ephedra, Gnetum, Welwitschia)
VI Angiospermae (flowering plants)	Green vascular mainly terrestrial plants, herbs, shrubs and trees; dispersal by fruits or by seeds. Include the bulk of modern plants species which are grouped in two classes i.e. Dicotyledons and Monocotyledons.

affinities. The natural systems remained dominant before the idea of evolution was accepted. The most important and the last of these systems was **Bentham and Hooker's System** of classification (1862-1883), according to them the seed plants were classified into **Dicotyledons, Gymnosperms** and **Monocotyledons**. But gymnosperms are a distinct group from the angiosperms and their placement between the dicotyledons and monocotyledons is inconsistent as per the current knowledge of this group.

Bentham and Hooker's System

Flowering plants are divided into dicotyledons and monocotyledons (number of cotyledon in seeds).

A. Dicotyledons

Dicotyledons (having two cotyledons), plants are herbaceous or woody; Stem well developed in comparison with the leaves; vascular bundles forming a ring in cross section of stem; secondary thickening present; leaves with net venation, petiolate; floral parts in five or fours.

1. Polypetalae (Petal present: separate)

Series I : Thalamiflorae - Flowers hypogynous ovary superior. This include six orders:

(i) Ranales

(ii) Parietales

(iii) Polygalineae

(iv) Caryophyllineae

(v) Guttiferales

(vi) Malvales

Series II : Disciflorae - Flowers hypogynous with conspicuous nectiferous disc, surrounds the base of the superior ovary. It contains four orders:

(i) Geraniales

(ii) Olacales

(iii) Celastrales

(iv) Sapindales

Series III : Calyciflorae - Flowers perigynous or epigynous; ovary superior or inferior. It contains five orders:

(i) Rosales

(ii) Myrtales

(iii) Passiflorales

(iv) Ficoidales

(v) Umbellales

2. Gamopetalae (Petals present: united)

Series I : Inferae - Ovary inferior. It contains three orders:

(i) Rubiales

(ii) Asterales

(iii) Campanales

Series II : Heteromerae - Ovary superior, stamens as many as the corolla lobes or twice, carpels more than two. The three orders are:

(i) Ericales

(ii) Primulales

(iii) Ebenales

Series III : Bicarpellatae - Ovary superior, stamens as many as the corolla lobes or fewer, carpels usually two. It has the following four orders:

(i) Gentianales

(ii) Polemoniales

(iii) Personales

(iv) Lamiales

3. Monochlamydeae (Petals absent)

Series I : Curvembryae (embryo curved round the endosperm, ovule usually one). These include families such as Chenopodiaceae, Amaranthaceae and Polygonaceae.

Series II : Multiovulatae acquaticae (aquatics with numerous ovules). It includes families such as Podostemaceae.

Series III : Multiovulatae terrestris (terrestrials plants with numerous ovules). They include families such as Nepenthaceae and Aristolochiaceae.

Series IV : Microembryeae (embryo very small in copious endosperm). They include families such as Piperaceae and Chloranthaceae.

Series V : Daphnales (ovary usually with one carpel and single ovule). They include families such as Lauraceae and Proteaceae.

Series VI : Achlamydosporeae (ovary usually inferior, unilocular and one to three ovuled). They include families such as Santalaceae and Loranthaceae.

Series VII : Unisexuales (flowers unisexual). They include families such as Euphorbiaceae and Urticaceae.

Series VIII : Ordines anomali. The families of uncertain relationship (Salicinae, Empetraceae and Ceratophyllaceae) were placed here.

B. Gymnospermae

They include Gnetaceae, Coniferae and Cycadaceae.

C. Monocotyledons

As the name indicate, monocotyledons have an embryo with one cotyledon. Many members are herbs, usually with parallel veined leaves. The stele has scattered closed vascular bundles. The flowers are usually trimerous.

Series I : Microspermae (ovary inferior, seeds very small). They include families such as Orchidaceae and Burmanniaceae.

Series II : Epigynae (ovary usually inferior, seeds large). They include families such as Iridaceae and Amaryllidaceae.

Series III : Coronarieae (perianth petaloid, ovary superior). They include families such as Liliaceae and Commelinaceae.

Series IV : Calycinae (perianth sepaloid, ovary superior). They include families such as Juncaceae and Palmae.

Series V : Nudiflorae (perianth mostly lacking, ovary superior). They include families such as Typhaceae and Pandanaceae.

Series VI : Apocarpeae (carpels free). They include families such as Alismaceae and Najadaceae.

Series VII : Glumaceae (perianth small, scale like or chaffy). They include families such as Cyperaceae and Gramineae.

Phylogenetic System

In this system of plant taxonomy genetic and phylogenetical relationship was reflected.

The most widely used systems of classification of the phylogenetic period are those of Engler (1886-1892) and Hutchinson (1926, 1934, 1948, 1959, 1969, 1973) and two modern systems Takhtajan (1969, 1980) and Cronquist (1969, 1981).

Engler's system

Like Bentham and Hooker, Engler accepts the primary division of the flowering plants into **Dicotyledons** and **Monocotyledons**. The dicotyledons are further divided into two division The **Archichlamydeae** and **Sympetalae**.

The **Archichlamydeae** are further divided into **37 orders** and about **226 families** and the sympetalae into **11 orders** and about **63 families** (Table 7.2).

Engler's system became popular because it was applied by him and his associates in their numerous publications to the whole plant kingdom, at all levels of the taxonomic hierarchy. It thus provided a universal reference system and as such became standard in Europe and North America.

CHEMOTAXONOMY

The application of chemistry to systematics is chemotaxonomy or chemical taxonomy.

Natural systems of classification should be based on the analysis and harmonization of evidence from all organs, tissues and parts. The external morphological study alone is not adequate and other branches of study are of considerable value in proper assessment of the systematic status of a taxon and its phylogeny. Hence the contribution to systematic from any branch of botany, vegetative anatomy, floral anatomy, palynology, embryology and cytology have played a significant role in plant taxonomy. The taxonomic contributions of cytogenetics and **chemotaxonomy** have made an equally great help to support the ideas of classification and phylogeny.

The concept that plant can be classified on the basis of their chemical characters is not new and it has a long been of practical value e.g. aroma from the crushed leaves and fruits (which is due to the presence of characteristic essential oils) of the Apiaceae (Umbelliferae) and Lamiaceae are the characteristic points for the identification of the members of these two families and the two subfamilies of the Asteraceae; the **Tubiflorae** (latex vessels are absent) and **Liguliflorae** (latex vessels are present) are distinguished on the basis of presence and absence of latex respectively (The both subfamily belong to companulales order). As compared to morphological characters, chemical constituents are more definable and of more fundamental significance for the plant taxonomy.

The earliest attempts to correlate chemistry with the phylogenetic level of development was that of **Abbott** (1886), who reported **saponin** containing plants occupied the middle level of Hackel's scheme of plant evolution. **Greshof** (1909) suggested that chemical characters should be included in natural classification. He was also of the opinion that every description of a new genus or species should include a short chemical description of that taxon.

The first successful attempt to combine chemical and morphological evidence in the study of a

Table 7.2. Engler's system of classification

Orders	Families
(A) MONOCOTYLEDONS	
Perianth absent or rudimentary	(*Gramineae*)
Perianth present	(*Liliaceae*)
(B) DICOTYLEDONS	
Petals absent or if present separate (I. *Archichlamydeae*)	
Casuarinales	Casuarinaceae
Juglandales	Myricaceae, Juglandaceae
Salicales	Salicaceae
Fagales	Betulaceae, Fagaceae
Urticales	Ulmaceae, Moraceae (including Cannabinaceae) and Urticaceae
Proteales	Proteaceae
Santalales	Olacaceae, Santalaceae, Loranthaceae, Balanophoraceae
Polygonales	Polygonaceae
Centrospermae	Phytolaccaceae, Nyctaginaceae, Molluginaceae, Aizoaceae, Protulaceae,
	Caryophyllaceae, Chenopodiaceae, Amaranthaceae
Cactales	Cactaceae
Magnoliales	Magnoliaceae, Winteraceae, Annonaceae, Eupomatiaceae, Myristicaceae, Cancellaceae, Schisandraceae,
	Illiciaceae, Monimiaceae, Calycanthaceae, Lauraceae, Hernandiaceae
Ranunculales	Ranunculaceae, Berberidaceae, Menispermaceae, Nymphaeaceae
Piperales	Piperaceae, Chloranthaceae
Aristolociales	Aristolochiaceae
Guttiferales	Paeoniaceae, Dipterocarpaceae, Theaceae, Guttiferae, Ancistrocladaceae
Sarraceniales	Sarraceniaceae, Nepenthaceae, Droseraceae
Papaverales	Papveraceae (including Fumariaceae), Capparaceae, Cruciferae, Resedaceae
Rosales	Hamamelidaceae, Crassulaceae, Saxifragaceae, Pittosporaceae, Rosaceae,
	Leguminosae, Krameriaceae
Geraniales	Geraniaceae, Zygophyllaceae, Linaceae, Erythroxylaceae, Euphorbiaceae, Daphniphyllaceae
Rutales	Rutaceae, Cneoraceae, Simaroubaceae, Burseraceae, Meliaceae, Malpighiaceae, Vochysiaceae,
	Polygalaceae
Sapindales	Anacardiaceae, Aceraceae, Sapindaceae, Hippocastanaceae, Melianthaceae
Celastrales	Aquifoliaceae, Celastraceae, Buxaceae, Icacinaceae
Rhamnales	Rhamnaceae, Vitaceae
Malvales	Elaeocarpaceae, Tiliaceae, Malvaceae, Bombacaceae, Sterculiaceae
Thymelaeales	Thymelaeceae, Elaeagnaceae
Violales	Flacourtiaceae, Violaceae, Turneraceae, Passifloraceae, Cistaceae,
	Bixaceae, Tamaricaceae, Caricaceae, Datiscaceae, Begoniaceae
Cucurbitales	Cucurbitaceae
Myrtiflorae	Lythraceae, Trapaceae, Myrtaceae, Sonneratiaceae, Punicaceae, Lecythidaceae, Rhizophoraceae,
	Combretaceae, Onagraceae
Umbelliflorae	Alangiaceae, Cornaceae, Garryaceae, Araliaceae, Umbelliferae
Petals united (II. *Sympetalae*)	
Ericales	Ericaceae
Primulales	Myrsinaceae, Primulaceae
Plumbaginales	Plumbaginaceae
Ebenales	Sapotaceae, Ebenaceae, Styracaceae
Oleales	Oleaceae
Gentianales	Loganiaceae, Gentianaceae, Menyanthaceae, Apocynaceae, Asclepiadaceae, Rubiaceae
Tubiflorae	Polemoniaceae, Convolvulaceae, Boraginaceae, Verbenaceae, Labiatae, Solanaceae, Scrophulariaceae,
	Globulariaeae, Bignoniaceae, Acanthaceae,
	Pedaliaceae, Gesneriaceae, Orobanchaceae, Myoporaceae
Plantaginales	Plantaginaceae
Dipsacales	Caprifoliaceae, Valerianaceae, Dipsacaceae
Campanulales	Campanulaceae (including Lobeliaceae), Compositae

single genus was the work of **Baker & Smith** (1920) on the essential oils of *Eucalyptus*. They suggested that the level of relationship should be reflected in chemical similarities (primitive plants are also chemically primitive). According to the morphological and chemical data collected on 176 *Eucalyptus* species, they divided the genus into three groups differing in both morphological structure and chemical constituents. They concluded that primitive species are those which have feather-veined leaves and high **Pinene** content in their essential oils, while more advanced types have intermediate venation and contain **Pinene & Cineole**. According to their system, the most advanced taxa show butterfly wing venation and contain oils with **Phellandrene**, **Piperitone and geranyl acetate**. The work of Baker and Smith was the first comprehensive chemotaxonomic-morphological study of a complex genus and in general their conclusions have been a significant contribution to the taxonomy of *Eucalyptus* (Fig. 7.1).

Phytoconstituents Useful in Plant Taxonomy

The occurrence and distribution of various types of chemical constituents present in plants; form the taxonomic evidence. However all kinds of chemical substances do not reveal information useful to the taxonomist.

Primary metabolites (constituents) are the parts of vital metabolic pathways and most of them are of universal occurrence, or at least occur in a very wide range of plants. They include proteins, nucleic acids, chlorophyll and polysaccharides e.g. Aconitic acid (first isolated from *Aconitum*) or citric acid (from *Citrus*), participate in the Kreb's (tricarboxylic acid) cycle and are present in all aerobic organisms; the presence or absence of such compounds is therefore not of much systematic value. The same is true with the amino acids which are known to be constituents of plant proteins or any of the sugar which is a part of the photosynthetic carbon cycle and so on.

In some cases, however, the **quantities of such metabolites vary considerably between taxa** and this in itself can be taxonomically useful. For example, taxa in which universally occurring substances were first detected (such as the two above) often possess particularly large quantities of the molecules concerned well above the amounts which participate in the essential metabolic pathways often as food-storage materials. Sometimes such compounds are stored in a different form other than that in which they are metabolized, e.g. **Sedoheptulose**, a sugar constituting the carbohydrate food reserve of the genus *Sedum*, which as sedoheptulose diphosphate is a part of the photosynthetic carbon cycle.

The development of biochemical methods for comparing the amino acid sequences of homologous proteins from different taxa has provided a powerful tool for systematic studies.

Secondary metabolites (or secondary plant constituents) perform non-vital (or at least non universally vital) functions and are therefore less widespread in plants. This restricted occurrence

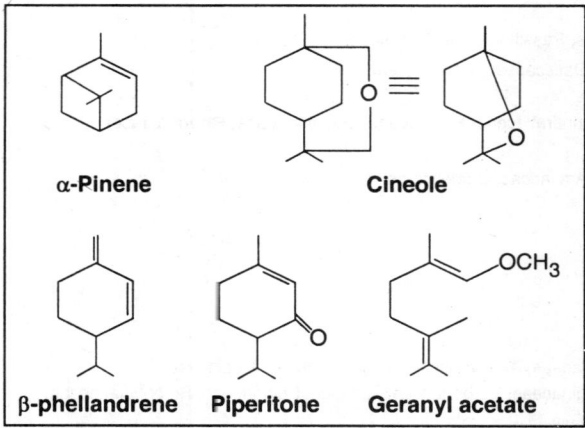

α-Pinene   Cineole

β-phellandrene   Piperitone   Geranyl acetate

Fig. 7.1. Chemical Constituents present in three groups of Eucalyptus species.

Table 7.3. Phytoconstituents useful in plant taxonomy

Compound grouping	Comments on botanical distribution
Terpenoids	Widely distributed
Monoterpenes	Widely distributed, of taxonomic value primarily below the generic level
Sesquiterpenoids	Rather wide distribution, but particularly important and useful in the taxonomy of the Compositae
Asperulosides and Aucubins (Iridoid glycosides)	Rubiaceae, Scrophulariaceae, and related families, Plantaginaceae, Cornaceae, and others
Ranunculins	Found only in the Ranunculaceae
Cyanogenetic compounds	Ranunculaceae and other families
Polyalcohols	Widely distributed but have taxonomic potential
Sulfur compounds	A chemically diverse grouping of compounds which in their various forms are widely distributed, the isothiocyanate-producing glycosides are characteristic of families in the Rhoeadales
Amino acids	Liliaceae and related (non-protein) familes, Leguminosae (particularly Papilionatae, and other groups)
Alkaloids	a chemically and biosynthetically diverse group of compounds rarely found in the lower vascular plants and irregularly distributed among the angiosperms, highly useful in the taxonomy of some groups.
Betacyanins and betaxanthins	Centrospermae ("Betanales")
Alkanes (fatty acids and waxes)	Widely distributed, possibly of use in classification below the genus level, and of use in organic geochemistry
Fatty acid epoxides	Found in seven families
Acetylenes	Distributed in the basidiomycetes and at least 13 angiosperm families, of particular use in the link between the Compositae and the Umbelliflorae
Assorted compounds	Ferns
Diterpenes	Rather wide distribution in the seed plants, taxonomicaly useful in specific groups such as the conifers
Triterpenes	Wide distribution in living organisms, taxonomically useful in several angiosperm families such as the Cucurbitaceae, and in the fungi
Carotenoids	The universally distributed photosynthetic carotenoids useful in algae classification; the nonphotosynthetic carotenoids in fruits of possible limited value as taxonomic markers in the angiosperms
Flavonoids	Very large number of diverse compounds found throughout the vascular plants and in nearly, if not all, angiosperms; of great taxonomic value below the genus level and of possible use in the classification of higher categories.
Lignins and Lignans	Useful in the classiciation of higher categories
Quinones	Widely distributed among living organisms, but compounds of this type with limited distribution have potential value in the classification of number of angiosperm families
Polysaccharides	Universally distribued, probably useful in the classification of higher categories particularly among the algae, comparative data mostly lacking
Plant glycosides	Great chemical variation in the non-sugar portion of the molecule, varyingly of great usefulness in taxonomy
Assorted compounds	Lichens
Wide range of chemical approaches	Umbelliferae
Wide range of chemical approaches	Leguminosae

among plants renders them valuable as taxonomic information. The most well-known groups of constituent which have been utilized in this way include **Carbohydrates (rare sugars), glycosides, alkaloids, phenolics comp. (flavonoids), glucosinolates, amino acids, terpenoids, oils and waxes**.

Secondary plant products are largely waste substances, food stores, pigments, poisons, scents, structural units or water repellents etc. In many cases they obviously do have an essential function but of a general nature so that the precise molecular configuration of the compound is not vital. Thus a yellow pigment with absorption maximum at 477 nm (which presumably defines its function) might be a Betalin or Anthocyanin and a poison might be an alkaloid or a glycoside (Table 7.3).

Principles of Chemotaxonomy

The principle of "chemical taxonomy" consists of the **investigation of the distribution of chemical compounds**, or groups of biosynthetically related compounds in **series of related or supposedly related plants**.

Chemical contributions to the classification of plants are based on their chemical constituents, i.e. on their **molecular characteristics"**. These characteristics are **genetically controlled** and have the advantage over morphological ones, that they can be very exactly described in terms of definite structural and configurational chemical formula. In this way it helps in understanding of their biosynthesis, which is a matter of fundamental systemic importance.

This can be due to many factors, which are not necessarily genetic, but include other factors like the organ analysed, the stage of development of plant and the particular plant population analysed.

The greatest virtue of the chemical method is

that it is entirely independent of the classical biological methods. It will therefore be possible for organic chemist not only to assist the botanist but also to check their conclusion and to point out problems, which may occur to them.

When considering chemosystematics and plant evolution it is the **biosynthetic pathway** which is important as the same type of metabolite can be the product of two quite different pathways e.g. an alkaloid with tetrahydroprotoberberine skeleton, biogenetically different from Canadine (= tetrahydroberberine) a tetrahydroprotoberberine alkaloid (member of the benzylisoquinoline family of alkaloid) and desacetylipocoside; (a secoiridoid isoquinoline alkaloid glucoside). **The enzyme catalysing metabolic reactions are of great importance than the product of the reactions as evolution depends on changes in enzyme characteristics.** The plants, which are similar morphologically and chemically, should have the same ancestor. This is not always true, however, due to convergent parallel evolution. For instance both *Crotalaria* (Leguminosae) and *Senecio* (Compositae) produce pyrrolizidine alkaloids by similar pathways, but these genera are not related morphologically (Fig. 7.2).

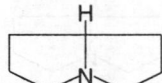

Fig. 7.2. Pyrrolizidine.

It is reported that when such criteria are applied to the results of chemical surveys obtained so far, it is found that most fall far short of these ideals. However rapid progress in these fields can be expected in the near future owing to the availability of powerful analytical methods. For example chromatographic, electrophoretic, counter current distribution technique and availability of highly efficient columns for fractional distillation of mixtures of volatile oils and the other modern instrumental technology of UV, IR, NMR and X-ray crystallography.

Many substances such as proteinogenic amino acids, some fatty acids and sugars occur in almost all plants and are therefore of little or no taxonomic interest. Compounds found only in one single species are also taxonomically useless if not biosynthetically related to plant constituents of intermediate distribution. It is among the later substances that we may expect to find compounds of the highest taxonomic value.

Identical compounds are often found in quite un-related plants and this has frequently puzzled chemists interested in the use of chemical characteristics in plant classification. This phenomenon is not as serious as it seems to be. It is easy to conceive that during evolution, conditions for the production of some compounds or group of biosynthetically related substances have been developed separately in many plants. However, it is highly improbable that totally unrelated plants would be in possession of enzymatic prerequisites for synthesizing several chemically unrelated compounds of intermediate distribution (Fig. 7.3).

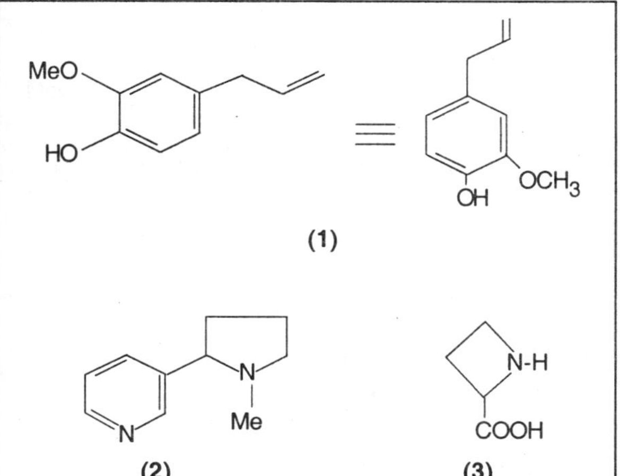

Different plants sometimes contain secondary constituents belonging to different classes of compounds but biosynthetically appear to be analogous (Fig. 7.4). Such plants probably having similar enzymes but the production of secondary chemical constituents may indicate relationship between the relevant plants. Sometimes identical compounds are found in quite unrelated plants.

Moreover "chemical divergence" caused by mutation, can also give rise to large differences in the production of secondary chemical constituents, such chemically abnormal plants creates great difficulties to chemotaxonomist.

One of the difficulties encountered in determining the chemical features of a plant species, is the variations found in contents of secondary metabolites. Chemotaxonomic studies should therefore include the investigation of the pattern of compounds occurring in plants and preferentially in all the various individual parts of plant such as the bark, wood, leaves, roots, cuticles and seeds. The chemical constituents generally vary considerably from one organ to another. Such integrated investigations are necessary in order to obtain really convincing evidence for the relationship or non-relationship of plants. It is always dangerous to draw taxonomic conclusion from the occurrence or non-occurrence of a single compound in a single part of a plant. Although compounds of considerable taxonomic value may be found in any part of a plant, it is reasonable to assume that the most important ones occur in phylogenetically old, conservative, little specialized organs. Thus, before any important conclusions are drawn about the presence or absence of a particular compound adequate sampling of a large

Fig. 7.3. Example of Identical Compounds found in quite un-related plants.

(1) Eugenol; Stored here and there in essential oils or as a glycoside wide spread in trace amounts; **(2)** Nicotine and Nornicotine stored in taxa of Solanaceae and Compositae; **(3)** Azetidine-2-carboxylic acid; stored as defensive compound by part of Liliaceae (green parts) and some Leguminosae - Caeselpinloideae (seeds; seedlings).

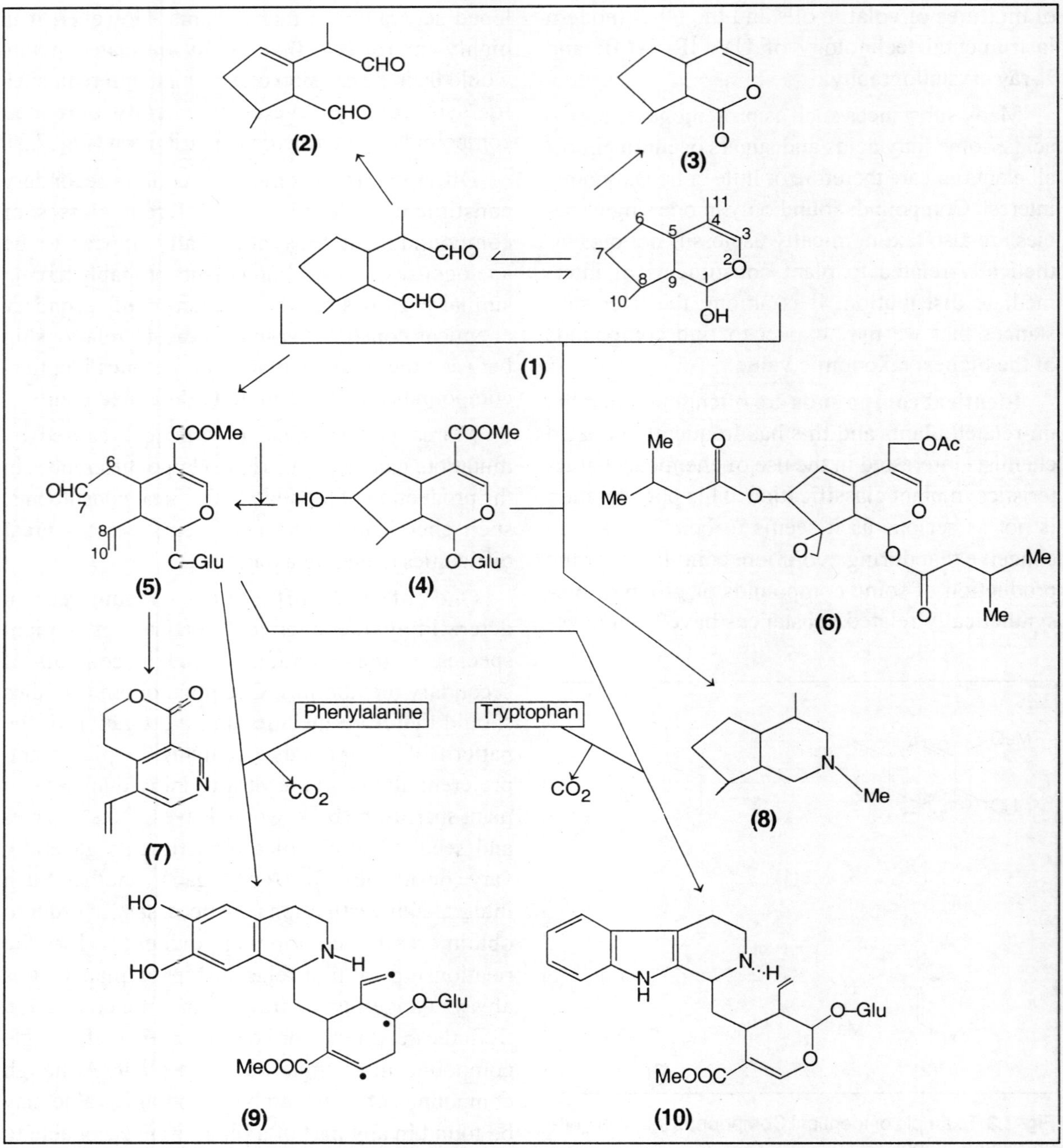

Fig. 7.4. The Biogenetically homologous, but structurally highly diverse class of iridoid compounds.

(1-3) Steam-volatile compounds, iridodial, dehydroiridodial and nepetalactone; (4) iridoid glycosides, loganin and 8-epiloganin; (5) a secoiridoid glucoside, secologanin; (6) an ester iridoid, valtratum; (7) a secoiridoid pyridine alkaloid, gentianine; (8) an iridoid piperidine alkaloid, skytanthine; (9) a secoiridoid isoquinoline alkaloid glucoside, desacetylipecoside; (10) a secoiridoid indolic alkaloid, strictosidine; precursor of many so-called complex indole alkaloids.

number of members of the species at different stages of development and growing in different environments should be made. Also, when applying analytical results to systematics all species in a genus should be investigated.

The early classification of plants was artificial and designed to serve practical purposes. It is thus important when classifying plants from biochemical data to consider all secondary metabolites and not just one class, as often have been done in the past. After Darwin, "Natural systems" founded on real relationship were proposed but even today one is still unable to construct a true **"phylogenetic" system**. The main reason for this is that vast majority of extinct species are unknown. **The natural systems are essentially based on comparative studies of the genetically controlled morphological and anatomical** (i.e. supermolecular) **characteristics of plants**. Some of these characters are of a very **general nature** and serve for the separation of **large systemic categories such as divisions, class and orders.** Others are less general but suitable for the **delimitation of smaller** groups of plants; **families, genera, subgenera** etc. The classification of plants thus rests upon very thorough considerations of many different biological characteristics.

Evolution depends upon a combination of internal and external factors such as mutation, recombination of genic differences and selection. During evolution it may happen that unrelated group of plants give rise to morphologically similar ones. (**Convergence or Parallel Development**). Conversely, related plants may give rise to very dissimilar descendants (**"divergence"**). Such phenomena cause considerable taxonomic difficulties.

The special value of the chemotaxonomic approach can be seen when chemical characters correlate well with data obtainable from other sources. To take just one example, the fact that there is chemical discontinuity among the families of the order **Rhoeadales** as defined by Wettstein (1935) has been used by modern taxonomists as a reason for dividing this assemblage of six or seven families into two orders, the **Capparales** and the **Papaverales**. Other reasons for making this split lie in the differences in anatomy (presence or absence of latex system) and in morphology (position of stamens). This new division has also been suggested by recent serological and palynological studies of the relevant families.

It should be pointed out in this case that there are many morphological similarities between the separated groups; for example common floral features (e.g. perfect hypogynous flowers, compound ovaries with parietal placentation). Thus, the additional chemical evidence may have been crucially decisive in the acceptance of this newer grouping. In this instance, the chemical data is unusually good in the sense that relatively wide chemical surveys have been conducted in the relevant families. It is reported that 300 crucifer species have been examined for glucosinolates with positive results and all the papaveraceae studied have shown to have complex mixture of alkaloids in their tissues.

Role of Secondary Metabolites in Chemotaxonomy of Medicinal Plants

Carbohydrates in Chemotaxonomy (Fig. 7.5)

Carbohydrates are universal constituents of living organisms and are widely spread in the plants and thus having little taxonomic significance but some rare sugars (**6-deoxyhexose, 2,6-dideoxyhexoses, Gentiobiose and gentianose, Polyols, Cyclitols, Polysaccharides**) have taxonomic significance.

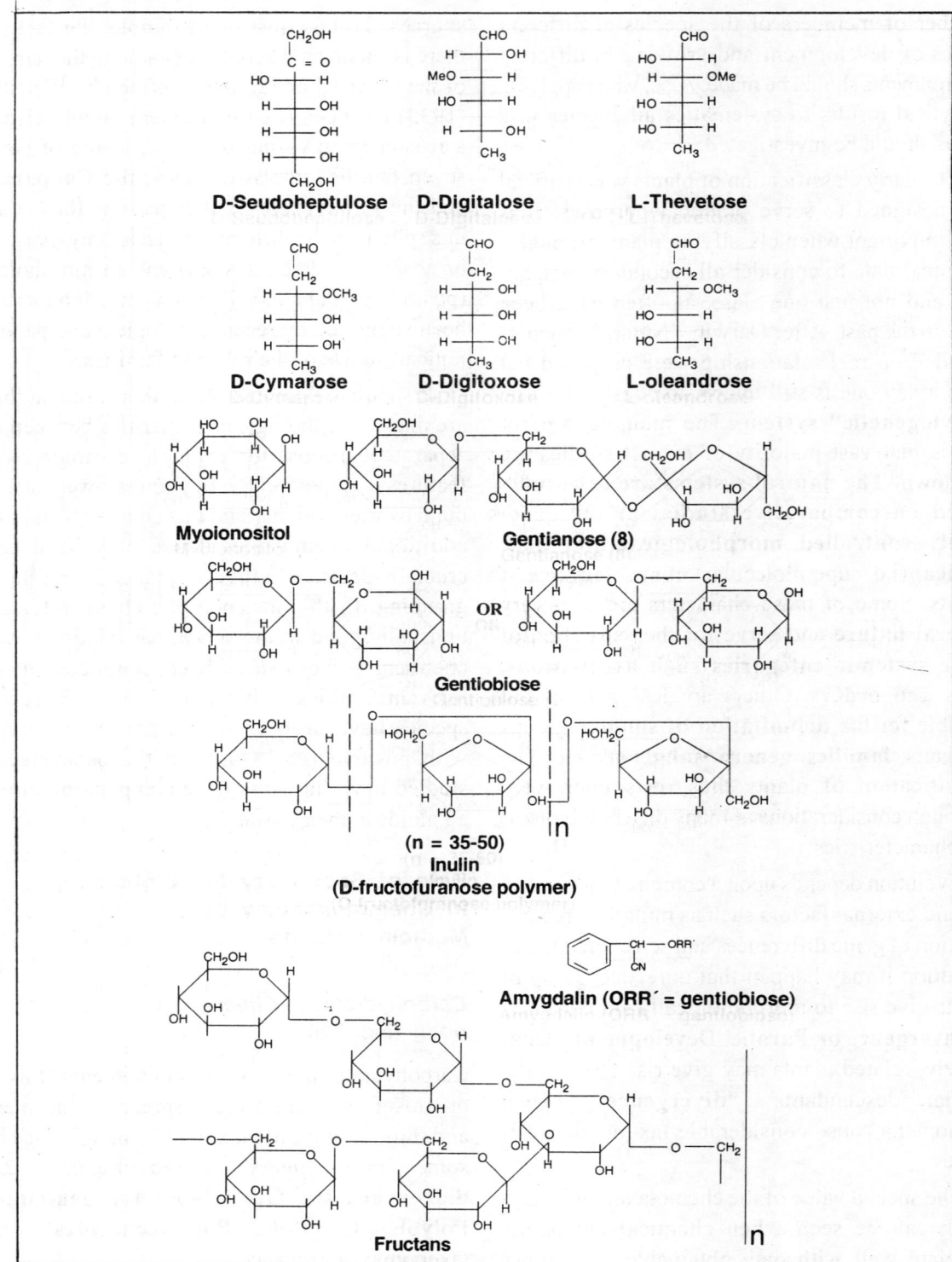

Fig. 7.5. Carbohydrate in Chemotaxonomy.

(i) **6-deoxyhexose** (occurs as methyl ethers) have restricted distribution and thus presence and absence can be utilized to understand the phylogenetic relationship. For example **L-thevetose** (=6-deoxy-3-O-methyl-L-glucose) and **D-digitalose** (=6-dexoy-3-O-methyl-D-galactose) are specific to cardiotonic glycosides.

(ii) **2,6-dideoxyhexoses** are often methylated and specific to cardiac glycosides, including **D-digitoxose** (=2,6-dideoxy-D-allose), **L-oleandrose** (=2,6-dideoxy-3-O-methyl-L-mannose) and **D-cymarose** (=2,6-dideoxy-3-O-methyl-D-allose). Cardenolides containing such sugars (deoxymethylpentose) are particularly abundant in the related **Apocynaceae** and **Asclepiadaceae**, although they appear in the groups of unrelated families.

(iii) **Gentiobiose and gentianose** (uncommon sugars) are present in **amygdalin** (cyanogenic glycoside) characteristic of the Rosaceae family and Gentiana genus family Gentianaceae, respectively.

(iv) *Polyols* : Among the **monosaccharide derivatives (D-sorbitol, D-mannitol and meso-xylitol)** D-sorbitol occurs naturally in the fruits of various Rosaceae. The presence and absence of this sugar alcohol in the Rosaceae can be utilized to identify the subfamilies. It is reported that the sorbitol is present in all species belonging to **Spiraeoideae, Pomoideae and Prunoideae** but in species (Ulmaria) belonging to Rosoideae it is absent and the absence of this chemotaxonomic marker confirms the removal of this genus (on morphological grounds) from Spiraeoideae to Rosoideae. Similarly the presence of sorbitol in the three genera *Rhodotypos*, *Kerria* and *Neviusia*, confirm their relationship with Spiraeoideae rather than to Rosoideae.

(v) *Cyclitols* : **Cyclohexanehexol** or **inositol** plays a fundamental biological role and L-ionositol occurs in several unrelated members of the large compositae family hence it is not of much significance from chemotaxonomic point of view but the presence of rare cyclitol, **L-leucanthemitol and L-viburnitol** are the characteristic of the compositae tribe.

(vi) *Polysaccharides* : Polysaccharides (or glycans) are arbitrarily defined as high molecular weight polymers resulting from the condensation of a large number of monosaccharides molecules. As natural molecules, polysaccharides are virtually universal in the energy storage forms (Starch, dextran, fructans, cellulose and inulin). Among these carbohydrates **inulin** is characteristic of the **Compositae** family while the **fructans** is present in **Gramineae**. Thus the polysaccharide are also utilized in confirming the phylogenetic relationship. For example the tropical and subtropical species of grasses accumulate starch in their leaves while temperate grasses belonging to the tribes, *Hordeae*, *Avenea* and *Festuceae*, accumulate fructans.

Glycosides in Chemotaxonomy
(Fig. 7.6)

Glycosides are compounds in which one or more sugar (**glycone**) is combined with non-sugar compound known as **genin or aglycone**. On the bases of linkage they are **O-glycoside** (sugar is linked with aglycone through oxygen atom of alcohol or phenol) e.g. Rhein (Rhubarb); **C-glycoside** (sugar is linked with aglycone through C-atom) e.g. Aloin. Similarly **N-glycoside** (Nitrogen atoms) e.g. Adenosine and **S-glycoside** (sulphur atom) e.g. Sinigrin.

O-glycosides and their occurrence is so widespread as to be of little chemotaxonomic value.

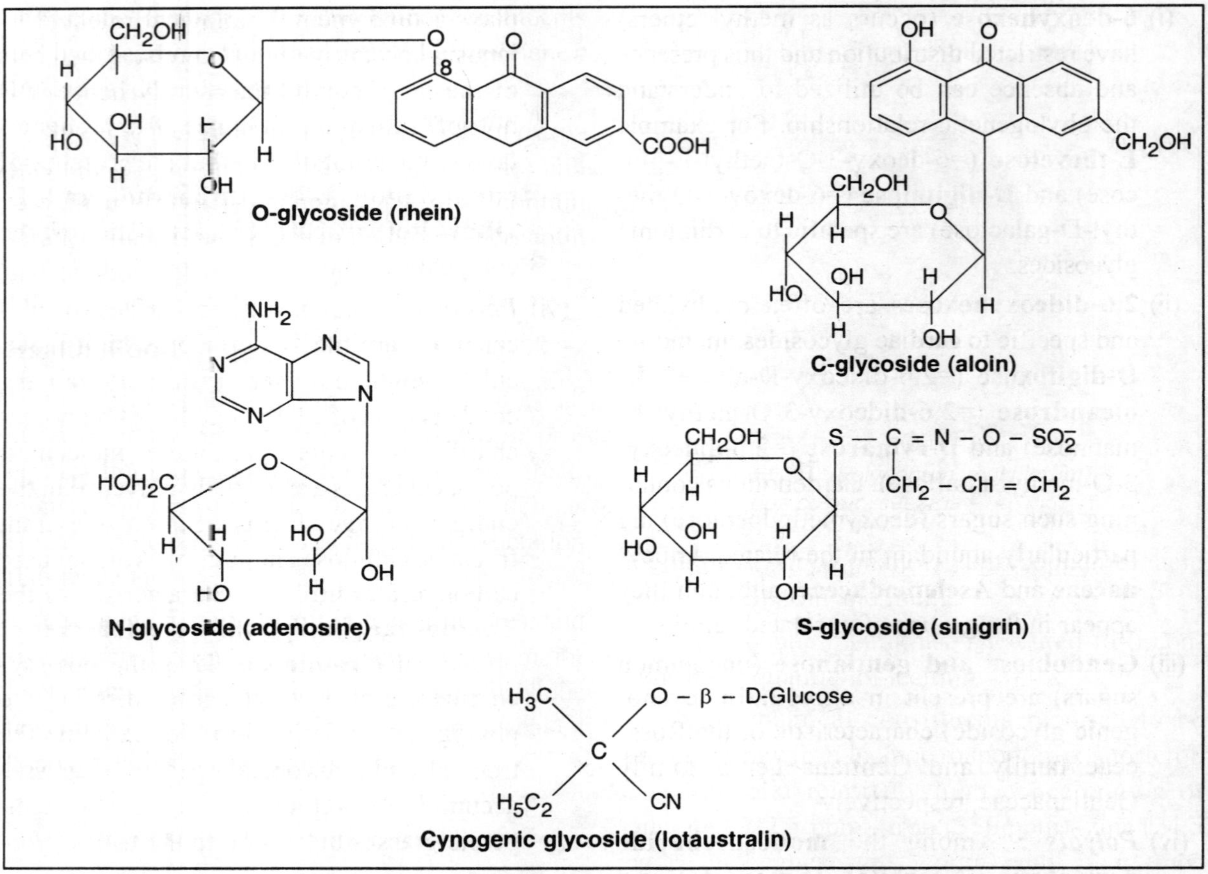

Fig. 7.6. Glycosides in Chemotaxonomy.

C-glycosides, which possess a direct carbon linkage between sugar and the aglycone, are rare in nature. They are found in some plants containing **anthraquinone** derivative e.g. Aloin in aloes (liliaceae) and the cascarosides of cascara (**Rhamnaceae**). About 25 C-glycosides of flavonoids group are known most are flavone a few isoflavone and flavanones.

S-Glycosides in which **sulphur** replaces oxygen in the sugar linkage are exemplified by those **furnishing isothiocyanates** on hydrolysis. These compounds are the family characteristic of the **cruciferae** and related families, Capparaceae, Moringaceae and Resedaceae.

Cyanogenic Glycoside as Chemotaxonomic Marker

About 100 plant species have the ability to produce hydrogen cyanide by enzyme hydrolysis. This property is particularly common in the **Rosaceae, Passifloraceae, Leguminosae, Sapindaceae and Gramineae families**. It seems that all these plants have ability to synthesize cyanogenetic glycosides from different amino acids (phenylalanine, tyrosine, valine, leucine and isoleucine). Synthesising cyanogenic glycoside based on leucine is restricted to South African acacia species (**Leguminosae** and members of **Sapindaceae**).

On the basis of **amino acid precursors** some conclusion for chemotaxonomy can be derived. For example, at the family level Cyanogenetic glycoside (amygdalin) synthesised from phenylalanine is restricted to the **Rosaceae** and such compounds synthesised from aliphatic valine or isoleucine is restricted to **leguminosae** (papilionoideae).

The accumulation of cyanogenetic glycosides is also significant in confirming the position of certain families for example suborder **Flacourtineae** (in Engler's Syllabus) of the violales possess a number of families (e.g. **Flacourtiaceae, Turneraceae and Passifloraceae**) rich in cyanogenetic compounds. The violaceae, a family of this order having doubtful positions on morphological grounds, reported to contain no genera having these compounds. The other suborders of the violales are reported to be without cyanogenetic compounds.

Glucosinolates as Chemotaxonomic Marker

Glucosinolates also known as thioglucosides are responsible for the characteristic flavours of various plants of **Brassicaceae** (mustard, radish and cabbage) and numerous species of botanically related families (e.g. Capparidaceae, Tropaeolaceae and Resedaceae) as shown in the Table 7.4.

From the above available **glucosinolates** it seem that these compounds occur abundantly in **Cruciferae** and the related **Capparidaceae**.

Glucosinolates are useful taxonomic markers within *Iberis* and *Arabis genera* (Cruciferae).

On the basis of **alkyl component** of glucosinolate compound *Brassica* species can be differentiated for example when mustard *Brassica juncea*, was examined it was found that those from Indian subcontinent contained **3-butenyl glucosinate and allylglucosinate** while those from **Asiatic Countries** contained only the **allyl compound** as the major component. *B. juncea* is thought to be a hybrid between *B. nigra* (which contain allylglucosinate) and *B. compestris*, (which contain 3-butenyl-glucosinate), but the artificially produced hybrids between these two species contain the allylglucosinate exclusively, hence ancestry of Indian species is in some doubts.

Table 7.4. Glucosinolate $R - C \begin{array}{c} S - Gluc. \\ \\ +NOSO_3^- \end{array}$

Glucosinolate	R. in Figure	Precursor	Occurrence
Glucocapparin	CH_3	Alanine	Capparidaceae
Sinigrin	$CH_2 = CH–CH_3$	Serine	Cruciferae
Gluconapin	$CH_2 = CH–CH_2–CH_3$	Serine	Cruciferae
Glucotropeolin	⬡–CH_3	Phenylalanine	Several families
Sinalbin	HO–⬡–CH_3	Tyrosine	Cruciferae
Gluconasturtin	⬡–$CH_2–CH_3$	Phenylalanine	Cruciferae
Glucobrassicin	(indole ring)–CH_3	Tryptophan	Brassica spp.

Like cyanogenetic glycoside most of the plants have the ability to synthesise glucosinates, but in most of them they are metabolized but not accumulated.

Chemotaxonomy of Medicinal Plants containing Phenolic Compounts
(Fig. 7.7)

Phenolic compounds are present in medicinal plants in considerable number, variety of chemical structures and quantities.

Compounds of restricted occurrence may have chemotaxonomic value; thus trihydroxy derivative of benzoic and cinnamic acids are more interesting than the commonly mono and dihydroxy compounds. For example, ellagic acid is absent in the ferns, gymnosperms and monocotyledons, but is infrequently found in the dicotyledons. It is a useful chemotaxonomic marker in the subfamily Rosoideae (Rosaceae); out of the seven tribes, only Kerrieae does not contain ellagic acid, hence on chemosystematic ground the removal of Kerrieae from Rosoideae can be confirmed. More over none of the remaining subfamilies of Rosaceae contains ellagic acid. 4-hydroxy benzoic acid and 4-hydroxy phenyl acetic acid have been reported in eight genera of the Saxifragaceae family but in Astilbe these compounds are replaced by 2-hydroxyphenylacetic acid. Thus this acid is chemotaxonomic significant marker for the genus Astilbe.

Coumarins are common volatile constituents contributing to odour of many plants. The hydroxylated derivatives are being restricted in distribution can be utilized as a chemotaxonomic marker. Umbelliferone occurs widely in the umbelliferae family while in compositae it is characteristic of the hawkweed genus (Hieracium) and proved to be useful taxonomic marker. The few species of Hieracium has been removed and grouped with Pilsoella genus on morphological and phylogenic grounds are confirmed on the basis of Umbelliferone.

The Flavonoids are potentially one of most useful taxonomic marker being its solubility and easy separation by paper chromatography.

Flavonoids are the largest group of phenolic compounds. They are mostly found in the vacuole of higher plant cell and absent from bacteria and majority of algae. The various types of flavonoids include flavones, flavanones, isoflavanones and isoflavonoids. Flavonols, anthocyanidins, chalcones and aurones. Flavonoids from vegetative parts and seed provide more reliable taxonomic evidence than the flower pigments.

Plant flavonoids patterns have given useful correlations with established morphological taxonomy in a number of instances. For example two tribes, Plumbagineae and Staticeae of the Plumbaginaceae family are designated on the bases of characteristic difference in leaf and flower flavonols and anthocyanins.

Quercetin-3-gentiobioside is restricted to member of the Tribuleae (Zygophyllaceae) tribe, which supports to the suggestion made on morphological grounds that this tribe should be treated as a separate family. Flavonoid C-glycosides such as Vitexin are considered primitive chemical characters which have often been lost in more highly developed taxa within subfamily Spiraeoideae of Rosaceae, only Quillaja contains C-glycosides and it has been suggested that this genus is a relict of the now extinct ancestors of the Pomoideae within the latter subfamily. The occurrence of C-glycoside in Aronia and their absence in Sorbus argues against cytological and morphological evidence that the two genera should be united.

In some genera flavonoid pattern in each species can be used as a fingerprint. The Baptisia genus (Leguminosae) contains about 62 flavonoids

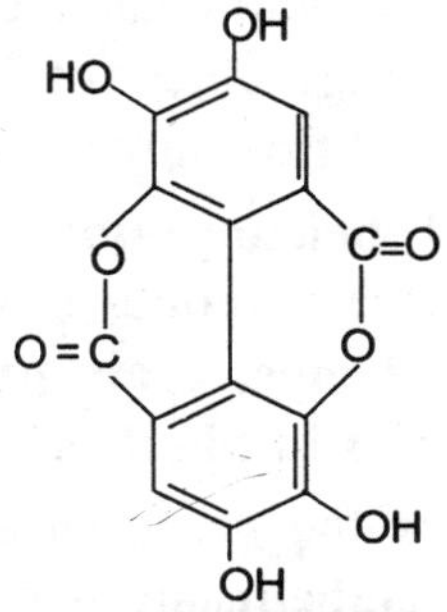

Ellagic acid

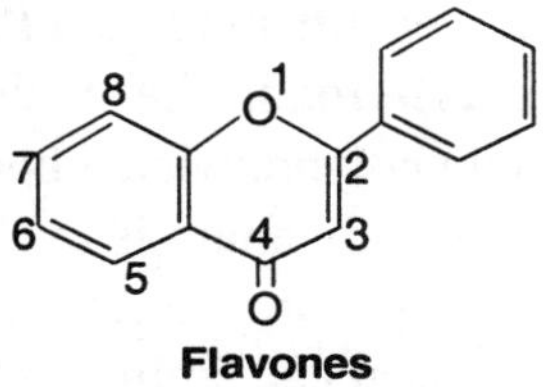

Coumarin

Flavanone

Flavones

Isoflavonoid

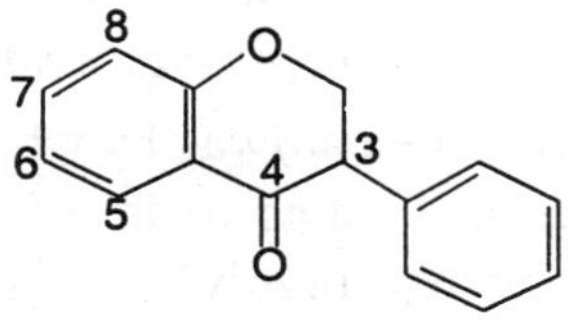

Isoflavanone (3-phenyl-γ-chromone)

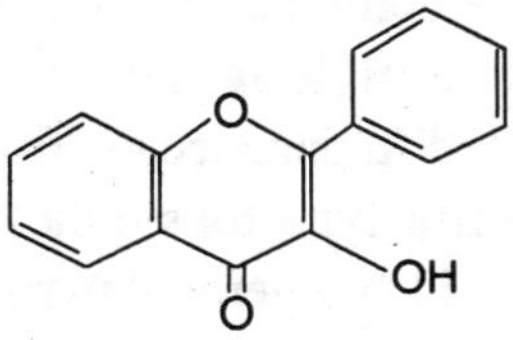

Anthocyanins

Flavonol

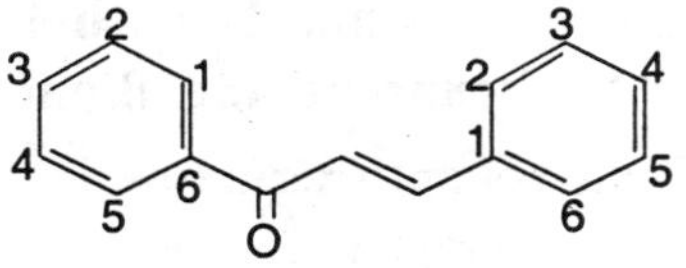

Chalcones

Aurones

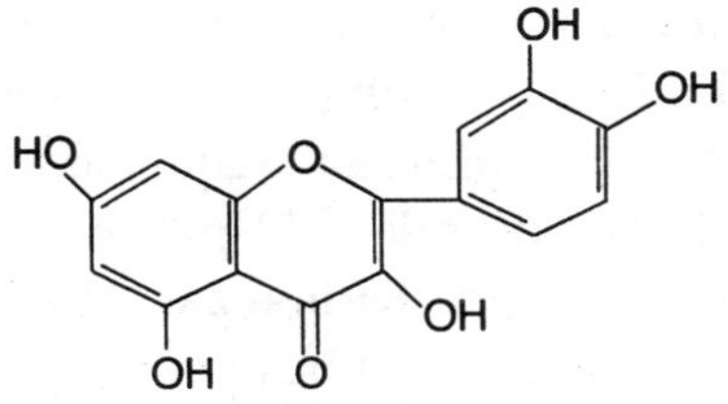

Quercetin R = H
Rutin R = rhamano-glucosyl (Flavonols)

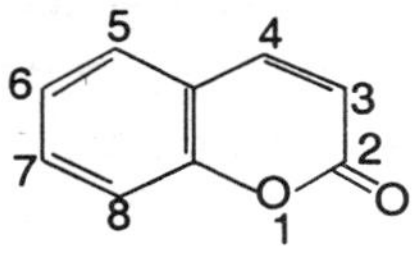

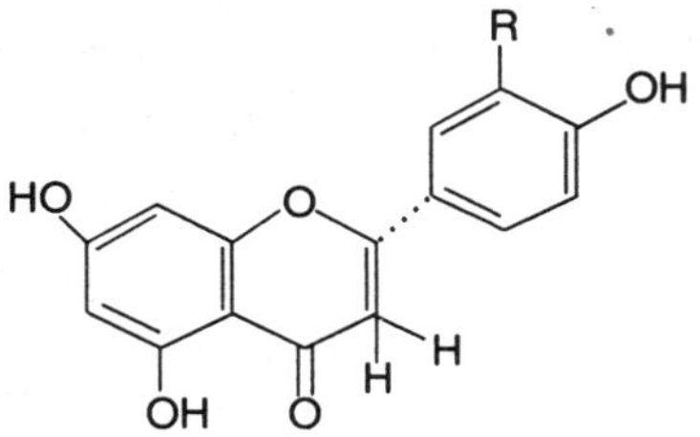

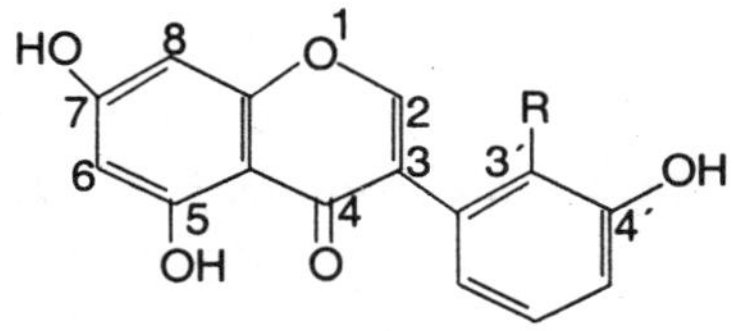

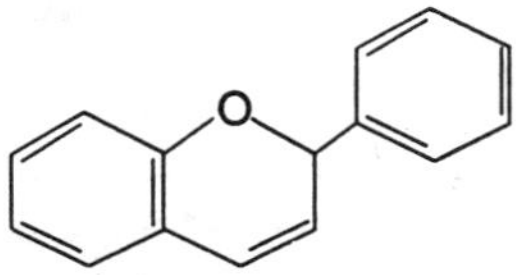

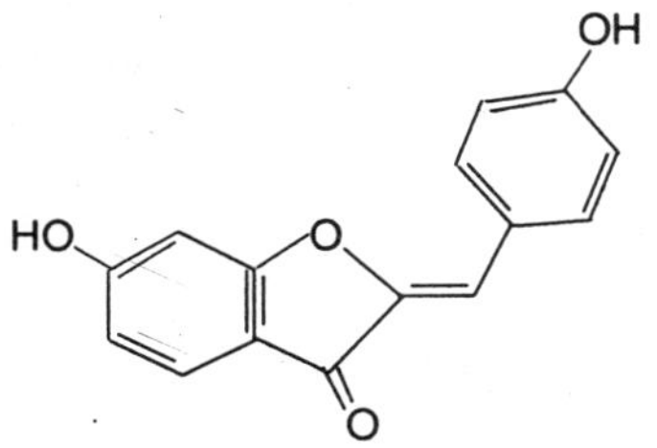

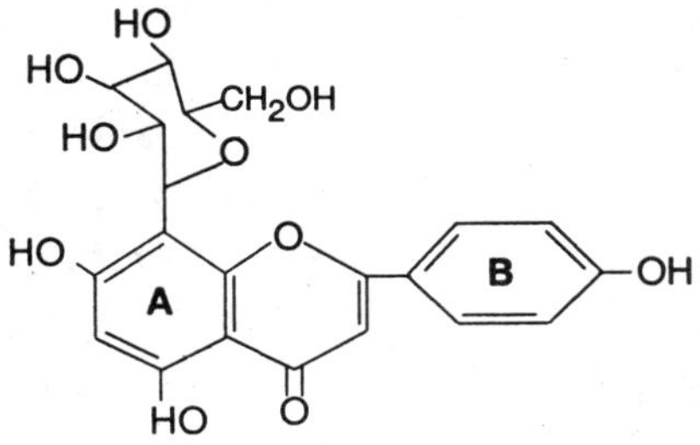

Vitexin

Fig. 7.7. Phenolic compounds in chemotaxonomy.

and each of 17 species has a characteristic pattern, however in closely related *Thermopsis* genus with 31 flavonoids, 13 species have almost identical patterns.

On the basis of **flavones** present in the heartwood of *Pinus* genus, subgenera *Haploxylon* were differentiated from *Diploxylon*, which do not contains flavone in the heart wood.

Woody plants are considered to be more primitive than the herbaceous plants. Woody plants contain leuco-anthocyanins (colourless flavonoids), while herbaceous plants are devoid of it. They were detected in 60% of the woody families examined and 15% herbaceous families. Thus nearly all woody dicotyledons families from Casuarinaceae (*magnoniales*) to **Ebenaceae** (Ebenales) contain leucoanthocyanins, but in herbaceous families, from **Aristolochiaceae** to **Compositae** are lacking. In monocotyledons all species of woody **Palmae** family contains leuco-anthocyanins and such compounds are extremely rare in herbaceous Gramineae and Orchidaceae.

Isoflavone Iridin is known only in the *Progonivis* section of *Iris*, *Iris flavissima*, which was originally placed in section. Progonivis does not contain Iridin and on the other hand resembles species of Regelira section in phenolic characters. Hence the transfer of Iris flavissima to regelina section has been suggested.

Quinones in Chemotaxonomy
(Fig. 7.8)

The glycoside formation involving hydroxyanthraquinone is frequent; hydroxybenzoquinone (e.g. 2, 6-dimethoxyquinone from **Adonis vernalis**, Ranunculaceae) and hydroxynaphthaquinone (plumbagin, **5-hydroxy-2-methyl-1, 4 naphthaquinone** from plumbago spp. **Plumbaginaceae**) have been obtained in free state only. The **naphthaquinone alkannin** and its reduction product alkannan are particularly characteristic of the subfamily, **Boraginoideae** of Boraginaceae; has not been obtained from any other family.

A number of benzoquinones, naphthaquinones and anthraquinones have a restricted distribution; hence, their presence can be potentially useful in plant taxonomy.

In **dicotyledons** the polyprenylated benzoquinones such as **embelin** are good taxonomic markers for **Myrsinaceae**, while **primitin** with shorter side chain occurs in related **Primulaceae**. In the **monocotyledons**, the Sedges (Cyperaceae) also contain polyprenylated **benzoquinone**, but in majority the side chain is cyclised to form **furan** rings as in **cyperaquinone**, a characteristic compound of **Cyperaceae** family and used within the family for classification which is otherwise difficult on the morphological grounds.

Acetate malonate pathway by which quinones are biosynthesised seems to be more primitive than the pathways involving shikimic acid. However **plumbagin** occurs in the Droseraceae and Plumbaginaceae family, **7-methyljuglone** in **Droseraceae and Ebenaceae** family. While the shikimic acid derived **juglone** is characteristic of the less highly evolved Juglandaceae. **Naphthaquinone of the alkannin** type biosynthesised from 4-hydroxybenzoic acid and geranyl pyrophosphate have only been found on the advanced *Tubiflorales*. However alkannin being characteristic of the *Boraginaceae*, while **Lapachol** is widespread in the **Verbenaceae and Bignoniaceae**.

The distribution of **anthraquinone** in the dicotyledons has more phylogenetic relevance, as these compounds such as **emodin** biosynthesised by the **acetate-malonate** pathways are found mainly in **Leguminosae, Polygonaceae and Rhamnaceae** families, while anthraquinone derivatives derived from **shikimic acid pathway** are found in more advanced **Rubiaceae, Verbenaceae and Bignoniaceae** families.

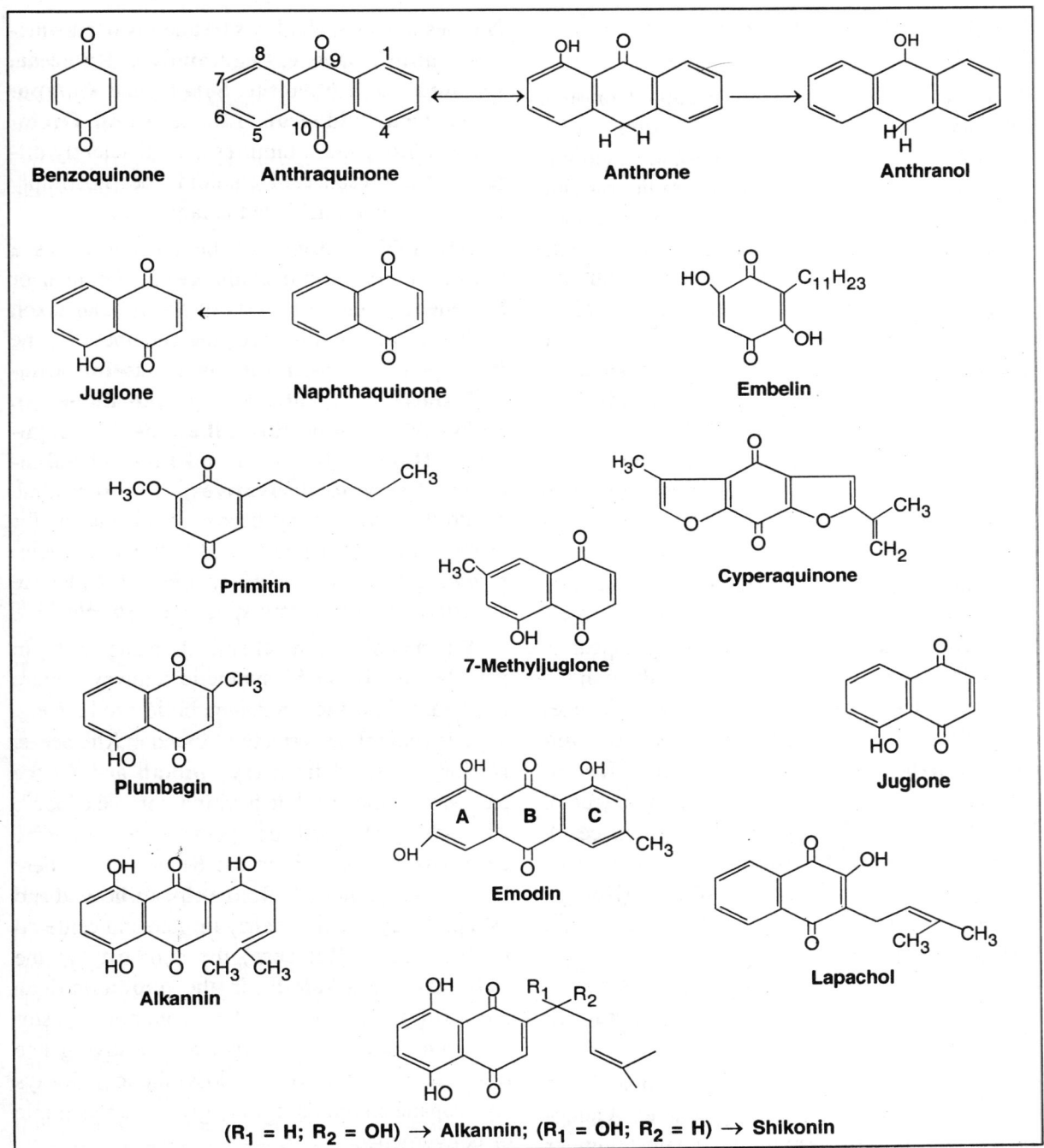

Fig. 7.8. Quinones in Chemotaxonomy.

Alkaloids in Chemotaxonomy
(Fig. 7.9)

Alkaloids are heterogeneous group of organic nitrogen containing bases, often with heterogeneous ring. Plants synthesising alkaloids are worldwide and occur in many families ranging from primitive mosses to highly complex Gramineae, although these secondary metabolites are most abundant in dicotyledons. **True alkaloids** have nitrogen containing heterocyclic nucleus derived from a biogenetic amine and they can be related structurally to **parent bases such as pyridine, piperidine, quinoline, isoquinoline and tropane etc.** True alkaloids are of rare occurrence in lower plants. In the fungi the lysergic acid derivatives and in gymnosperms and pteridophytes, the lycopodium, ephedra and taxus alkaloids are the best known.

Alkaloids distribution in Angiosperms is uneven. The **dicotyledon orders Salicales, Fagales, Cucurbitales and Oleales** at present appear to be alkaloid free. Alkaloids are commonly found in the order **Centrospermae** (Chenopodiaceae) **Magnoliales** (Lauraceae, Magnoliaceae) **Ranunculales** (Berberidaceae, Menispermaceae, Ranunculaceae), **Papaverales** (Papaveraceae), **Rosales** (Leguminosae sub-family Papilionaceae), **Rutales** (Rutaceae), **Gentianales** (Apocynaceae, Loganiaceae, Rubiaceae), **Tubiflorae** (Boraginaceae, Convulvulaceae, Solanaceae) and **Campanuales** (Campanulaceae subfamily **Lobeliodeae**, Compositae-subfamily Senecioneae) in the dicotyledones and the **Liliales and Orchidales** in monocotyledons.

Among the individual families probably the **Papaveraceae** and the totally unrelated **Apocynaceae** will prove to contain the greatest number of these secondary metabolites. Every species belonging to Papaveraceae reported to contain alkaloids, while the Apocynaceae exhibit great diversity of **complex indole alkaloids.** Other families in which alkaloids frequently occurs include **Ranunculaceae, Leguminosae, Rutaceae, Loganiaceae, Rubiaceae, Solanaceae, Compositae, Amaryllidaceae, Liliaceae and Orchidaceae.** Since these families are sufficiently different, the presence of alkaloid does not imply taxonomic relationship at the family level.

Alkaloid content can be considered as a source of **taxonomic evidence** as chemical or biogenetic group of species of a particular taxon is the same. For instance, the members of the **Papaveraceae synthesise isoquinoline alkaloids those of the Fabaceae; (Lupin alkaloids), Rubiaceae; (Quinoline alkaloids), Apocynaceae; (Indole alkaloids) and those of Solanaceae; (tropane derivatives).** But sometime alkaloids have a very narrow distribution, for example morphine is restricted to *Papaver somniferum*, **coniine** to a few species of Apiaceae and strychnine to a few species of *Strychnos*.

When applying the chemical characteristic in plant taxonomy, the biosynthetic pathway is more important than the final metabolic product e.g. quinine (quinoline derivative) found in Rubiaceae, is biosynthesised from **tryptophan** and by the pathway similar to that forming complex indole alkaloids characteristic of Apocynaceae. Quinoline derivative also occurs in the Rutaceae, but here they are biosynthesized from **anthranilic acid** and by a pathway which is fairly limited and centered in this family (Rutaceae) the similarity of the **quinolizidine alkaloids** in the **papilionoideae and ranunculaceae** indicates a common ancestor but some time the convergence and divergence may also effect the normal biosynthetic pathways e.g. tropane alkaloids from hygrine is an example of convergence.

Distribution of alkaloids has proved useful in the **taxonomy of the Fabaceae**. Three genera of Fabaceae *Genista*, *Ammodendron* and *Adenocarpus* contain ammodendrine (hysterine) alkaloids.

Out of these *Genista* and *Adenocarpus* were included in the Genisteae, whereas *Ammodendron* was placed in Sophoreae, a tribe characterized by the presence of **matrine** alkaloids. This suggests the transfer of Ammodendron to the tribe Genisteae.

The tribe *Sophoreae, Genisteae* and *Podalyrieae* of the subfamily *Lotoideae* of the Fabaceae are characterized by the presence of **Lupin alkaloids** and this suggests that these tribes may have originated from common ancestral stock.

The accumulation of **isoquinoline** alkaloids in the families **Fumariaceae and Papaveraceae** indicate very close relationship between two families.

There are instances where **alkaloid biosynthesis can be helpful** to chemotaxonomist for arranging the species within the genus according to their alkaloidal content. For example, in the genus Argemone, which is difficult to classify purely on the basis of morphological grounds, the species can be arranged into three groups on the basis of their alkaloidal content. **Group I** contains alkaloids of **protopine and berberine** type but not of **pavine type**. **Group II** contains all three types. **Group III** contains only the **pavine type**.

Although specific alkaloid can be said to be characteristic of an order, genus or family, it does not mean that same alkaloids are not synthesised in plants belonging to totally different order, family or genera. However frequency of occurrence may be much higher in the former. Some characteristic alkaloids are the **Protoberberines** [(quaternary or tertiary tetracyclic alkaloids) (isoquinoline)] of the Ranunculaceae, lycorine (isoquinoline C_6C_2-N-C_1C_6 type) of the Amaryllidaceae family, spiroamine alkaloids of Erythrina and α, α'-substituted **piperidines** characteristic of Lobelia species (Lobeliaceae). This criteria of characterisation to be used carefully; previously thought to be unique to a particular family genus or species have now

been found in totally unrelated plant and even **morphine**, once classical example of an alkaloid unique to a single species has been found in second *Papaver* species *P. setigerum* Albeit one that is closely related to *P. somniferum*.

Tropane Alkaloids

Tropane alkaloids have in common nitrogen bicyclic structural element named as **azabicycles (3,2,1) octane**, i.e. [1, 8-methyl-8-azabicyclo; 3,2,1] octane, derived from ornithine.

About 200 alkaloids are known, which are distributed in the angiosperm families:

(1) *Solanaceae :* About twenty genera of the family solanaceae are reported to have tropane alkaloids e.g. Atropa, Brugmansia, Datura, Mandragora, Physalis, Schizanthus, Scopolia, Solandra, Withania);

(2) *Erythroxylaceae* (Erythroxylum);

(3) *Proteaceae* [Bellendena, Darlingia, Knightia, (pyranotropanes)];

(4) *Convolvulaceae* [Convolvulus, calystegia (aromatic ester of tropanol and calystegines)] and also found distributed sporadically in few isolated genera

(5) *Bruguiera* (Rhizophoraceae)

(6) *Phyllanthus*,

(7) *Peripentadenia* (Euphorbiaceae);

(8) *Cochlearia* (Brassicaceae) and

(9) *Heisteria* (Olaceae).

Most representative structure of tropane alkaloid is given in Fig. 7.9.

Terpenoids and Steroids in Chemotaxonomy (Fig. 7.10)

All terpenoids are multiples of the isoprene unit (C_5) . These compounds are considered as groups rather than individual compounds based upon the isoprene units (i.e. hemiterpenoids $C_{5 \times 1}$,

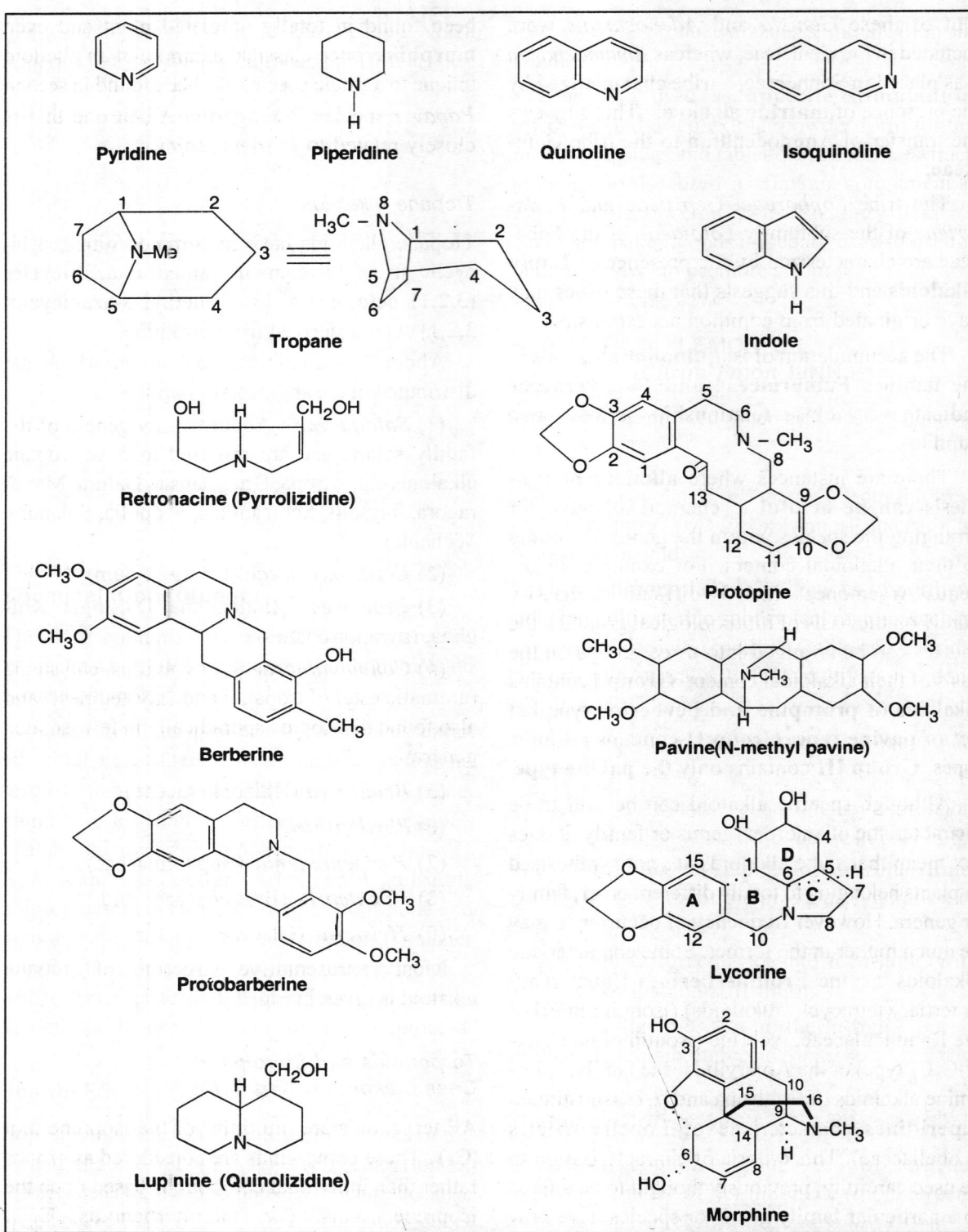

Fig. 7.9. Alkaloids in Chemotaxonomy.

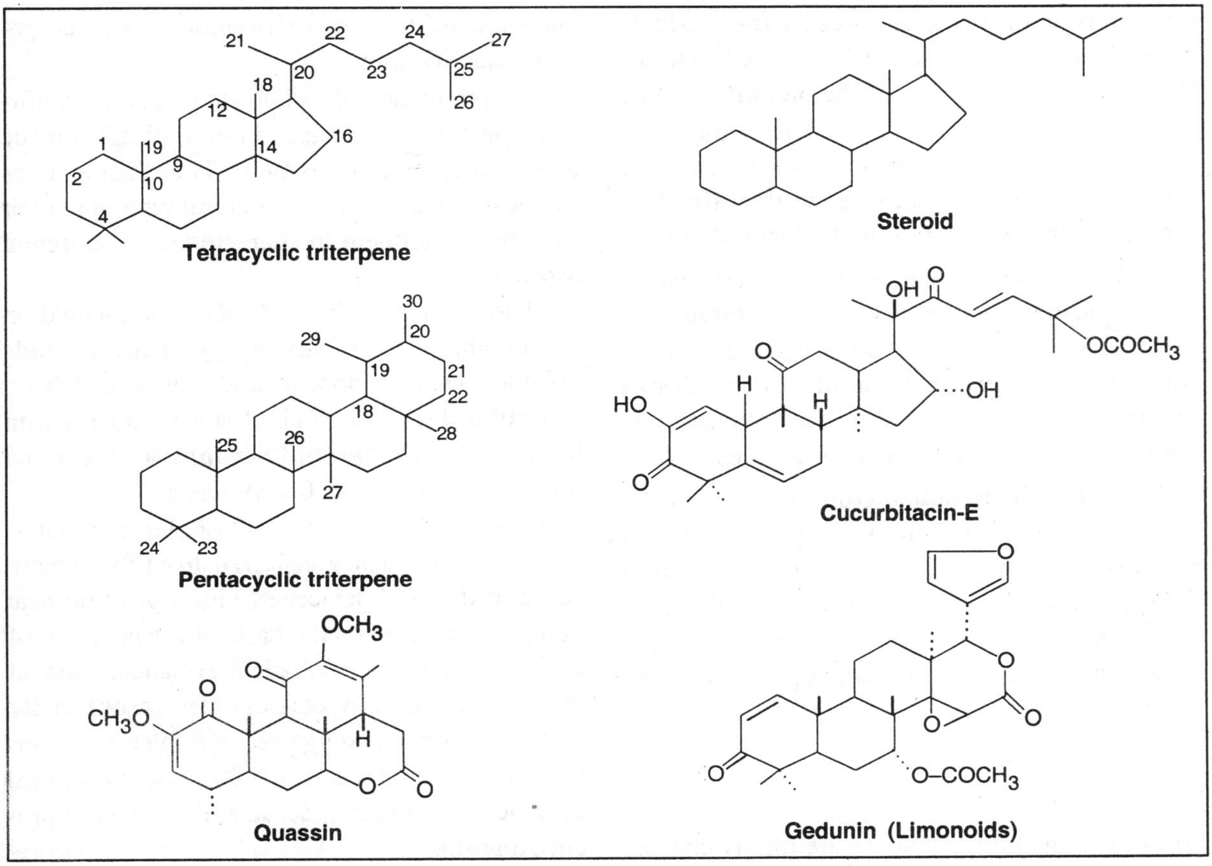

Fig. 7.10. Terpenoids and Steroids in Chemotaxonomy.

monoterpenoid $C_{5\times2}$, sesquiterpenoid $C_{5\times3}$, diterpenoids $C_{5\times4}$ triterpenoids $C_{5\times6}$ and carotenoids $C_{5\times8}$).

The **steroids** have the same ring structure as the **tetracyclic triterpenoids**, but are distinguished from these compounds by their **lack of methyl group at C4 and C14**.

The wide variety of terpenoids and steroids in plants together with their diverse occurrence make these compounds of little value in chemotaxonomic point of view.

The **triterpenoids saponins** are also too widely distributed to have taxonomic value when considered alone. However, in combination with other phytoconstituents such as phenols and flavonoids, they can play role in confirming the relation of **Pittosporaceae**. This family has more affinity with **Araliaceae than Saxifragaceae** hence it should therefore be included in the order **Araliales** (Umbellales) rather than in the **Rosales**.

The **steroidal saponins** have a much narrower distribution as it is being restricted to the **monocotyledonous** families like **Liliaceae, Dioscoreaceae, Amaryllidaceae, Agavaceae and Bromeliaceae** although they also occur in the dicotyledonous families **Solanaceae** and **Scrophulariaceae**.

The **Solanaceae** is characterised by **alkaloidal saponins**, which have not been found outside this family, while the related **veratrum alkaloids** are confined to the Veratril tribe of the Liliaceae. **Diterpenoid alkaloids of the aconitine type** are characteristic of the related *Aconitum* and *Delphinium* genera of the Ranunculaceae. They also occur in the Garryaceae, a family difficult to classify on the base of morphological grounds.

Oxidised terpenoid derivatives are useful taxonomic markers, as the **Cucurbitacins** are the characteristic of the Cucurbitaceae family while the **Meliacins, Limonoids and Quassins** are found in the closely related **Meliaceae, Rutaceae and Simaroubaceae** families.

The **monoterpenoids composition** of the *Pinus genus* (Pinaceae) has been useful in tracing hybridisation between species and the migration of the genus while the cultivators of the blue spruce (*Picea pungens*, family Pinaceae) have been identified from their monoterpenoid composition.

Iridoids (Fig. 7.11)

Iridoids in the broadest sense are highly characteristic metabolites, which occur mainly in a number of assumed phylogenetically related dicotyledonous plant families. The detection of iridoids in Callitrichaceae, Eucommiaceae, Fouquieriaceae, Hippuridaceae, part of Icacinaceae, *Liquidambar*, part of Loasaceae, Theligonaceae and other often mono- or oligotypic taxa

made a considerable contribution to their appropriate classification.

The production of iridoids in plants has confirmed some recent changes in classification made on morphological basis only. These compounds can be divided into five structural types and their occurrence can help to characterize the different tribes of Compositae.

Bate-smith and Swain (1966) commented on the possible value of **taxonomy of the Iridoids** (monoterpenoid cyclopentanoid lactones), of these, **asperuloside** is found in **Rubiaceae** and **aucubin** occurs in **Cornaceae and Scrophulariaceae** and also in **Buddleia and Garryaceae**.

In the 12th edition of Engler's syllabus **Buddleia** has been transferred from the loganiaceae to the Buddleiaceae (with a position near Scrophulariaceae) on the basis of the presence of aucubin and on morphological evidence, removal of Garryaceae from Apetalous orders to the vicinity of the Cornaceae is suggested in Engler's syllabus and this treatment receives support from chemical evidence as both Garryaceae and Cornaceae produce **aucubin**.

Thus aucubin occurs in Cornaceae and Scrophulariaceae and also in Buddleia and Garryaceae, Buddleia was once included in loganiaceae but has now been moved to Buddleiaceae which is placed near scrophulariaceae while Garryaceae has been removed from apetalous orders to the family of *Cornaceae*.

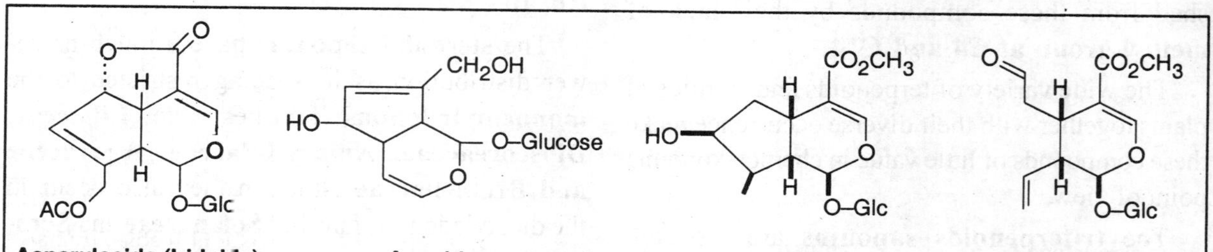

Fig. 7.11. Iridoids in Chemotaxonomy.

Sesquiterpene lactones have been isolated from all tribes except Asterae, Arctotideae and *Mutisieae*. The closely related *Heliantheae* and *Helenieae*, being particularly rich in these compounds, are the only tribes to synthesise a variety of **ambrosanolides** (Guaianolide, Eudesmanolide, Eremophilanolide) (Fig. 7.12). These compounds are characteristic of *Ambrosia*. On the basis of this lactone distribution the removal of *Ambrosia* and related genera from the tribe *Heliantheae* is suggested. These genera should be recognised as a separate tribe. Such sesquiterpene lactones are often very bitter and sometimes taste acrid, which occur in Hepaticae, Cupressaceae, Magnoliaceae, Lauraceae, Umbelliferae & Compositae (Table 7.5).

The *Cynareae* is characterised by a lack of

Table 7.5. Sesquiterpene lactones in the Compositeae

Tribe	Germacranolide	Santanolide	Eremophilanolide	Guaianolide	Ambrosanolide
Vernonieae	+	+	–	–	–
Eupatorieae	+	–	–	+	+
Astereae	–	–	–	–	–
Inuleae	–	+	–	+	+
Heliantheae	+	+	–	+	–
Helenieae	–	–	+	–	–
Anthemideae	–	–	+	–	–
Senecioneae	–	–	–	–	–
Calenduleae	+	–	–	–	–
Arctotideae	–	–	–	–	–
Cynareae	+	–	–	+	–
Mutisieae	–	–	–	–	–
Cichorieae	–	+	–	+	–

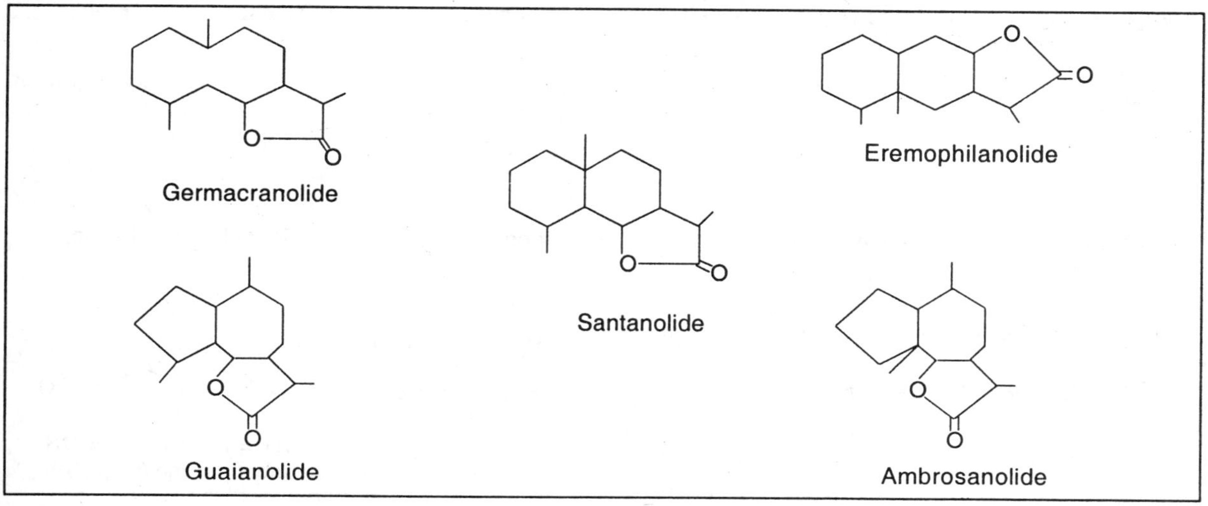

Germacranolide

Santanolide

Eremophilanolide

Guaianolide

Ambrosanolide

Fig. 7.12.

tricyclic lactones only, guaianolides occurring rarely. Thus, it seems that most species belonging to this tribe have not evolved the enzymes necessary for the further cyclisation of germacranolides.

The *Senecioneae* is distinguished from all other tribes by its content of **eremophilanolides** and the occurrance of such compounds in *Adenostyles* indicates that this genus should be included in the Senecioneae and not the *Eupatorieae* as in earlier classification.

Essential Oils in Chemotaxonomy (Fig. 7.13)

Essential oils are the complex mixtures of odorous and steam volatile compounds deposited by plants in the subcuticular space of glandular hairs, in cell organelles, in idioblast, in excretory cavities and canals or exceptionally in heartwoods.

Chemically the essential oils are heterogeneous mixture of hydrocarbons, terpenes (mono, sesqui and diterpene), phenylpropanoids, alcohol, aldehyde, ketones, ethers and esters.

Presence or absence of essential oils regardless of their compositions provides a very valuable taxonomic character. As per the definition the essential oil is a complex one, it is a combination of excretory structures (anatomical side) and production of steam-volatile excretion (chemical side).

The bulk of essential oil bearing plants belongs to the seed plants. In **Thallophytes** true essential oils occur in some fungi (e.g. in the genus Lactarius) and in a number of *Chlorophyta*, *Rhodophyta* (Red Algae) and *Phaeophyta* (Brown Algae); in these plants essential oils are deposited in specialized cells (Excretory hyphae

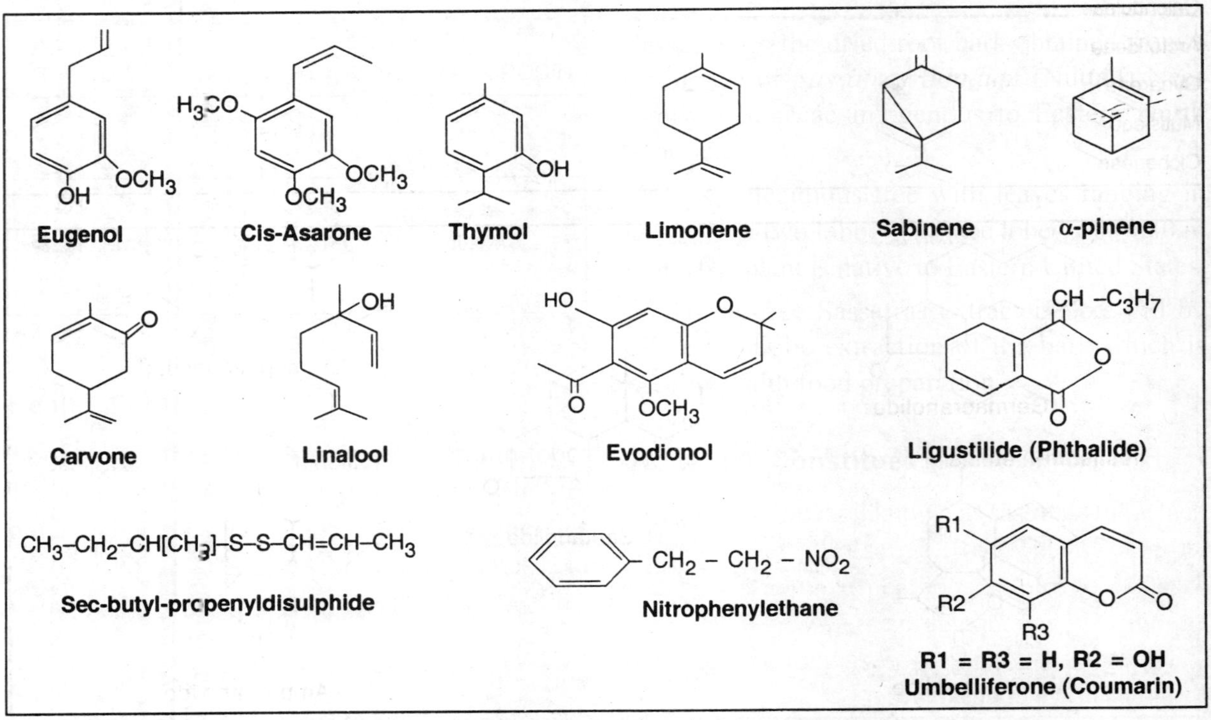

Fig. 7.13. Essential oil Component in Chemotaxonomy.

or cells of idioblastic nature). In **Bryophyta** essential oil are restricted to Liverworts. In **Pteridophytes**, only rarely noticable amount of essential oils are produced. In **Spermatophytes** (seed plants) the essential oils ubiquitous in **Coniferopsida and Taxopsida** (Gymnosperms), which possess schizogenous cavities and canals. In **Coniferopsida** the essential oils seems to be restricted to *Ginko biloba* (Lysigenous cavities). Chlamydospermae seems to be devoid of essential oils. In angiospermae (flowering plants) the most of them having essential oils. These are classified in 62 orders (Engler's syllabus, Vol. 1964).

From the chemotaxonomical point, the bulk of well known constituents of essential oils occurs in many taxonomically unrelated taxa e.g. **Eugenol, cis-asarone, thymol, limonene, sabinene, α-pinene. Carvone and Linalool**. Such compounds are taxonomically useful only at the **generic level**. Other oil constituents can be termed **taxon specific** because they seem to occur in only a few species, for example: **Sec-butyl-propenyl-disulphide** (component of the oleoresin of a few species of *Ferula* (Umbilliferae) and **Nitrophenylethane** (Cinnamon-scented constituents of the essential oils of Aniba and Ocotea-taxa family Lauraceae).

On the basis of chemical constituents of essential oils, the medicinal plants can be classified into following groups.

(i) Rutaceae

(ii) Myrtaceae

(iii) Umbelliferae

(iv) Compositae

Rutaceae

Rutaceae family plants are chemically characterised by the synthesis and accumulation of essential oils, furanocoumarins, anthranilic acid derived alkaloids and limonoids. Prenylations of aromatic compounds is common in this family; example of this tendency are furano and dimethylpyrano-coumarins and a number of essential oil constituents such as **Evodionol** (a phloracetophenone derived 2, 2'-dimethylchromene. Similar tendencies are perceptible in Umbelliferae (coumarins) and Compositae (Precocene and 6-desmethoxy derivative).

Myrtaceae

Myrtaceae family consists of tannin-rich essential oil plants. Methylated, prenylated and (or) acetylated phloroglucinol derivatives occurs frequently in their essential oils; production of this very characteristic type of acetogenesis (Torquatone, a phloroglucinol derivative; present in some species of *Eucalyptus*) represent a chemical trend of this family.

Umbelliferae

Umbelliferae family constitute the plants with furano and dimethylpyrano-coumarins and essential oils which tends to contain phthalides. For example **Ligustilide** (phthalide occurring in the essential oils of species of *Angelica, Cinidium, Conioselinum, Levisticum* and *meum*) (Umbelliferae) ferulol type monoterpenoids and acetylenic compounds like falcarinone. The latter link the family chemically with **Araliaceae, Pittosporaceae and Compositae**.

Compositae

Compositae plants are chemically characterised by synthesis and accumulations of many classes of natural compounds. In Asteroideae (= Tubiflorae) essential oils are common. They often contains acetylenic compounds e.g. matricaria ester (an ester of a C-10 polyacetylenic carboxylic acid occurring in essential oils of many compositae plants) and tend to comprise complex derivative of thymol; in some genera and tribes, e.g. Nematicidal, thymol derivatives occurring in several species of *Helenium* (Compositae). As indicated by many metabolic trends in the synthesis of series of essential oils, an evolution line from Rutales → Umbelliferae (Umbelliferae and Araliaceae only) → Asterales can be drawn.

Non-Protein Amino Acid in Chemotaxonomy (Fig. 7.14)

Betalains (betacyanins and betaxanthins - amino acids derivatives) are vegetable pigments characteristic of some fungi but after the detection of betalains in **Cactaceae and Didiereaceae** the centrospermous affinities were more or less generally accepted for these taxa. The occurrence of betaxanthins in the fungus *Amanita muscaria* by no means invalidates their importance in angiosperms classification.

Non-protein amino acids are sufficiently restricted in distribution and hence useful as taxonomical markers. Thus branched chain and cyclopropane derivatives related to **hypoglycin A**; have only been isolated from closely related **Sapindaceae and Hippocastanaceae**; Azeti-

dine-2-carboxylic acid is characteristic of closely related **Liliaceae, Amaryllidaceae and Agavaceae.**

Non-protein amino-acid characteristic of two genera

LATHYRUS :
- Homoarginine
- 2,4-diaminobutyric acid
- N^3-oxalyldiaminopropionic acid
- Lathyrine

VICIA :
- Canavanine
- 3-cyanoalanine

Canavanine has only been isolated from Papilionoideae and has never been found in any plant belonging to the **Caesalpiniodeae** or **Mimosoideae** subfamilies of the Leguminosae.

Non-proteins amino acids have been found to be systematically significant within some families or genera. Thus the tribes of the **Cucurbitaceae** family can be differentiated according to their non-proteins amino acid content and the presence or absence of substituted asparagines, m-Carboxyphenylalanine or 3-pyrazol-1-yl-alanine has helped to place several genera or species whose morphological relationship was unclear.

$$H_2N-OC-CH_2-CH(NH_2)-COOH \text{ (Asparagine)}$$

The presence or absence of certain characteristic non-protein amino acids confirm the identification between two genera Lathyrus and Vicia of the **Papilionoideae**, which otherwise is not possible to identify the isolated seeds purely on the basis of morphological grounds.

Polyketides in Chemotaxonomy

Large class of compound found in fungi and to a lesser extent in higher plants. Chemically the majority are aromatic derivatives but also as allylic compounds.

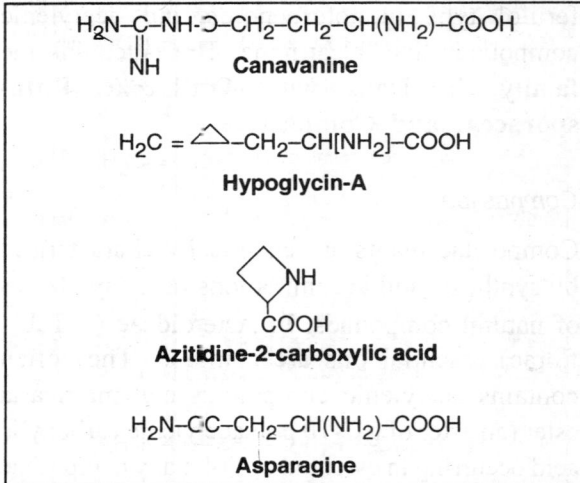

Fig. 7.14. Amino Acids in Chemotaxonomy.

-CO-CH$_2$-CO-CH$_2$-CO-CH$_2$-CO-CH$_2$-

(Polyketide chains)

Note : There is no relationship between families of higher plants biosynthesising of polyketides.

Quinones are biosynthesised in higher plants by several pathways, polyketides derived naphthaquinone does not play much characteristic role in chemotaxonomy of higher plants.

Anthraquinones biosynthesised by acetate malonate pathways are found in **polygonaceae, Leguminosae and Rhamnaceae** families.

Other polyketides with taxonomic significance include Vesicant, long-chains phenols such as **Urushiol**, which are characteristic of the family Anacardiaceae.

Amines in Chemotaxonomy

The wide spread of amines in plants limit the usefulness of amine in chemotaxonomy. In general plants with flowers synthesising volatile aliphatic amine are common amongst the **Caprifoliaceae, Cornaceae, Rosaceae and Araceae families, while the Papilionoideae and Labiatae** are almost devoid of such flowers.

The di and polyamines occurs widely but monoamine and 3-aminopropionitrile has been found only in three species of Lathyrus (Leguminosae), *L. odoratus, L. hirutus* and *L. roseus.*

Some of **heterocyclic amine**, such as noradrenaline, ephedrine and histamine have an erratic distribution while **mescaline** appears to be restricted to members of the **Cactaceae.**

APPLICATIONS OF CHEMOTAXONOMY

Plant Division

Chemical characters always advantageous over morphological character being more precise and easily identifiable/detectable as example **Flavonoids** are generally found in Bryophyta except

one or two reports where it has been reported the isolation of crystalline anthocyanin from a red Bryum species (which on hydrolysis produce luteolinidin) was being reported. Similarly, **Lignin** that no plant lower than mosses contains a substance like lignin. Hence **lignin and flavonoids** are common in almost all plants groups higher than the **bryophytes.** It is found that lignin from gymnosperms, mono and dicotyledons usually exhibit characteristic chemical differences.

All the **Centrospermae** (except caryophyllineae) contain betacyanins (betanin) this betacyanins also occur in the order *Opuntiales* (Cactaceae), which further supports to the botanists assumption that the order Centrospermae and *Opuntiales* are phylogenetically related.

There are few others chemical substances which confirms relations between those two orders - Isoquinoline alkaloids, **Salsoline** in a Salsola species (**Chenopodiaceae**) and Carnegine in a Cactaceae; Corypalline from a Corydalis species (**Papaveraceae**) having the similar isoquinoline nucleus in their structures.

Related Genera having similar Enzyme System producing Analogous Metabolites

The pyrrolizidine alkaloids (Senecio) are analogous with quinolizidine (Lupin), although their precursors are ornithine and lysine respectively but they have similar enzyme system. However it has also been observed that both type of alkaloid have been found to occur in botanically related genera e.g. "Senecio alkaloids" reported to occur in **Crotalaria** (Leguminosae, Papiolionatae) and "Lupin alkaloids" have been isolated from **Lupinus and Cytisus** (Pepilionatae) both belonging to Genistae genera, which also cover crotalaria, other examples is of **"furo"** and pyranoquinolines which belong to family Rutaceae and Amaryllidaceae respectively also have similar enzyme systems.

Complex Metabolic Products are Good Chemotaxonomic Marker

The occurrence of complex secondary metabolites like biflavonoids and complex alkaloids are helpful in the classification of medicinal plants.

The **Biflavonoids** are plant polyphenols, widely distributed in the plant kingdom with over 4000 different structures. Structurally, they are divided into several subclasses; **Flavanol, Anthocyanins and Chalcones**.

They are biosynthesised through a combination of the shikimic acid and the acylpolymalonate pathways. They are omni present in vascular plants but more **rarely in bryophytes**. Some biflavonoids classes have a restricted distribution; e.g. isoflavonoids occur predominantly in the **Fabaceae** family. The **biflavonyls** have mainly been reported in **leaves of gymnosperms**.

It has been reported that the **Biflavonyls** are absent in the **genera of Pinaceae**, hence the inability to synthesize biflavonyls can be used as a characteristic of the order **Pinales** hence the complex structure compounds like biflavonyls are very important for the chemical classification of the gymnosperms.

Complex Alkaloid Structure

The total number of Indole alkaloids of known structure amount to about 1100. The most important subgroup of indole alkaloids is formed by the **aspidospermine** type and related bases with about 250 representatives. In this subgroup about fifteen types of nucleus are reported. These alkaloids are present in Apocynaceae, Euphorbiaceae and Rubiaceae but the **Plumerane** (subgroup of Indole) alkaloids occur only in one plant of family Apocynaceae. In this sub group the three types of nucleus are isolated (Fig. 7.15).

1. Tetrahydrosecodine
2. (–) Quebrachamine
3. (+) Dihydrocleavamine

The family Apocynaceae can be subdivided into three subfamilies:

1. Plumieroideae
   • Alstonieae
   • Rauwolfieae
   • Allamandeae
2. Cerberoideae
   • Skytantheae
   • Thevetieae

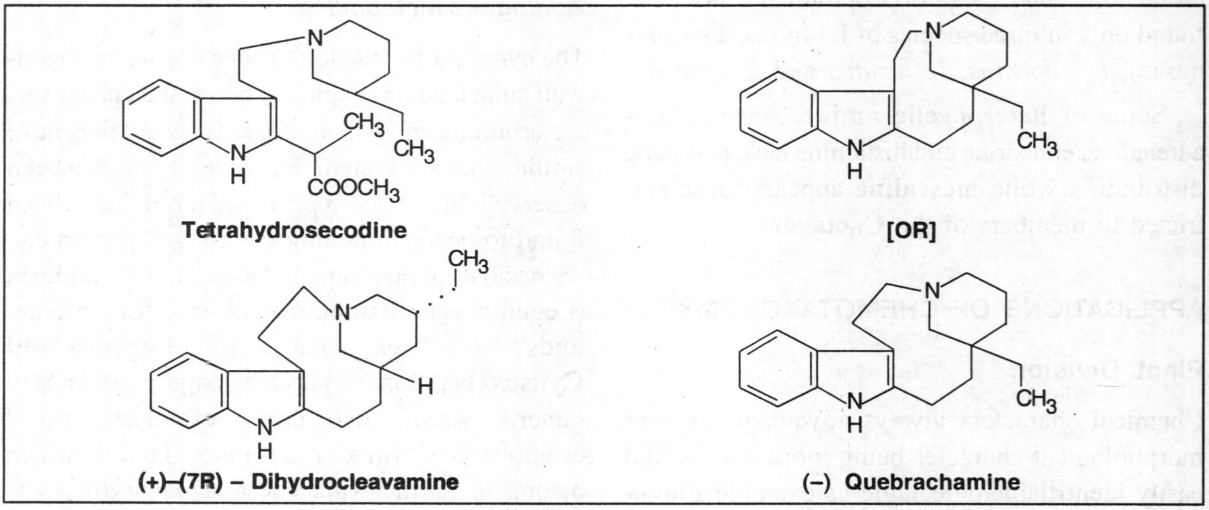

Tetrahydrosecodine

[OR]

(+)–(7R) – Dihydrocleavamine

(–) Quebrachamine

Fig. 7.15. Alkaloids of Pulmerane group.

3. Echitoideae
   - Parsonsieae
   - Nerieae
   - Ecdysanthereae
   - Ichonocarpeae

A large number of different alkaloids have been reported from species belonging to these three subfamilies. **Indole** alkaloids (gramine), however, have been found in the subfamily **Plumieroideae** only, apart from indole alkaloids – the **steroidal** alkaloids (solasodine), monoterpenoid **piperidine** alkaloid of the **skytanthine** type (α-skytanthine, coniine and piperine) and **spermidine** alkaloids

(inandenine) as well as the dimeric piperidine derivative **carpine**. Skytanthine bases are the sole alkaloid type, which have been found in the **Cerberoideae**. Steroidal alkaloids have been isolated only from plants of the subfamily **Echitoideae** and from those of the genus *Holarrhena*, which belongs to the first subfamily **Plumieroideae**. There is a striking relationship between this genus and the subfamily **Echitoideae** based on taxonomic criteria, which suggests the classification of Apocynaceae into three subfamilies, which is further confirmed on the basis of different structures of indole alkaloids (Fig. 7.16).

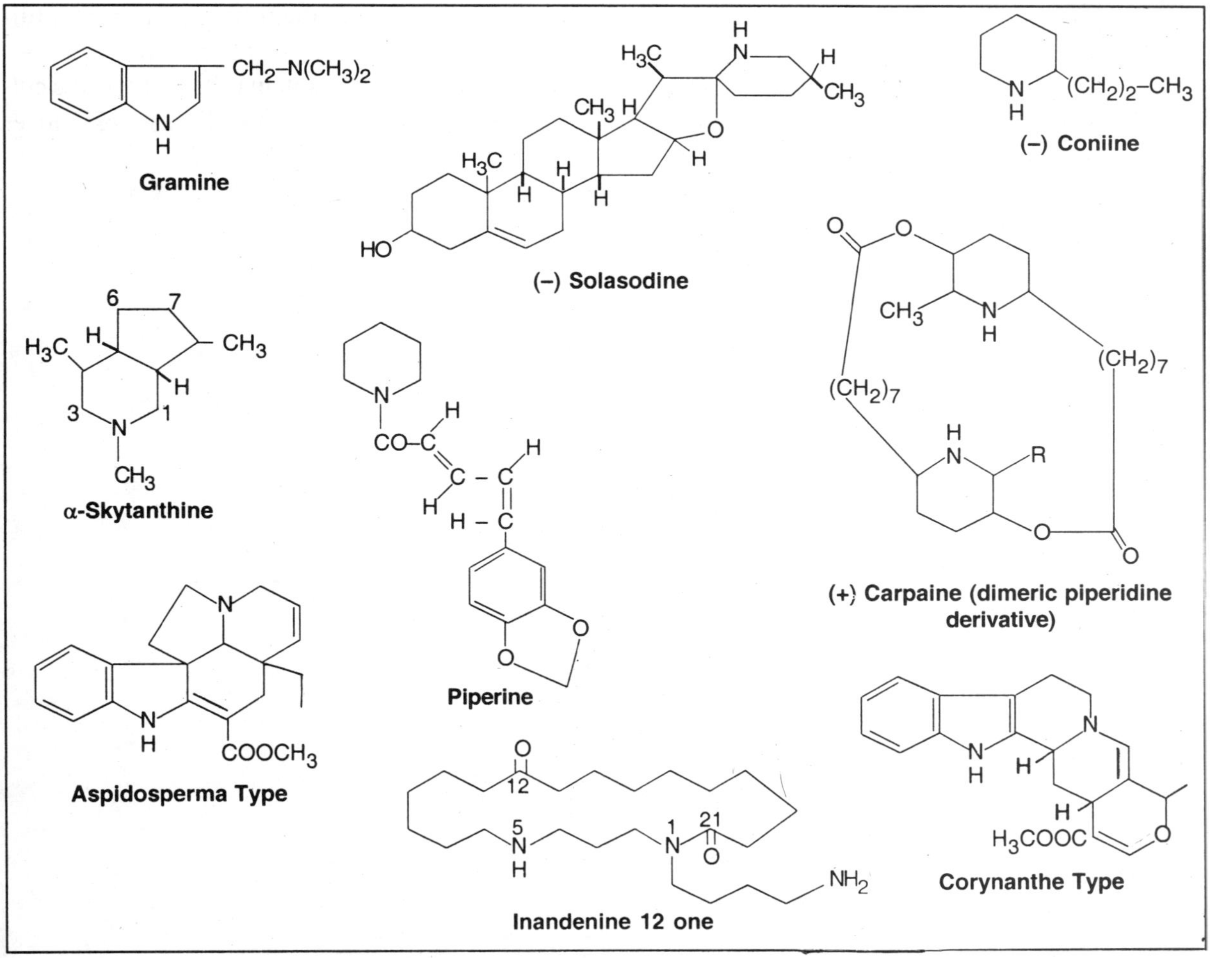

Fig. 7.16. Complex Alkaloids in Chemotaxo

CHEMOTAXONOMY AND ECONOMIC AND MEDICAL BOTANY

Phytochemists and economic botanists are often looking for new sources of important chemical compounds (examples: colchicine, quinine, reserpine, digitoxin) or classes of constituents (examples: tanning materials, complex indole alkaloids). Generally they will be most successful when they follow the lead of natural classification supplemented by phytochemical knowledge, i.e. if they use the chemotaxonomic approach. There are many examples, the few given suffice, however, to illustrate the fact that comparative phytochemistry combined with an adequate plant classification is an excellent guide for chemical exploration of the plant world.

The same is true for prevention and treatment of plant poisoning of animals and man. If poisoning is caused by a plant species related to *Colchicum autumnale*, for instant by *Gloriosa superba* from a bunch of flowers or by *Bulbocodium vernum* cultivated in a garden, it will be wiser to suspect colchicine poisoning and to act accordingly. The same holds for the many types of plant contact dermatitis. **Tuliposide-A** and its allergenic product of hydrolysis, **tulipalin-A**, not only occur in all species of the large genus Tulipa, but also in related liliaceous genera such as Erythronium, Gagea and Alstroemeria. Very recently Hausen et al reported that species of Lilium and Allium triquetrum, but not Asparagus officinalis, contain moderate amounts of 1-tuliposide-A. These authors suggested that breeding of the above mentioned ornamental liliaceous taxa for high tuliposide-B and low tuliposide-A content could result in mildly allergenic cultivators retaining a reasonable disease resistance.

Marine Pharmacognosy
(Novel Medicinal Agents from Marine Source)

INTRODUCTION

Marine Pharmacognosy is a sub-branch of pharmacognosy, which is mainly concerned with the naturally occurring substances of medicinal value from marine. It is not a new area for pharmacognosy, even the early civilizations of Greece, Japan, China and India have explored marine life as a source of drugs. In the western medicine **agar, alginic acid, carrageenan, protamine sulphate, spermaceti and cod & halibut** liver oils are the marine medicinal established products.

The oceans cover more than 70% of the earth's surface and contain over 200,000 invertebrates and algal species.

Macroalgae or seaweeds have been used as crude drugs in the treatment of iodine deficiency states such as goitre etc. Some seaweeds have also been utilized as sources of additional vitamins and in the treatment of anaemia during pregnancy. Marine products have also been used for the treatment of various intestinal disorders as vermifuges, hypochloesterolaemic and hypoglycemic agent e.g. *Cystoseria barbata*; *Sargassum confusam* and *Jania rubens*.

Seaweeds have also been employed as dressing materials, ointments and in gynaecology. For example, *Porphyra atropurpurea* have been used in Hawaii to dress wounds and burns; and *Durvillaea antractica* to treat scabies in New Zealand. Prepared, sterilized stripes of *Laminaria digitala* in conjunction with prostaglandins have been used to dilate the cervix, as the strips swell up to several times to their original diameter when moistened.

During the last 30-40 years numerous novel compounds have been isolated from marine organisms having biological activities such as antibacterial, antiviral, antitumour, antiparasitic, anticoagulants, antimicrobial, anti-inflammatory and cardiovascular active products.

Marine flora and funa play significant role as a source of new molecular entity. The oceans of the world contain over 5 million species in about 30 phyla. Because of the diversities of marine organism and habitats, marine natural products enclose a wide variety of chemical classes, including **terpenes, shikimates, polyketides, acetogenins, peptides, alkaloids** of varying structures and a multitude of compounds of mixed biosynthesis.

While terrestrial sources have yielded numerous drugs, marine natural products represent a relatively untapped resources for new drug development. The marine environment may contain over 80% of the world's plant and animal species. During the past 30-40 years, numerous novel compounds have been isolated from marine organisms and many of these have been reported to have biological activities, some of which are of interest from the point of view of potential drug development. On the other hand some of the compounds pose potential risk to human health. In this latter category are the **paralytic or diarrhetic and amnesic shellfish toxins**. The former can be fatal, but the latter, although producing very unpleasant effects, are not fatal. Both paralytic and diarrhetic shellfish toxins are produced by dinoflagellates, while amnesic shellfish, poisoning result from the ingestion of shellfish contaminated with diatoms. The ingestion of other marine organisms which can also lead to serious poisoning, include the potent neurotoxin, tetrodotoxin, resulting from eating pufferfish and ciguatoxin, associated with ingestion of tropical fish which have fed on the dinoflagellate, *Gambierdiscus toxicus*.

MARINE ORGANISM AS POTENTIAL SOURCE OF DRUGS

Knowledge of biological activities and/or chemical constituents of marine organisms is important not only for the discovery of new therapeutic agents but such informations may also be of immense value in exploring, new sources of economic materials, precursors for the synthesis of complex chemical substances and compounds of novel chemical structure. thereby prompting the chemist for the synthesis of a series of modified compounds of therapeutical importance. Thus, in recent years, considerable importance is attached to the discovery of new biodynamic agents from marine source to search new source of drugs from sea.

A survey of literature indicated that extracts from marine organisms had been evaluated for various biological activities. This has led to the isolation of substances possessing antimicrobial, antibiotic, antiviral, anticancer, cardioactive, anti-inflammatory, anthelmintic, anticoagulant neurophysiological and insecticidal activities.

Although, numerous compounds have been isolated from marine organisms and the biological activities attributed to many of them; but still very few of them have been marketed or are under development. There are number of reasons that is why more number of compounds originating from marine plants and animals have not been developed. There is no doubt that much of the work undertaken in the 1960s, 1970s and probably the early 1980s was driven by an interest in the chemistry of new compounds rather than in their biological activities. The earlier studies on chemistry of marine natural products were limited to the isolation, structure elucidation and phylogenetic relationship of specific substances, such as quinonoid pigments and sterols. Now this field attracted the attention of not only the natural product chemists but also those of marine biologist, biochemist, pharmacologist etc. The invention of the aqualung and the advent of new technology in the past few decades led to the awareness that the oceans may be a new frontier of biomedical research, as it has a vast resources for the discovery of marine derived medicine. Increasing sophistication of the tools available to explore the deep sea has expanded the habitats, which can be sampled; and has greatly improved the opportunities for discovery of novel metabolites.

Much of the earlier work limited the biological testing to antimicrobial activity, but this was often extended later to testing for cytotoxic properties, which may provide useful leads for anticancer drugs. This latter area is one that most of the compounds in various stages of clinical trials are located. Screening for other activities has of course, also been undertaken, for example for antiviral, anti-inflammatory, anticoagulant, antiparasitic and prostaglandins.

Many of the marine compounds have shown promising biological properties but have complicated chemical structures, the synthesis of which would be hard and expensive. These organisms are valuable as source of new biologically active chemical structures, but unless either the compounds or a derivative of them can be readily synthesized they are of little commercial interest to the pharmaceutical industry.

CONOTOXIN

Conotoxin (Conus venom) present in marine are used to develop new moiety drugs for producing receptor mediated effects without much side effects e.g. CNS drugs, antihypertensive, antiasthamatic and neurovascular blocking agents.

The active principle site of action of these toxins are peptide with disulphide linkage. About four conotoxins are of therapeutically importance.

Marine Algae

Four types of marine algae reported:

1. Cyanophyceae (Blue green algae)
2. Chlorophyceae (Green algae)
3. Phacophyceae (Brown algae)
4. Rhodophyceae (Red algae)

These algae are of significant importance in therapy. They are being used as CNS drugs, antimicrobial agents, antifouling, antiviral, anticoagulant, hypotensive, diuretic and hypoglycemic agents.

ANTIMICROBIAL COMPOUNDS

Cephalosporins : Discovered in the 50's from a marine fungus, Cephalosporium acremonium Cephalosporin C (Fig. 8.1) was isolated. The modification of the original cephalosporin (cephelothin sodium), has been widely used as an

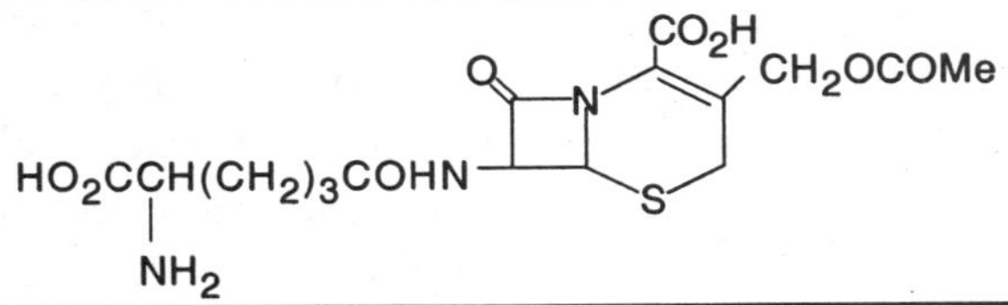

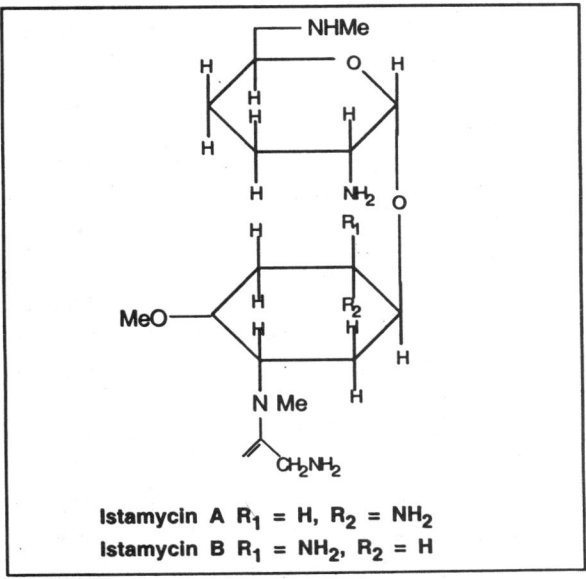

Fig. 8.1. Cephalosporin C.

antibiotic drug active against microbes insensitive to penicillin and ampicillins.

Marine organisms, which can be grown in culture labs to yield valuable compounds, would be of interest to the pharmaceutical industry. Istamycin is one of the compounds, which have been obtained by fermentation of marine organism.

Istamycins (Fig. 8.2) : These are the fermentation products of marine microoganism, Streptomyces lenjimariensis SS-939. These compounds are reported to have in vitro activity against both gram-negative and gram-positive bacteria, including those with known resistance to the aminoglycoside antibiotics.

Istamycin A R_1 = H, R_2 = NH_2
Istamycin B R_1 = NH_2, R_2 = H

Fig. 8.2. Istamycin.

Marine sponges are colourful and have resistance for bacterial decomposition; they can be the potential source of novel antimicrobial agent. On screening of sponges, it was observed that sponges of family Verongidae contain a series of antimicrobials and closely related compounds.

A list of few antibacterial or antimicrobial, agents isolated from sponges given in Table 8.1.

Novel series of **sesquiterpenes** have also been isolated from sponges such as **nitenin** and **furospongin** from *Spongia nitens* and *Spongia officinalis* respectively.

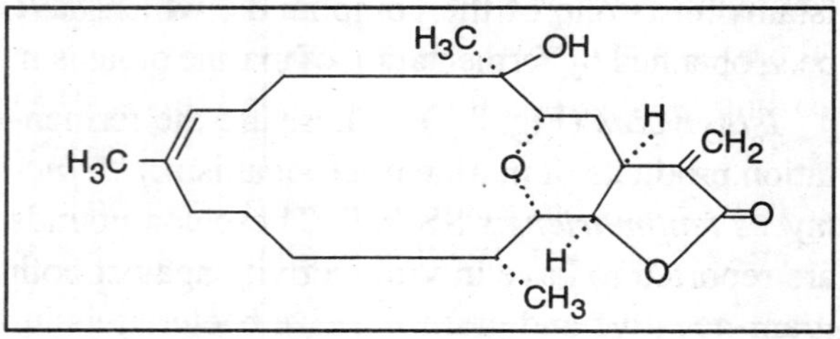

Antimicrobial agents are obtained from *Gorgonian corals* belonging to phylum Cnidaria.

Eunicin (Fig. 8.3) – a macrocyclic cembrenoid compound has been isolated from gorgonian *Eunicia mammosa* with antibacterial activity.

ANTIMICROBIAL AND ANTIBIOTIC ACTIVITY FROM ALGAE

Zonarol and Isozonarol (Fig. 8.4) obtained from brown algae *Dictyopteris zonariodes* have fungicidal properties.

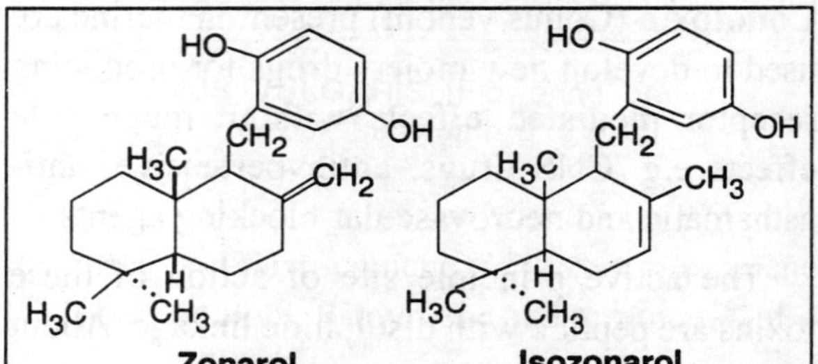

Fig. 8.3. Eunicin.

Fig. 8.4. Zonarol and Isozonarol.

Table 8.1. Antibacterial, antimicrobial and antibiotic agents isolated from marine sponges

Name	Structure (see page 167, from no.1 to 14)	Source	Biological Activity
3,5, dibromo-1-hydroxy-4-oxo-2, 5-cyclo-hexadiene-1 acetamide	(1)	*Verongia cauliformis, V. fistularis, V. aerophoba, V. thiona*	Antibiotic
3, 5-dibromo-1-hydroxy-4, 4-dimethoxy 2, 5 cyclo-hexadiene-1-acetamide	(2)	*V. cauliformis*	Antibacterial
Aeroplysinin-1 (+)	(3)	*Verongia aerophoba*	Antimicrobial
Aeroplysinin-1 (–)	(4)	*Lanthella aridis*	Antimicrobial
2-cyano-4, 5 dibromopyrrole	(5)	*Agelas oroides*	Antimicrobial
5, 6-dibromo-1H-indole-3-ethanamine	(6)	*Polyfibrospongia maynardii*	Antibacterial
5, 6-dibromo-1-H- ndole-3 (N-methyl ethanamine)	(7)	*Polyfibrospongia maynardii*	Antibacterial
3-Bromo-2-(4-bromophenoxy)-phenol	(8)	*Dysidea herbacea*	Antibacterial
Monobromo and Dibromophakellin	(9)	*Phakellia flabellata*	Antimicrobial
Acanthellin-1	(10)	*Acanthella acuta*	Antibacterial
Nitenin (sesquiterpene)	(11)	*Spongia nitens*	Antibacterial
Furospongin-1	(12)	*Spongia officinalis*	Antibacterial
Ircinin-1	(13)	*Iricinia oros.*	Antibacterial
Variabilin	(14)	*Iricinia variabilis*	Antibacterial

Antibacterial, antimicrobial and antibiotic agents from marine Sponges

Tetrabromo heptanone (Fig. 8.5) has shown antimicrobial properties against large number of micro-organisms. It is obtained from red algae *Bonnemaisonia hemifera*.

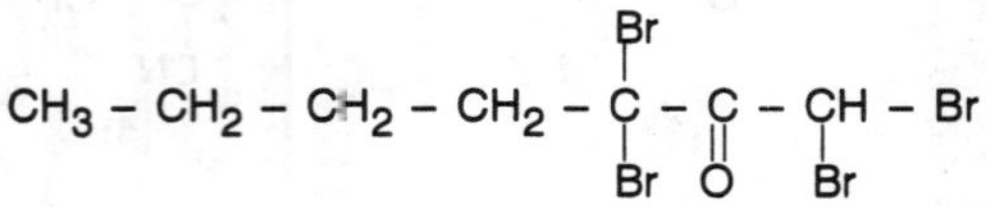

$$CH_3 - CH_2 - CH_2 - CH_2 - \underset{\underset{Br}{|}}{C} - \underset{\underset{O}{||}}{C} - \underset{\underset{Br}{|}}{CH} - Br$$

Fig. 8.5. Tetrabromo heptanone.

Polyhalo-acetones (Fig. 8.6) and its isomers and four *polyhalo-3-butene-gone* obtained from red algae *Aspargopsis taxiformis*, possess antimicrobial properties.

Sargassum species (brown algae) contain brominated polyphenol, which is used as antimicrobial agent as well as antifouling agents.

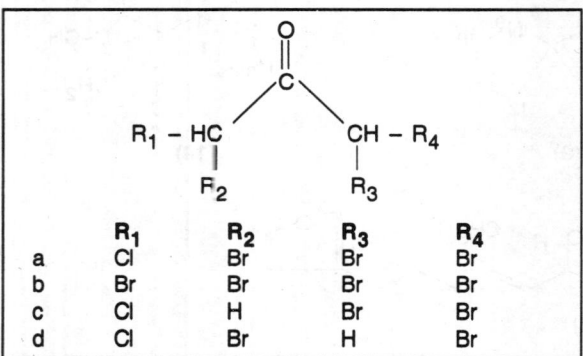

	R_1	R_2	R_3	R_4
a	Cl	Br	Br	Br
b	Br	Br	Br	Br
c	Cl	H	Br	Br
d	Cl	Br	H	Br

Fig. 8.6. Polyhalo acetone.

ANTIVIRAL COMPOUNDS

Many marine micro-organisms have been screened for antiviral activity and wide range of active compounds have been reported, but only few compounds are reported to have significant therapeutic activity and these are:

Anti viral and Anti HIV agents : Laminaran species from brown algae are reported to have anti viral, anti HIV and anti coagulant activity.

Ara-A (Fig. 8.7) : It is a semi-synthetic compound based on the arabinosyl nucleosides isolated from the sponge *Tethya crypta*.

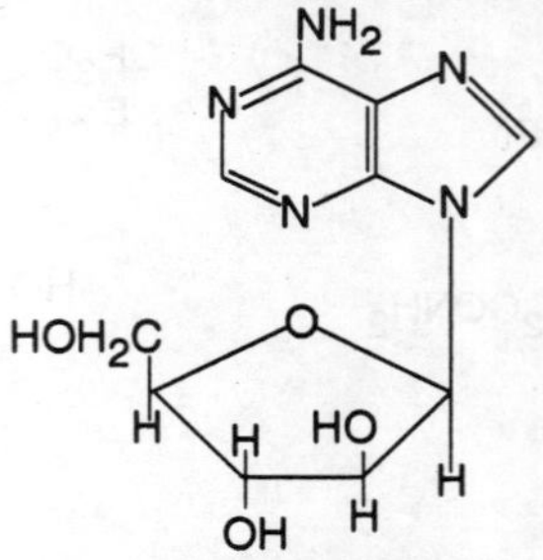

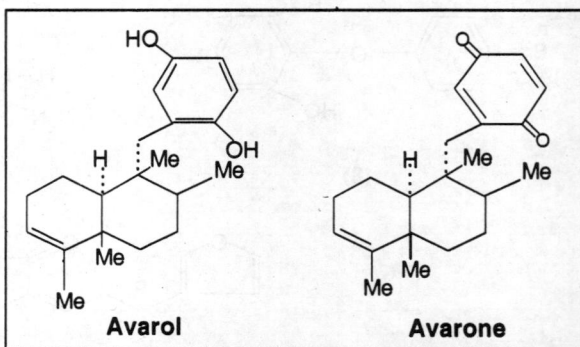

Fig. 8.7. Ara-A.

Avarol and Avarone (Fig. 8.8) : These compounds are isolated from a sponge, *Disidea avara*. These compounds inhibit the **immunodeficiency** virus, have high therapeutic indices and the ability to cross blood brain barrier.

Avarol

Avarone

Fig. 8.8. Avarol and Avarone.

Didemnins : These are cyclic depsipeptides isolated from tunicate, *Trididemnum* species.

Eudistomin A (Fig. 8.9) *and β-Carbolines :* This is also isolated from tunicate, *Eudistoma olivaceum*.

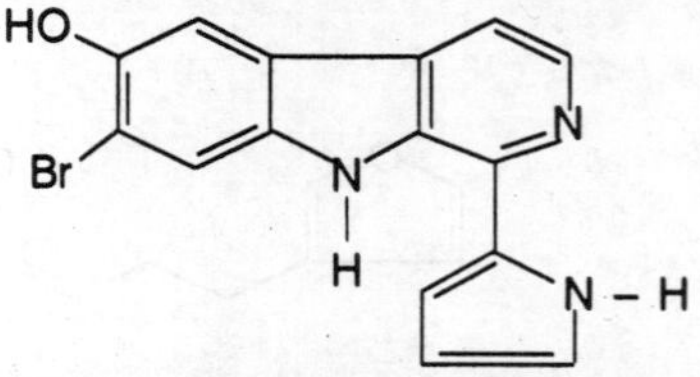

Fig. 8.9. Eudistomin A.

Laurenterol (Fig. 8.10) possessing antibacterial activity against gram-positive bacteria obtained from *Laurencia* spp. (*Ophioderma variegatum*) and from the sea hare *Aplysia catifornica*.

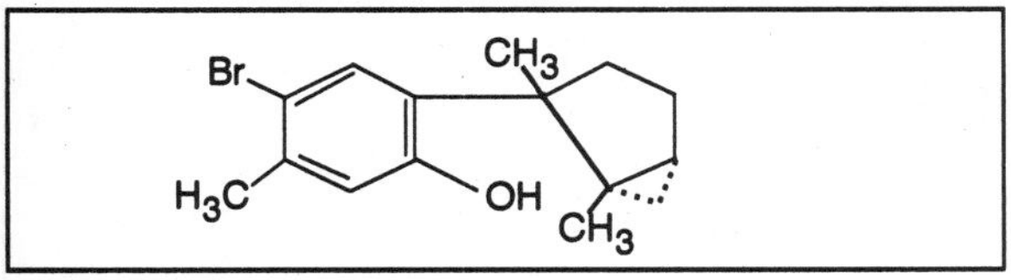

Fig. 8.10. Laurenterol.

Oppositol [Fig. 8.10(a)] antibacterial agent from Laurencia suboppostia; against *Staphylococcus aureus*.

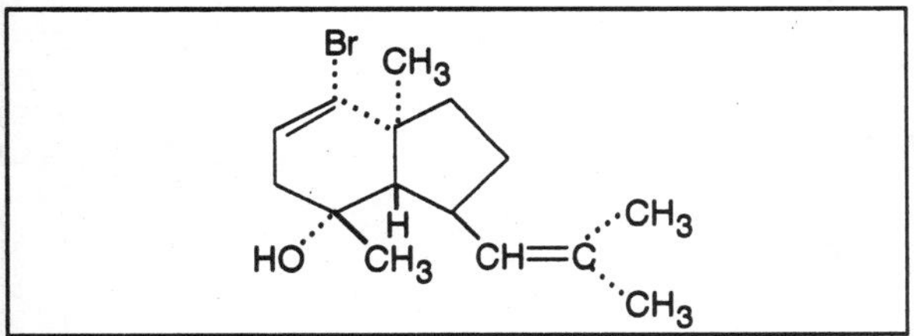

Fig. 8.10(a). Oppositol.

Patellazol B (Fig. 8.11) isolated from the tunicate, *Lissoclinum patella* has very potent *in vitro* activity against Herpes simplex viruses.

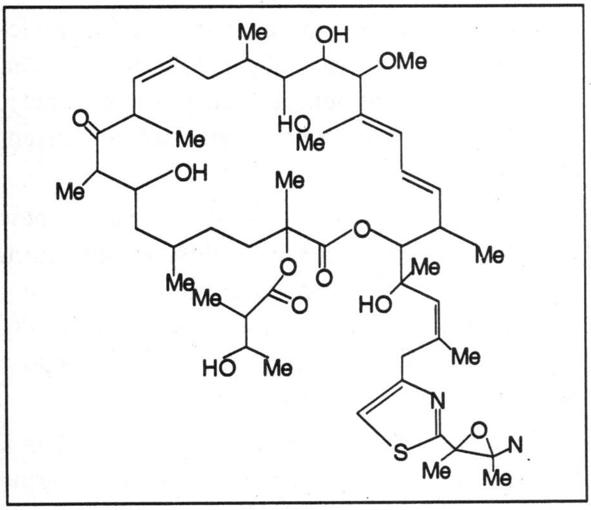

Fig. 8.11. Patellazol B.

CYTOTOXIC COMPOUNDS

Large number of compounds isolated from marine organisms have been tested for cytotoxicity in the search for drugs active against cancer. Among all, the best known novel compounds with high potential as anticancer drugs are found to be macrolides, known as **bryostatins** isolated primarily from the **bryozoan**, *Bugula neritina* and later some have been extracted from sponges and tunicates.

Many Bryostatins (1-18) are reported to have antileukaemic activity but only Bryostatin-1 and Bryostatin-2 have undergone phase 2 clinical trials.

Bryostatin (Fig. 8.12) triggers activation and differentiation of peripheral blood cells from Lymphocytic leukemia patients. It also causes activation of protein Kinase C and arachidonic acid metabolite release. Both Bryostatin 1 and 2 enhance the efficiency of interleukin-2, in initiating the development of **in vivo** primed cytotoxic T-lymphocytes.

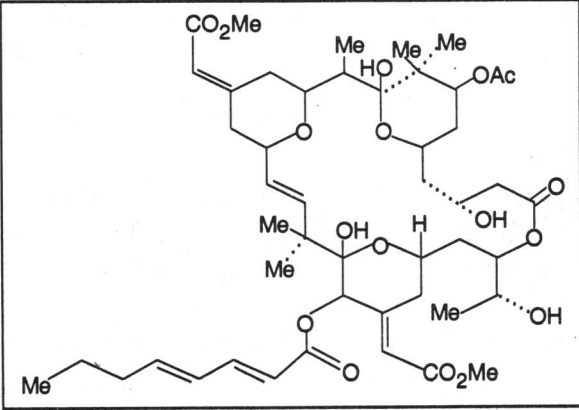

Fig. 8.12. Bryostatin-I.

Dolastatins is a family of cyclic and linear peptides and depsipeptides; isolated from the sea hare, *Dolabella auricularia*. The highly cytotoxic compounds are Dolastatin-10, Dolastatin-H and Isodolastatin-H (Fig. 8.13).

In addition to the peptides, the polypropionate,

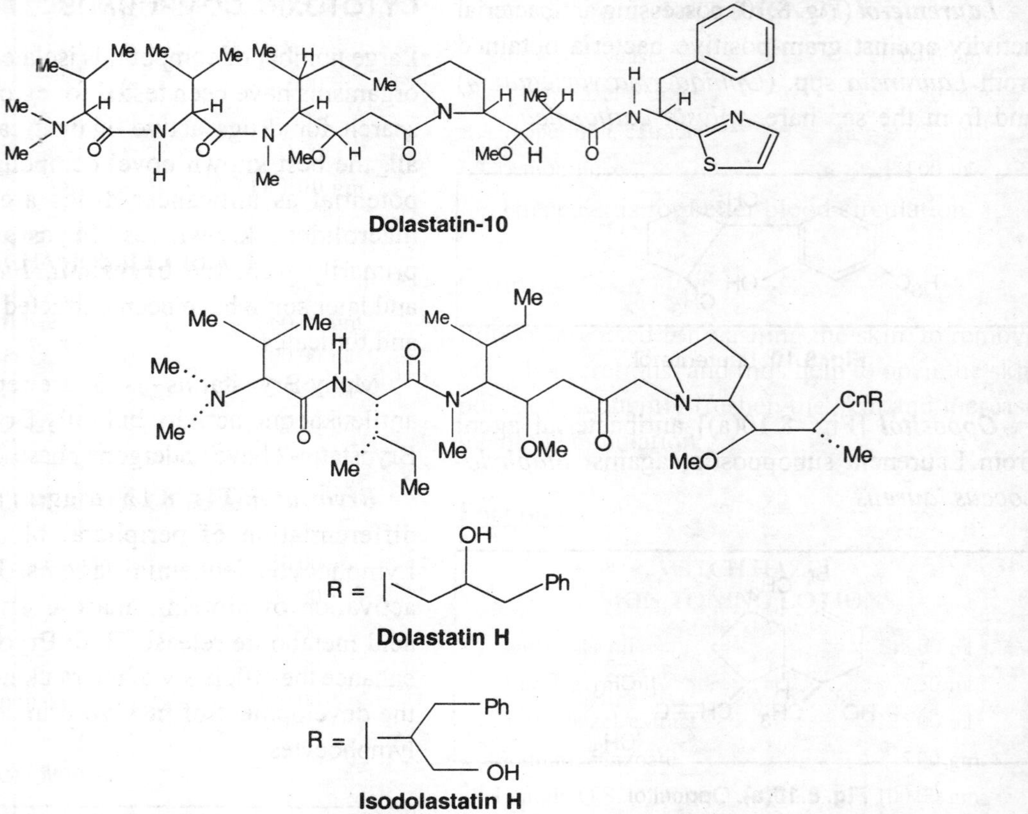

Fig. 8.13.

Antipyrone A and B have also been extracted from *D. auricularia*.

Eleutherobin is a compound obtained from a marine encrusting gorgonian *Erythropodium caribaeorum*. It is extremely potent for inducing *in vitro* tubulin polymerization and is toxic to cancer cells with an IC-50 similar to that of taxol.

Xenia a novel diterpene called xenicane isolated from the soft coral *Xenia elongata*. This compound has shown some effectiveness in inhibiting mitochondria respiration in cancer cells.

Nephthea : The soft Coral Nephthea reported to contain a bioactive compound **Lemnabourside** which is 5 alpha-reductase inhibitor. It is quite active in prostate cancer cells, as they tend to be androgen dependent. The drug possess ability to inhibit the conversion of testosterone into more potent dihydrotestosterone.

Halimide : A low molecular pectin like molecule isolated from green algae *Helimeda opuntia*, used in the treatment of early stage cancer, particularly breast cancer resistant to current chemotherapy.

Ecteinascidin 743 (ET-743), a natural new product isolated from the *Caribbean* sea squirt. It is totally novel and different from existing anticancer drugs. ET-743 have shown high activity in cases of advanced sarcoma, that had relapsed or were resistant to conventional therapy.

Yondelis TM (ET-743) : Yondelis TM is a new anti-tumour drug derived from the marine organism *Ecteinascidia turbimata* a "Sea Squirt" or tunicate found in the Caribbean and Mediterranean sea. It is still at the stage of being an investigational drug and it has been suggested (USA) that drug is quite useful in the treatment of patient with advanced STS after failure of conventional chemotherapy.

Aplidine : Spanish biotechnology firm Zeltia, developed this drug from a marine organism, Mediterranean tunicate *Aplidium albicans*, against medullary thyroid carcinoma.

It is reported that Aplidin, **a novel antitumour** agent of marine origin undergoing phase II clinical trials, induces growth arrest and apoptosis in human MDA-MB-231 breast cancer cells at nanomolar concentrations.

Ara-C a potent inhibitor of tumour such as Sarcoma-180, Erlich carcinoma and L-1210 leukaemia in mice. It is also reported to be active against acute myelogenous leukaemia and human acute leukaemia. It is one of the standard drugs used in the treatment of **acute leukaemia**; both in children and adults.

Ara-C is a semi-synthetic drug originated from the *Caribbean sponge*, the basic compound was **spongothymidine**, which led to the synthesis of **1-α-D-arabinofuranosyl** cytosine (Ara-C), developed and marketed by Upjohn Pharmaceutical Company as **Cytosar**.

Ara-A : It is another synthetic analog to adenine arabinoside, of Ara-C compound. The reports says the compound to be effective for the treatment of *Herpes encephalitis*.

Asperidol : It is a non-lactonic cembranoid obtained from gorgonian coral, have **anti-cancer** activity.

Aplysistatin (LSV) an **antileukaemic** agent obtained from sea hare *Aplysia angasi*.

Dola-triol (LIV) : Active **antileukaemic** agent possessing different diterpenoid ring system has been reported from the Indian Ocean sea hare *Dolabella auricuiaria* **Holuthurin**. It is a toxic

triterpenoid glycoside obtained from sea cucumbers belonging to phylum *Echinodermata* (*Actinopyga agassizi*) are reported to inhibit the growth of sarcoma-180 and adenocarcinoma in mice.

Thelothurin A and thelothurin-B : These both are cytotoxic saponin obtained from sea cucumber *Thelonata anasas*.

Spongouridine isolated from Caribbean sponge *Cryptothya crypta*, has shown promising **antiviral** and antitumour activities.

Tocotrienol (Lx) : An antitumour compound, isolated from water soluble extract of *Sargassum tortile*, (Brown algae).

CARDIOVASCULAR AND NEUROPHYSIOLOGICAL AGENTS

Anthopleurin-A is a heart stimulant possessing four times more activity than natural cardiac glycosides (digitalis and strophanthus). It is a polypeptide in nature, isolated from sea anemone *Anthopleura xanthogrammica*.

Eledoisin is a peptide obtained from posterior salivary glands of eledone spp. *Eledone moschata* and related species. It is fifty times more potent than acetylcholine, histamine or bradykinin ion provoking hypotension. It is a potent vasodilator and hypotensive agent.

Eptatretin is a potent cardiac stimulant, having direct action on mammalian myocardium as produced by epinephrine and digitalis glycosides. It is obtained from aneural bronchial heart of the Pacific hagfish *Eptatretus stoutii*.

D-octopamine is an amine found in salivary glands of octopus spp. *O-vulgaris, O-macropus* and *Eledone moschata*. It is a potent cardiotonic.

Laminin belongs to heterotrimeric glycoproteins and is obtained from marine algae *Laminaria angustata*.

It has potent hypotensive effect on mammals.

Tetrodotoxin is a toxin but possessing cardiovascular and neurophysiological activities. It is obtained from the skin and testis of Goby, *Gobius criniger*; and also from the skin of male and female Costa Rican frog, *Atelopus chiriquensis*.

α-Cintotoxin, ω-Iontoxin, μ-ionotoxin and κ-contotoxin

α-Conotoxin is obtained from *C. figulinus*. It is used in stroke, Parkinson's disease as muscle relaxant, antihypertensive agents and analgesic.

ω-Conotoxin is obtained from *C. geographus*. It is used to block neuronal calcium channels at pre-synaptic terminal of neuromuscular junction like nifidipine and nitradipine.

μ-Conotoxin is also obtained from *C. geographus* and used in ischemia.

κ-Conotoxins blocks potassium channel and is used in hypertension, arrythmia and asthma.

ANTI-INFLAMMATORY AGENTS

Pseudopterosins

These are the group of diterpene glycosides. The **pseudopterosins-1** and **seco-pseudopterosins-3** were isolated from *Caribbean octocorals* but are found in small quantity. Both have shown more potent anti-inflammatory activity in comparison to indomethacin.

Marine bi-indole

The bi-indole compound is obtained from *Rivularia firma* (Marine cyanobacterium) and is quite potent anti-inflammatory compound active in both, the carrageenan (Sulphated polysaccharide carrageenan) induced rat paw oedema and kaolin induced rat paw oedema (Non-immune inflammatory response).

Manoalide

It is a non-steroidal anti-inflammatory and pain killer compound obtained from marine sponge *Luffariella variabilis*.

Dendalone-3-hydroxy-butyrate

It is marine anti-inflammatory agent obtained from sponge *Phyllospongia dendyi*.

Tetrabromo heptanone has been isolated from red algae.

ANTHELMINTIC

Kainic acid ($C_{10}H_{15}NO_4$)

A valuable anthelmintic used clinically in Japan against parasitic round worm, tapeworm and for the treatment of ascariasis. It is obtained from red algae (dried) *Digenea simplex*.

Domoic acid ($C_{15}H_{21}NO_6$)

It is obtained from red algae **chondria armata**. It is also used in the treatment of ascariasis and is effective in expelling another parasite pinworm.

ANTICOAGULANTS

Acanthaphora from red algae contain Laminaran sulphate used as anticoagulant.

Carrageenan

Carrageenan isolated from species of *Chondrus*, *Eucheuma* and *Gigartina*, reported to have anti-coagulant activity.

Laminarin

A highly sulphated laminarin (polysaccharide from marine algae) has been reported to have anti-coagulant activity.

PROSTAGLANDINS

The term prostaglandlin is often abbreviated as

PG, PGE$_2$, denotes a protaglandlin of the E series with two double bonds.

Prostaglandins are a family of cyclic oxygenated, C$_{20}$ fatty acid (Prostanoic acid (Fig. 8.14)) derivative substances which consist of a cyclopentane ring with two side chains having 7 and 8

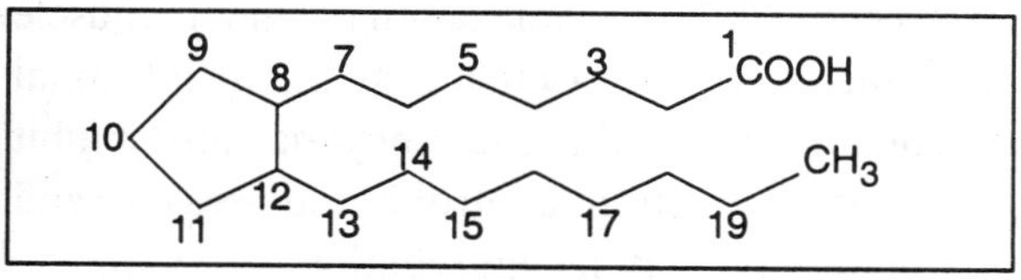

Fig. 8.14. Prostanoic acid.

carbon atoms, respectively. The carboxylic group is present on C$_7$ chain and a C$_8$ chain with methyl terminus. Prostaglandins are biosynthesised from three essential fatty acids, $\Delta^{8,11,14}$ eicosatrienoic (dihomo-γ-linolenic acids), $\Delta^{5,8,11,14}$ eicosatetraenoic acid (arachidonic acid) and $\Delta^{5,8,11,14,17}$ eicosapentaenoic acid, which yield prostaglandins of the 1-, 2- and 3- series respectively known as PGE$_1$, PGE$_2$ and PGE$_3$ (Fig. 8.15).

Name prostaglandins was given due to the fact that they were first discovered in seminal fluid, although later on, it was reported that they are not only produced in the prostate gland but

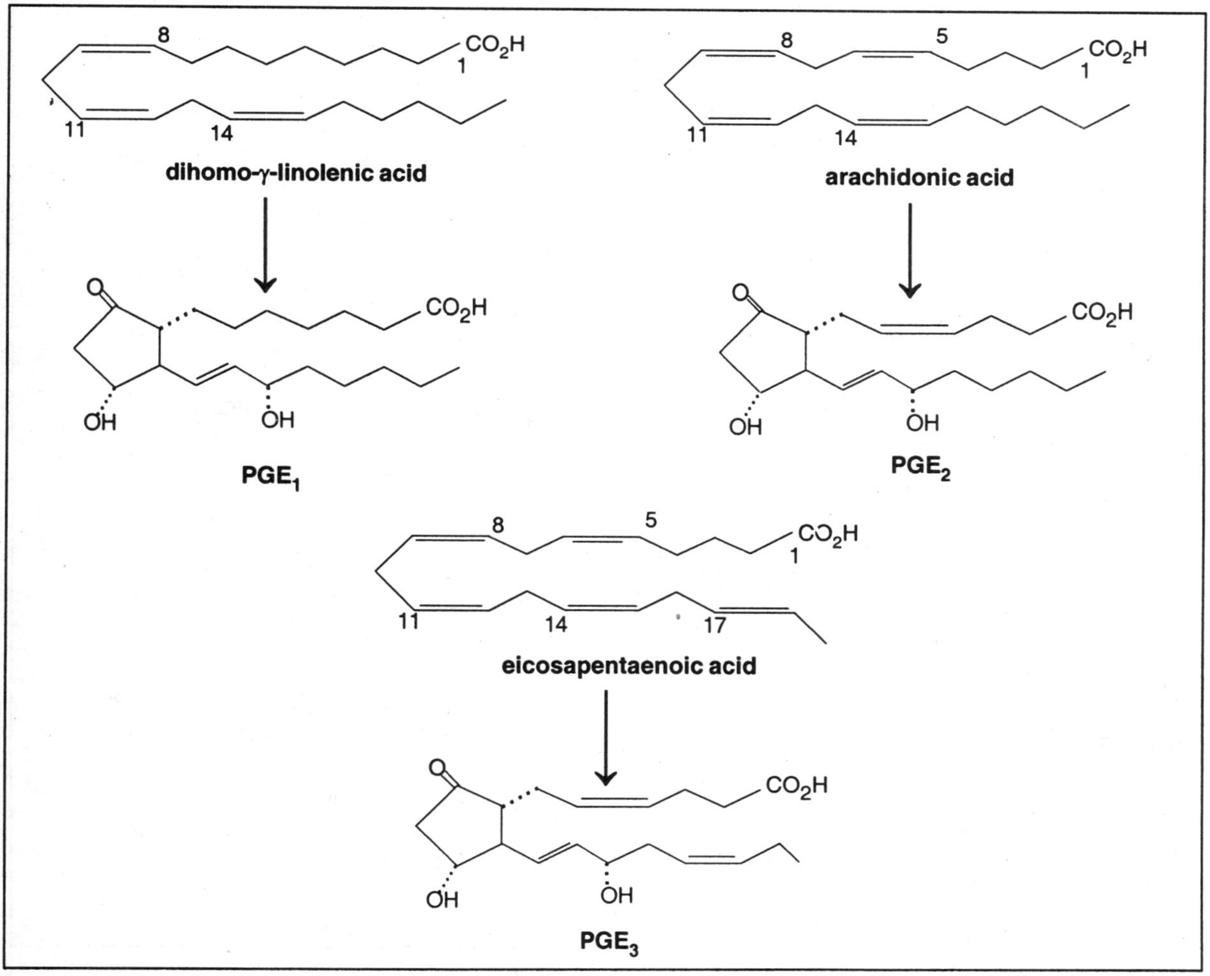

Fig. 8.15. Biosynthesis of PGE$_1$, PGE$_2$ and PGE$_3$.

occur practically in all mammal organs although in very small amounts. PGE$_1$ and PGF$_1$ were initially isolated from sheep seminal plasma but these compounds and PGD$_2$, PGE$_2$ and PGF$_{2\alpha}$ are widely distributed. Animal source can't supply sufficient amounts for drug usage. The soft Coral *Plexaura homomalla* (sea whip) from **Caribbean** has been reported to have very high (2–3%) level of prostaglandin esters, predominantly the C-15 epimer of PGA$_2$ (1–2%) with related structures. Prostaglandins of A-, E- and F- type (Fig. 8.16) are widely distributed in soft corals, especially

Plexaura. Although some synthetic prostaglandins are also available, but it is reported that biological activity is effectively confined to the natural enantiomers; the Unnatural enantiomers of PGE$_1$ had only 0.1% of the activity of the natural isomer.

Prostaglandins constitute a group of biologically potent substances of wide spectrum activity. It causes contraction and relaxation of smooth muscle of the uterus, cardiovascular system, the intestinal tract and of bronchial tissue. They may also inhibit gastric acid secretion, control blood pressure and suppress blood platelet aggregation.

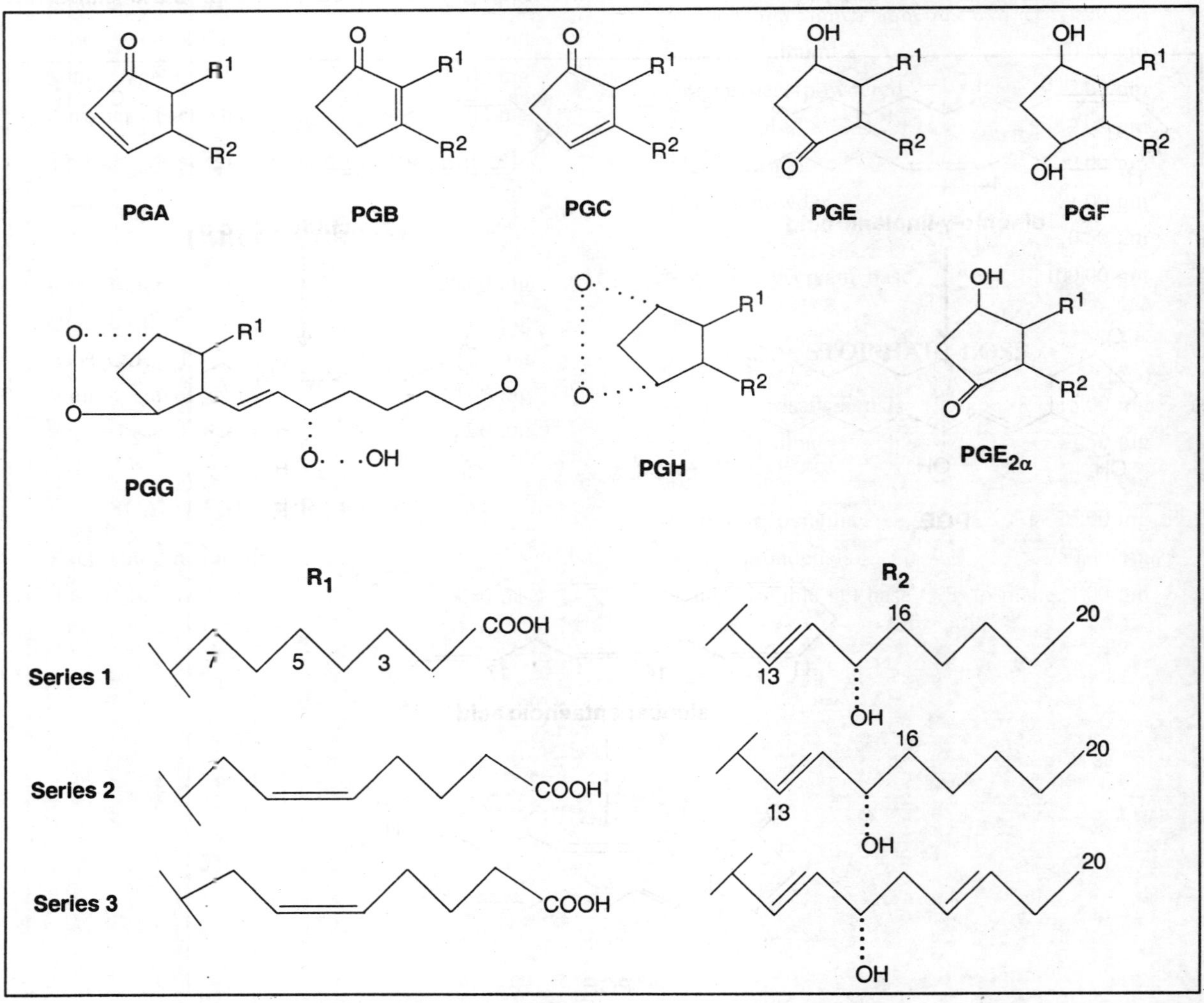

Fig. 8.15. Prostaglandins of A-, E- and F- type.

As such they are inactive but on modification, the inactive compounds become active. Six different series (A-E) produced by modification of the cyclopentane ring are now available as synthetic products. They can be useful in birth control, induced child birth, abortion, mensuration problem, peptic ulcers, treatment of asthma, regulation of blood pressure and tranquillising effect on CNS.

15-epi-PGA$_2$ acetate, methyl ester derivative, obtained from the caribbean gorgonial *Plexaura homomalla* in high concentration. **Some prostaglandins have also been isolated from red algae** *Gracilaria lichenoides* i.e. PGE$_2$, which have antitumor activity. The inactive 15-epi PGA$_2$ and its diester have been converted into useful prostaglandins (15s) PGA$_2$ and (15s) PGE$_2$. Active (15s) PGA$_2$ and (15s) PGE$_2$ identical to prostaglandins derived from mammalian sources has been isolated from *P. homomalla* collected from different location.

Natural Allergens

ALLERGENS

Allergens are inciting agents of allergy i.e. the substances capable of sensitizing the body in such a way that an unusual response occurs, in hyper sensitive person. Allergen may be of biologic, chemical or of synthetic origin. It is common to speak about the substances such as pollens, danders, dust etc. as natural allergens. Although the chemical identity of allergen is unknown but most known **allergens are protein or glycoprotein** and do not have much difference from other immunogens except perhaps being somewhat smaller in size (mol wt. 10,000-70,000). Most allergenic substances are mixture in composition. Allergens from related sources often are similar chemically and cross allergenic.

A number of low molecular weight chemicals (**allergenic haptens**) are partial immunogens and induce allergy after combining covalently with a suitable protein carrier viz. drug allergy.

WHAT IS ALLERGY

The allergy (**Hypersensitivity**) may be defined as a specific **immunologic reaction** to an immunogen, a normally harmless substance (allergen). It was first defined in 1906 by **von Pirquet** who described **allergy as changed or altered reaction in the body of an individual, in response to a substance or condition that is harmless to others.**

Sneezing is always considered to be a symptom of a cold but sometimes it is an allergic reaction to some thing in the air. According to reports available approximately 30% population suffers from some sort of allergic syndrome. However, few persons develop symptoms that are sufficiently severe to require the services of allergist or physician. The occurrence of allergic disease is determined by the characteristic of the individual as well as those of the allergen and even the condition of exposure.

Disease occurs only in those individuals who are previously sensitized by exposure to the allergen and become more sensitized on subsequent exposure but sometimes it is genetically determined in children of allergic parents who are more likely to develop allergies to the particular allergen even on first exposure, even if only one parent is allergic. Sensitization may also vary with the age of the individual, nature of the allergen, route and degree of exposure and many other factors.

The immunological processes involved in allergy results in tissue damage which otherwise do not differ fundamentally from those seen in the normal immune response.

Normally, the immune system functions as the body's defence against invading agents, such as bacteria and viruses. When an allergic person first comes into contact with an allergens, the immune system treats the allergens as an invader and mobilizes to attack. The immune system does this by generating large amount of a type of **antibody** (a disease fighting protein) called **immunoglobin E** or **IgE**. Each **IgE** antibody is specific for one particular allergenic (allergy producing) substance. In the case of pollen allergy, the antibody is specific for each type of pollen. One type of antibody may be produced to react against oak pollens and another against ragweed pollens. Thus, antibodies are considered to be specific and because allergenic substances do produce specific antibodies, each type of allergy is constitutionally different from other types. Allergy can be classified into **four types** on the basis of immune effectors, mediators and cell involved in the reaction (Table 9.1).

Most of the environmental allergens produce Type I allergies. Type II & Type III allergies are produced due to auto immune and in alloimmune diseases.

The IgE molecules are special because IgE is the only class of antibody that attached to the body's mast cells (Tissue, cells and to basophils). When the body is first subjected to the allergen (antigens) the condition is referred to as the primary exposure. Because no antibodies have been formed previously, hence no symptoms of the allergy are produced during primary exposure, however on subsequent exposure its specific IgE attach the allergens and **antigen antibody reaction occurs**; with the liberation of powerful inflammatory chemicals like histamine, cytokines, leukotrienes or SRS (slow-reacting substance) and bradykinin. These chemicals act on tissues in various parts of the body, such as the respiratory system and causes the symptoms of allergy.

Some people may develop asthma with allergy, the symptoms of asthma include coughing, wheezing and shortness of breath due to narrowing of bronchial passages in the lungs, production of excess mucus and inflammation. It can be fatal and requires immediate medical attention.

Table 9.1. Allergy manifestations and their mechanisms of action

Basis	Type I (Immediate Reagin-mediated)	Type II (Cytotoxic)	Type III (Immune complex Arthus type)	Type IV (Delayed : Cellular-mediated Tuberculin-type)
Immune effectors	IgE	IgG; IgM	IgG (IgM)	Effector T cells
Cells involved in inflammation	Mast cells Basophils	Macrophages (cell-mediated lysis) or	Neutrophils	Macrophages Lymphocytes
Mediators	Histamine Leukotrienes	Complement (C´-mediated lysis)	Lysosomal enzymes	Lymphokines
Time of onset in sensitized individuals	0–30 min	Immediate but may not be apparent for some time	2–24 hr	6–24 hr
Manifestations	Rhinitis Urticaria Angiodema Asthma Anaphylaxis	Hemolytic anemia Neutropenia Thrombocytopenia	Serum sickness Vasculitis Glomerulonephritis Extrinsic alveolitis	Contact dermatitis Allergy of many infections

Following are predisposing factors which make the person hypersensitive to allergens:

(i) Hereditary tendency to allergic response;

(ii) Dysfunction of the endocrine glands;

(iii) Increased excitability of sympathetic and parasympathetic nervous systems;

(iv) Absorption of metabolic and catabolic substances;

(v) Hepatic dysfunction; and

(vi) Psychic influences.

TYPES OF ALLERGENS

The allergens can be classified on the basis of types of symptoms, which depend on the shock organs affected by the particular allergens and its route of entry into the body;

- Inhalant allergens
- Ingestant allergens
- Injectant allergens
- Contactant allergens
- Infectant allergens
- Infestant allergens

Inhalant allergens

Inhalant allergens are air borne substances as chemicals, causing respiratory disease, inflammation in the nose and lungs. Inflammation in the nose is manifested by sneezing, lacrimation, itching and swelling of nose and eyes. The condition is known as **Sinusitis or hay fever**. The odour emanating from new-mown hay is often responsible for the 'fever' or stuffiness of the nasal passages. Inflammation of lungs is often expressed as **asthma**. Air pollution, both in-door and out-door, play a significant role in the aggravation of airway disease in the asthmatics and may contribute to the overall increase in asthma morbidity.

Symptoms of allergies to air borne substances are:

- Sneezing often accompanied by a runny or clogged nose.
- Coughing and post nasal drip
- Itching eyes, nose and throat.
- Allergic shiner (dark circles under the eyes caused by increased blood flow near the sinuses).
- The 'allergic salute' (in a child persistent upward rubbing of the nose that causes mark on the nose).
- Watering eyes, conjuctivitis (an inflammation of the membrane that lines the eye lids causing red-rimmed, swollen eyes and crusting the eyelids).

As soon as the allergens land on mucous membrane, an inside lining of the nose, a chain reaction occurs that leads the **mast cells** in these tissue to release histamine and other chemicals. These powerful chemical contract certain cells of some small blood vessels in the nose, that allow fluid to escape, which causes the nasal passage to swell resulting in nasal congestions.

The allergens that can cause air borne allergies (**inhalant allergens**) include pollens, dust, mites, mold spores and animal allergy (epidermis or dander).

The type of allergen can be identified from the symptoms which occurs in the patient-

Pollen allergen's symptoms

- Symptoms intensify in the morning and worsen on windy days.
- Symptoms flares on days with high pollen counts. Eyes may itch or swell.

Mold allergen's symptoms

- Symptoms intensify, during evening especially

as the day cools off when humidity is present.

- Symptoms intensify when mowing grass, raking leaves.
- Symptoms intensify with exposure to moldy foods such as blue cheese, mushrooms etc.

House dust/dust mite allergen's symptoms

Symptoms are worse inside a dusty building or house. Symptoms flare within 30 minutes after going to bed.

Itching of eyes is more in comparison to skin itching.

Pollen allergens

Pollens are the tiny, egg shaped, round, angular, square, rectangular or otherwise shaped male cells (organ) of flowering plants. These microscopic, powdery granules are necessary for plant fertilization. The average pollen particle size is less than the width of an average human hair.

Most pollen grains are single entities but some may be 2-compound, 3-compound, tetrad, or so forth. They may either have no germinal apertures as such (**acolpate**) or have many pores (**multicolpate**) or range in between (**dicolpate, tricolpate, tetracolpate**). The surface appearance of outer wall (**exine**) is characteristic, it may range from smooth (**psilate**) to spiny (**echinate**) with various intervening gradations (reticulate granulate, cophate).

These pollens can be further classified into two types:

- Anemophilous (wind pollinated);
- Entomophilous (insect pollinated).

Anemophilous

Anemophilous pollens are usually small 15-45 µ in diameter, light, non-adhesive and relatively smooth and are produced by plain looking plants e.g. **Trees** (oak, walnut); **grasses** (bermuda grass and timothy) and **weeds** (ragweed, plantain).

Entomophilous

Entomophilous pollens are usually larger in size (upto 200µ in diameter), heavier, adhesive and may be somewhat spiny. Plants are scented, with coloured flowers such as clover, hollyhock, honey suckle and rose.

Most common allergic reactions are produced by wind pollinated (anemophilous) pollens, because of their light weight and the dry nature these pollen grains are carried for long distances. It does little good to rid an area of offending plants, as the pollens can drift in from many miles away. In addition, most allergic pollen comes from plants that produce them in huge quantities. A single ragweed plant can generate a million of pollen grains a day.

The chemical composition of pollen is the basic factor that determines its likelihood cause hay fever. For example, pine tree pollen is produced in large amount by common tree, which makes it a good candidate for causing allergy. However, the chemical composition of pine pollen, appears to make it less allergic than other type; moreover, pine pollen is heavy, it tends to fall straight down and does not scatter, therefore they rarely reaches human noses.

The plants responsible for seasonal pollinosis have the following criteria:

1. The pollen must contain an excitant of hay fever.
2. The pollen must be anemophilous or wind born, with regards to its mode of pollination.
3. The pollen must be produced in sufficiently large quantity.
4. The pollen must be sufficiently buoyant to be carried to considerable distances.

5. The plant producing pollen must be widely and abundantly distributed.

Early Spring Pollinating Trees

Ulmus americana L. (american elm)	Acer Saccharinum (silver maple)
Ulmus rubra muohlenb (slippery elm)	Acer rubrum, (red maple)

List of plant or tree producing pollens (allergens) :

Alfalfa	Eucalyptus
Almond	Gladiolus
Apple, Acacia	Hazelnut
Barley	Juniper
Blue grass	Mulberry
Canary grass	Mustard
Cherry	Lemon & related species of citrus

Grasses

The following is the list of grasses that shed allergenic pollens:

- Cynodon dactylon (Linn.) Pers (Bermuda grass)
- Sorghum halepense (Linn.) (Johnson grass)
- Dactylis glomerata Linn. (Lockshoot) (Orchard grass)
- Phleum Pratensis Linn. (Timothy)
- Poa pratensis Linn. (Kentucky bluegrass)
- Agrostis alba Linn. (Red top)
- Anthoxanthum odoratum Linn. (Sweet vernal grass)

- Lolium perenne (Perennial rye)

The grasses pollinate throughout the year and no particular season is apparent.

Weeds

The weeds belonging to the family Chenopodiaceae, Polygonaceae, Plantiginaceae, Amaranthaceae and Compositae are responsible for shedding allergenic pollens.

Some weed plants pollinate in the beginning of summer while others pollinate later in the summer depending upon their geographical location extending into late fall. *Plantago major* L. (Common plantain) and *Plantago lanceolata* L. (English plantain) are cause to wide spread early summer weed pollinosis.

Following are other hayfever weeds that shed allergenic pollens:

- Rumex Crispus Linn. (Yellow dock)
- Rumex acetosella Linn. (Sheep sorrel)
- Chenopodium album Linn. (Lamb's quarters)
- Chenopodium ambrosioides Linn. (Mexican tea)
- Amaranthus palmeri wats (Palmer's amaranth)
- Amaranthus retroflexus Linn. (Pigweed)
- Acnida tamariscina (Nutt) wood (Western water hemp.)
- Salsola kali Linn. var. tenuifolia Mey (Russian thistle)
- Iva xanthifolia Nutt (Marsh elder)
- Franseria tomentosa Gray (False ragweed)

- Artemisia ludoviciana Nutt
  (Western mugwort)
- Artemisia tridentata Nutt
  (Sagebrush)
- Ambrosia species
  (Ragweed)
- Kochia scoparia L.
  (Burning bush)

The genus Ambrosia is responsible for approximately 90% of the pollinosis in the United States. The two species that may be found in greatest abundance are the **gaint or great ragweed** (*Ambrosia trifida* L) and the dwarf or **Common ragweed** (*Ambrosia artemisiifolia* Linn.). Although these vary considerably in the height, leaf structure and general habit, their pollens are practically indistinguishable. They range in size from 18-21 μ, are uniformly rounded, are tricolpate and have somewhat spiny exine.

Mold allergy

Along with pollens from trees, grasses and weeds, molds are an important cause of seasonal rhinitis or non-seasonal hay fever. Mold season often peaks from July to late summer. Unlike pollens, molds may persist after the first killing frost, some can grow at subfreezing temperatures, but most become dormant. After the spring thaw, molds thrive on the vegetation that has been killed by the winter cold in the warmest areas, however, molds thrive all year and can cause year-round (perennial) allergic problems. In addition, molds growing indoors can cause perennial allergic rhinitis even in the coldest climate.

Microscopic fungal spores or sometimes, fragments of fungi may cause **allergic rhinitis** (hay fever). Because they are so small, they (mold spore) may evade, the protective mechanisms of the nose and upper respiratory tract to reach the lungs. In some people, symptoms of mold allergy may be brought on or worsened by eating certain foods, such as cheeses, processed with fungi. Occasionally, mushrooms, dried fruits and foods containing yeast, soya, sauce or vinegar, will produce allergic symptoms.

Allergenic molds : Like pollens mold spores are also important air-born allergens, only if they are abundant, easily carried by air currents. Found almost everywhere, mold spore areas are numerous in number ever more than the pollens in the air.

The most common mold genera are Alternaria, Macrosporing, Helminthosporium, Hormodendrum (cladusporium), Aspergillus, Penicillium mucor, Rhizopus, Syncephalastrum, Curvularia, Brachysporium and Pullularia. Alternaria and Cladosporium (Hormodendrum) are the molds most commonly found both indoors and outdoors throughout the United States and in India.

House Dust and Dandruff Allergens

Dust is almost indefinable because it differs from one place to the next; but commonly it composed of mold spores; cotton linters, or fragments of cotton fibres that are light enough to float in the air, animal danders (epithelial scales), cat, dog, guniea pigs, chicken, rabbit, human hair and dandruff, chicken excreta, mice dandruff and house mites, cokroach excreta, odours and perfumes etc. In house dust, common allergens are particularly the acarine mite, dermatophagoides and specifically its species *D. pteronyssinus*. About 30% of patients with symptoms of asthma or hayfever are sensitive to disintegrating bits of insect, dust inhaled from air and soil; hence it is not possible to diagnose the sensitivity to dust.

House dust sensitivity differs from pollen allergy in several respects and suspected particularly when the patient's history includes one or more of the following factors:

Perennial symptoms that worsen when the

patient remains indoor, increased nocturnal symptoms increased symptoms when performing household chores and increased symptoms associated with turning on/off heating or air conditioning systems.

Dust mite allergy

Dust mite allergy is an allergy to a microscopic organism that lives in the dust and is found in all dwellings and work places. Dust mite is perhaps the most common cause of **perennial allergic rhinitis**. It produces symptoms similar to pollen allergy and can produce asthma.

The dust mites appear to be distributed universally and usually found in furnishings stuffed with vegetable fibres (e.g. cotton). It is generally believed that mite allergens are responsible for most dust allergy but there are some peoples who are allergic to dust but not the dust mites as it is not found in some dusts.

Ingestant Allergens

Allergens which are present in food stuff and swallowed are termed **ingestant** (Food allergy). **A food allergy is an immune system response to a food**. Once the immune system decides that a particular food is harmful it creates specific antibody to it.

The gastrointestinal symptoms are mainly effected by the food allergens but they also causes skin rash, puffed lips and tongue, migraine, rhinitis or other symptoms like severe eczema of hand and feet. The effects of food allergens are not localised to one organ or area of the body, but it may transferred to other organs by the blood. Thus, an **atopic dermatitis**, such as tomato rash, strawberry rash, or that caused by eating oranges, chocolate or shellfish, is developed by patients.

Some most common food allergens ingested by patients are:

Milk, egg, peanut, tree nut (walnut, cashew nut etc.), fish, shellfish, soy, wheat, orange juice, cod liver oil or other vitamins - containing fish liver oils. In addition to the above mentioned normal food there are food additive, which also could be allergic to any individual viz. mannitol, sorbitol, polysorbates, malt-dextrins, citrus, bioflavonoids, artificial preservatives, artificial colors, citrus pectin, talc, soy lecithin, gluten, soy flour, rice flour, alfalfa, potato starch and gum acacia.

Most satisfactory method of combating food allergens is elimination of the offending substance from the diet. Dairy milk allergy is a specific immunologic antibody-antigen reaction due to a lacto-albumin, because heating and boiling alter this protein. Milk allergy may result in severe dermatitis, recurrent rhinorrhea, bronchitis and asthma. Its antigenicity can be avoided by the use of commercial milk substitutes that are prepared from soyabean isolates.

Injectant Allergens

Injectant allergens causes symptoms similar to those of the antibiotics e.g. Penicillin, cephalosporin and semi-synthetic penicillin etc. Itching of the palms of the hands and the soles of the feet, erythema and peeling of the skin are characteristic. In severe cases anaphylactic shock may occur.

The natural sources of injectable allergens are produced by the sting of bees, hornets and wasps. The allergens injected by the stings of such insects can induce severe local and constitutional reactions sometimes causing death.

In addition to penicillin products, other injectable that may cause allergies are liver extract, antitoxins and the glandular products.

Contactant Allergens

A number of plants and their products have been

identified as the causes of contact allergies. The plant most responsible for contact dermatitis in North America belong to the *Ancardiaceae* family, primarily the genus **Toxicodendron** (Rhus) and include **poison ivy, oak and sumac**. The allergen component of these plants, called **urushiols** (a

OH
OH
R

Urushiol

R = C-15 aliphatic side chain (Poison oak)
R = C-17 aliphatic side chain
R = May possess 0, 1, 2 or 3 double bands

phenolic compound) are found in the oleoresin fraction and are derivatives of pentadecylcatechol or heptadecylcatechol. Many plants of compositae family, which include the ragweeds also cause contact dermatitis and the allergens responsible had been identified as **Sesquiterpenoids lactone**.

Allergen plants are responsible for considerable hazard in USA where **poison ivy** are widespread as a woody vine lacquer used for producing oriental type finish on furniture. Its use causes industrial hazard for the craftsman. Similar type of compounds have been isolated from fruit pulp of *Ginkgo biloba* and from the glandular trichomes of annual *Phacelia* spp. (*Hydrophyllaceae*) of the Californian Mojave desert. **The dermatitic action of these compound is due to the oxidation of the allergen to quinone, which then bind with protein nucleophile giving an antigenic complex.**

Another class of chemical compound, **Sesquiterpene lactone** isolated from plants of compositae, lauraceae and magnoliaceae and from Liverwort Frullania (*Jubulaceae*), causes allergic contact dermatitis in the hypersensitive individuals. **The α-methylene group exocyclic to the γ-lactone is the principle immunochemical responsible for the allergic reaction.** Such compound (*Pseudoguainolide parathenium*) is obtained from the plant *Parthenium hystero-*

phorus, an aggressive weed causing public health problems in parts of India.

Other plants species, which can give rise to contact allergic reactions are *Ruta graveolens*, asparagus, ornamental "dumb cane" (*Dieffenbachia seguine*), buck wheat, butter cups, catalpa leaves, chrysanthemums, ginkgo leaves, lobelia, marigolds, may-apple, osage orange, flowering spurge, snow on the mountains and smart weeds.

Aeroallergens, such as the various pollen grains containing oils, trichomes from various leaves, flowers and small fragments of plant tissue carried by smoke originating from brush fires, grass fires and burning leaves are also cause for contact (allergens) dermatitis.

A number of plant products used as additives in cosmetics and perfumes are irritants and cause skin allergy to some hypersensitive individuals. These types of allergens are termed as **Hypoallergenic Cosmetics**, to denote this fact, the cosmetic manufacturer add the brand names of Ar-ex, allercreme, almay and Marcelle are example of hypoallergenic cosmetics.

Certain natural products added to cosmetics such as talcum and perfume are chief source of contact allergy such as orris root, an ingredient to talcum powder.

Dibromofluorescein, commonly used in lipsticks.

Wool fat (lanolin) in cosmetics, soap and soap powders, plain detergents and enzyme detergents, nail polishes, hair dye and hair spray are also included among the major causes of contact dermatitis.

Infectant Allergens

Allergy caused by the metabolic product of living micro-organism in the human body. The continual presence of certain types of bacteria, protozoas, molds, helminths and other parasites in the body of human being are responsible for chronic infection for which patients are not aware but metabolic product of their growth causes some patient sensitized and the patient may exhibit allergic symptoms, which does not response positively to routine skin test for inhalant allergens. In such patient bacterial metabolic waste are considered to be infectant allergens.

The continuous presence of growth products and metabolic waste of parasitic organism such as hookworms, tape worms, pinworms, threadworms and dermatophytes are referred as **infectant allergens**.

ALLERGENIC EXTRACTS

Allergenic extracts are concentrated solutions or suspensions of allergens used for the diagnosis and therapeutic purposes. Extracts are **aqueous** (0.9% Sodium chloride used as diluent) or glycerinated (50% glycerin as diluent). Most preparations are buffered at pH 8 and contain phenol (<0.4%) as an antimicrobial preservative. They are sterilized by aseptic filtration and used as injectable products administered in the physician's office and for many years were prepared by the individual users. Commercial extracts have gradually replaced extemporaneous preparations as number of small speciality companies marketing allergenic extracts several decades ago have today disappeared with merger into larger. Pharmaceutical companies and the several other manufacturers of allergenic extracts are multinational corporations.

The manufacture of allergenic extracts intended for international export or import must be carried out in licensed laboratories as per the terms and condition laid down by section 351 of the Public Health Services Act.

Preparation

The preparation of allergenic extracts required same general procedure and precautions required with all parenteral products. In addition to the general aseptic condition the extraction process should be carried out in a cold room. The extracts are thermolabile and must be sterilized by aseptic filtration. Sterility test for both aerobic and anaerobic microorganism must be performed in guinea pigs particularly for autogenous extracts where unknown toxic constituents may be present.

In addition to general procedure used for the preparation of other extractives the following is the unique procedure for most allergenic extracts:

Materials

The allergenic substances to be extracted are obtained from commercial suppliers and only the most reliable source are selected. It should be free from adulteration and should not contain more than 1% of extraneous foreign matter, prompt and proper dehydration is important to prevent alteration of the allergens and prevent microbial contamination.

Grinding

The material to be extracted must be ground or subdivided for the efficient extraction of the allergens. Materials such as hair, feathers and textiles should be divided finely with shears.

Defatting

Many allergenic substances, including all pollens should be defatted before final extraction, ether and petroleum ether are most commonly used for this purpose. It provides clear final extract free from irritants (cotton seed, pepper, mustard and ginger etc.). This defatted extract can be used in the preparation of some patch testing substances.

Extraction

The extraction procedures are based upon the

assumption that allergens are water soluble proteins or glycoproteins. Extraction is carried out normally for 24-72 hours in cold room using sterile, pyrogen free buffered saline, coca's solution or similar aqueous menstrum of pH 8.

Buffered saline

Sodium chloride	5.00 g
Monobasic potassium phosphate	0.36 g
Dibasic sodium phosphate anhydrous	7.00 g
Phenol crystals	4.00 g
Water for injection USP to make	1000 ml

Coca's Solution

Sodium chloride	5.0 g
Phenol crystals	5.0 g
Sodium bicarbonate	2.5 g
Water for injection USP to make	1000 ml

After extraction, mixture is clarified by coarse filtration. Some extracts are dialyzed against saline or running tap water to remove irritants or colouring matter (e.g. house dust, mustard, potato, spinach, beets). The processed extract is sterilized by filtration through cellulose membrane filter.

Freeze-dried pollen extracts : These are prepared with the same procedure except that water rather than electrolyte solution is used as extracting medium.

Standardization

Most allergenic extracts carry the statement "No US standard of potency". The two most common measures of allergenic potency are weight/volume (w/v) and the Protein Nitrogen Unit (P.N.U.), unit of potency for allergenic extracts. 1 mg protein nitrogen equal 1,00,000 P.N.U. (Table 9.2).

Stability and storage

The potency of allergenic extracts start reducing within a matter of week or months after their preparation, very dilute solution tend to reduce potency by absorption to the surfaces of containers

Table 9.2. Units of potency for allergenic extracts

Unit	Description	Used
Weight/volume (w/v)	Allergen (g) per volume (mL) of extracting fluid	Worldwide
Protein Nitrogen Unit (P.N.U.)	1 mg protein N = 100,000 PNU	Worldwide
Allergy Unit (A.U.)	Skin testing to end point	US
Biological Unit (B.U.)	Skin testing relative to histamine	Europe

used for packing but the inclusion of Tween-80, Tween-20 or human serum albumin reduce this absorption.

All the allergenic extracts should be refrigerated at 2-8°C and freezing should be avoided.

Expiry Date

Aqueous extract	-	18 months
Glycerinated scratch test and bulk extract	-	3 years
Lyophilized products	-	4 year
After reconstitutions	-	18 month

Pollen extracts

Pollens are the most common cause of atopic disease in most parts of the country, but allergens vary somewhat with the region. Therefore allergen extracts prepared from some of the common pollens (e.g. rageweed, several grasses and tree) have been among the most widely studied and it has been reported that these products are reliable for both diagnosis and in several cases for therapeutic use when properly prepared (Table 9.3).

Dust Extracts

The allergens in house dust are not related to the inorganic dirt from outside but to the products of aging and decompositing materials in and around the house. The dust for commercial extracts generally is obtained from house cleaning or rug cleaning firms and is pooled to get some homogencity.

Table 9.3. Pollen extracts

TREES

Acacia	Elderberry	Osage orange
Alder, grey	Elm, American	Palo verde
Almond	Eucalyptus	Peach
Apple	Hackberry	Pear
Apricot	Hazelnut	Pecan
Arbor vitae	Hemlock	Pepper tree
Ash	Hickory	Pine
Bayberry	Hop-hornbeam	Plum
Beech	Ironwood	Poplar
Birch, spring	Juniper	Privet
Birch, white	Locust	Redwood
Bottle brush	Maple	Russian olive
Box elder	Melaleuca	Spruce
Carob tree	Mesquite	Sweet gum
Cedar	Mock orange	Sycamore
Cherry	Mulberry	Tamarack
Chestnut	Oak, white	Tree of heaven
Cottonwood	Olive	Walnut
Cypress	Orange	Willow

GRASSES

Bahia	Corn	Redtop
Barley	Fescue, meadow	Rye grass, perennial
Beach	Grama	Salt
Bent	Johnson	Sorghum
Bermuda grass	June grass	Sudan
Bluegrass, Kentucky	Koeler's	Sweet vernal grass
Brome	Oats	Timothy grass
Bunch	Orchard grass	Velvetgrass
Canarygrass	Quack	Wheat
Chess		Wheatgrass

WEEDS AND GARDEN PLANTS

Alfalfa	Fireweed	Poppy
Amaranth	Gladiolus	Povrtyweed
Aster	Goldenrod	Quailbush
Balsam root	Greasewood	Ragweed, giant
Bassia	Hemp	Ragweed, short
Beach bur	Honeysuckle	Ragweed, western
Broomweed	Hops	Rose
Burrow brush	Iodine Bush	Russian thistle
Careless weed	Jerusalem oak	Sagebrush
Castor bean	Kochia	Saltbrush
Chamise	Lamb's quarters	Scale
Clover	Lily	Scotch broom
Cocklebur	Marigold	Sea blight
Coreopsis	Marshelder	Sheep sorrel
Cosmos	Mexican tea	Snapdragon
Daffodil	Mugwort	Sugar beet
Dahlia	Mustard	Sunflower
Daisy	Nettle	Western waterhemp
Dandelion	Pickleweed	Winter fat
Dock	Pigweed	Wormseed
Dog fennel	Plantain, English	Wormwood

Dust mites are of more concern, as mites are more responsible for most dust allergy. Standardized extract of Dermatophagoides species are available. The dust mite is distributed universally and is usually found in furnishing stuffed with vegetable fibres (e.g. cotton) (Table 9.4).

Table 9.4. Dust extracts

House dusts	Dust mites
• House	• D. farniae
• Mattress	• D. pteronyssinus
• Upholstery	• Mite mix
	• Cedar and red cedar
	• Cotton gin
	• Oak
	• Grain elevator
	• Padauk
	• Wood dusts

Fungal extracts

Fungi are omni present and may be found in the home on textiles, leather goods, upholstered furniture, food and plants. Therapy should include efforts to create mold and fungi free environment. The allergenic extracts are prepared variously from mycellium, medium or both but little know how is available of fungal allergenic extracts preparation method. Some of the fungal and mold allergen extracts available are given in the Table 9.5.

Table 9.5. Fungal extracts

Altermaria	Mucor
Asperigillus	Mycogone
Botrytis	Nigraspora
Cephalosporium	Penicillium
Cephalothecium	Pullularia
Cladosporium	Rhodotorula
Curvularia	Rusts
Epidermophyton	Saccharomyces
Fusarium	Spomdylocladium
Gliocladium	Trichoderma
Helminthosporium	Trichophyton
Hormodendrum	Verticillium
Microsporium	

Insect extracts

Sensitivity testing and immunotherapy are commonly recommended and employed for the stinging insects. The venom extracts have been shown to be highly effective when properly employed. The list of the standardized extract is given in Table 9.6.

Table 9.6. Standardized extract.

INSECT EXTRACTS

Stinging insect : Whole body
- Ant black
- Ant red
- Ant carpenter
- Ant mix (black/red)
- Ant fire

Stinging insect : Venom protein
- Honey bee
- Yellow hornet
- Wasp
- White faced hornet
- Mixed verpid

INHALANT ALLERGY TO INSECT

Black fly	Horse fly	Spider
Butter fly	House fly	Sow bugs
Cockroach	Mosquito	Water fly
Daphnia	Moth	
Fruit fly	Mushroom fly	

Miscellaneous Inhalant Extracts

Miscellaneous allergens are those other than pollen, dust and molds that cause atopic allergies , these includes epidermal from domestic animals (cat, dog and horse). The number of other inhalant allergens is remarkable (Table 9.7).

Table 9.7. Miscellaneous inhalant extracts

MAMMALIAN EPIDERMAL/FEATHERS

Camel	Chicken	Pigeon
Cat hair	Dog	Goose
Cat pelt	Goat	Duck
Deer	Guinea pig	Parakeet
Canary	Hog	

MISCELLANEOUS INHALANT

Acacia	Hemp fibre	Orris root
Algae	Henna	Silk
Cartor bean	Guar gum	Sisal
Cotton seed	Jute	Tobacco leaf
Derris root	Leather	Tragacanth
Grain dust	Lycopodium	Wood dust

Photosensitizing Agents

INTRODUCTION

The word "photosensitizing" means which makes individual sensitive to light. It may be defined as the hypersensitivity to sunlight caused by the presence of **photodynamic** substance or **photosensitizer** in the skin. It was first observed in animals where it had caused considerable economic losses in livestocks for hundred of years. The syndrome occurs in animals with highly pigmented skin on exposure to sunlight. The syndrome is characterised by appearance of erythema and **pruritis**. The affected animal scratches and rubs the exposed skin and finding relief in the shade. Latter the animal develops swelling and oedema leading to cracking of the skin and exudation of oedmatous fluid.

The photosensitizing agent has property to fluorescence. On exposure to visible light it absorbs a quantum of energy and the molecule becomes activated. This energy is transferred to other molecules such as amino acids, histamine, tryptophan and tyrosine, which in turn become activated; subsequently decompose or undergo further chemical reactions. The observed inflammatory changes in skin are in response to these chemical processes only. A characteristic feature of these chemical reactions is that they require oxygen, differing them from sunburns, which are independent of oxygen supply.

PHOTOSENSITIZING REACTIONS

Three types of sensitive reactions can result from exposure to photosensitizing agents:

- Photoallergy;
- Photophobia and;
- Phototoxicity.

Photoallergy is an allergic reaction of the skin to UV light.

Photophobia is a fear or strong desire to avoid all light sources based on a painful sensitivity of the eyes to strong light.

Phototoxicity is an irritation of the skin after exposure to UV light. Immediate reactions may include itching, burning, swelling, scaling and rashes.

These types of reactions can be based on:

1. The amount of the photosensitizing agent ingested.
2. Factors such as the colour of skin, hair, eyes and the amount of base tan, as well as the strength and duration of exposure.
3. Medical condition.

4. Ingestion of photosensitizing agents in foods or drugs.

Not all individuals who ingest these agents will have a reaction, and if they do, it is not necessarily true that they will have the repeated reaction. The common photosensitizing agents are ingredients that may leave skin vulnerable to ultraviolet light exposure, causing erythema, itching, scaling, rashes or inflammation.

CLASSIFICATION OF PHOTO-SENSITIZER

Photosensitizer can be divided into two main groups:

- Photodynamic
- Photosensitizing

Photodynamic Photosensitizer

Photodynamic agents require oxygen for their action. This group include photodynamic dyes, hermatoporphyrin, **hypericin**, phagopyrin, bengal

rose, erythrosin, anthracene, acridine dye, methylene blue, quinine, chlorophyll, buck wheat and porphyrin. These substances photooxidize terpenene, blood serum and cause haemolysis. They are topically inactive but on intradermal injection causes immediate photoreaction of short durations. The decrease in temperature of irradiation inhibits the photosensitization effect.

Photosensitizing Photosensitizer

Photosensitizing agents do not require oxygen for reaction. These photosensitizing agents include **furanocoumarins** and their **derivatives**. These compound neither cause photo-oxidation of terpenene or haemolysis, nor photooxidize blood serum protein to any appreciable extent, but provoke dermatitis characterized by latent period erythema followed by pigmentation on epicutaneous application and intradermal injection. Temperature of irradiation has no effect on photosensitization activity of these compounds. These compound have therapeutic value in leucoderma.

Photosensitizers combined with ultraviolet light may also contribute to other health problems, including skin cancer, photoaging and allergic reactions. Remember that the effect of photosensitizers will change from person to person.

As regards the photosensitizing effect of photodynamic compounds and of furanocoumarin on the skin is concerned, it is reported that effect is quite different, in case of photodynamic compounds (toluidine, methylene blue etc.) erythema appears immediately after irradiation and disappears after a few hours whereas that produced by photosensitizing agent (e.g. Furanocoumarins etc.) appears only after latent period of few hours and last several days, and is succeeded by the increased pigmentation, thus both the classes have different mechanism of action (Table 10.1).

Hypericin

Pseduohypericin

Table 10.1. Difference between photodynamic and photosensitizing agents

Photodynamic	Photosensitizing
1. Naturally occurring or may be synthetic pigments and dyes, which require oxygen for their action e.g. erythrosin, rose bengal, rhodamin, anthracene; Acridine dye, methylene blue, chlorophyll, quinine, hypericine, buckwheat and porphyrin.	Furanocoumarins naturally occurring in plants belonging to family Umbelliferae and Rutaceae e.g. psoralen, bergapten, xanthotoxin, imperatorin
2. Photodynamic agents may arise in the body in the following way: (a) *Primary photosensitization :* The photodynamic substances are ingested and absorbed unchanged into the body. (b) Photosensitization due to the synthesis of unusual pigment. (c) *Hepatogenous photosensitization :* The photosensitizing is due to accumulation of phylloerythrin in the body due to liver damage of the ruminants.	Furanocoumarins on application on the skin make complex with DNA and on irradiation produces pigmentation of the skin.
Photodynamic agents : They photooxidize terpene to ascaridol, they haemolysis RBC, oxidise serum protein and unsaturated fatty acid	Furanocoumarin do not photooxidize the terpenene, neither haemolyse RBC or oxidize serum protein and unsaturated fatty acid.
Photosensitizing effect : Erythema produced by photodynamic compound appears **immediately after irradiation** and disappear after a few hours.	Erythema produced by furanocoumarin appears **after a latent period of several hours**, last for several days and in following by an increased pigmentation.
Effect of temperature : Lethal photosensitization of bacteria produced by photodynamic compounds dyes strongly inhibited by a decrease in temperature of irradiation.	Temperature practically has no influence on lethal photosensitization of bacteria, produced by Furanocoumarin.

PHOTOSENSITIZING SUBSTANCES

Photosensitizing substances (agents) are ingredients that may leave skin vulnerable to ultraviolet light exposure, causing erythema, itching, scaling, rashes or inflammation. These substances combined with ultraviolet light also may contribute to other health problems including skin cancer, photoaging and allergic reactions. The following are common photosensitizing agents:

- Medications
- Porphyrin
- Herbal supplements

(i) Medications and Other Agents that Increase Sensitivity to Light Introduction

Many medications, herbal and over the counter supplements contain ingredients that may cause photosensitivity i.e. chemically induced change in the skin that makes an individual unusually sensitive to light. An individual who has been photo-sensitized may develop a rash, sunburn or other adverse effect on exposure to light of an intensity or duration that would normally not affect that individual (Annexure I).

(ii) Porphyrins and their Analogues as Skin-photosensitizing Agents

Porphyrins and their analogues (chlorins, phthalocyanines and porphyrenes) possess several physicochemcial and photobiological properties, which make them particularly adequate to act as skin-photosensitizing agents. Thus, their level of hydro-/lipo-philicity can be modified by selecting the nature of the metal ion coordinated at the centre of the tetrapyrrolic macrocycle, as well as by controlling the peripheral substituents departing from the meso positions of the individual pyrrole or isoindole moieties. Moreover, the presence of various light absorption bands located in different regions of the UV/visible spectrum (from the near UV to the far red) allows one to photoexcite these compounds by a variety of wavelengths, thereby modulating the degree of light penetration into the cutaneous tissue, hence the extent of the photodamage. In particular, a suitable formulation for the topical deposition of porphyrins/ phthalocyanines limits their penetration to the epidermal skin layers thus avoiding the entry of the photosensitizer into the general blood circulation and minimizing the risk of systemic effects. These possibilities will be illustrated by the results obtained using a synthetic phthalocyanine, namely Zn(II)-octadecyl-phthalocyanine (ZnODPc), topically administered to healthy mice, as well as to ex-vivo obtained human skin. In both cases, the irradiation (600-700 nm light; 100 mW/cmsq) of skin areas loaded with 10-20 µg/g ZnODPc caused a cutaneous damage, which was restricted to the epidermis with no apparent photosensitivity in distal skin areas. Maximum efficiency was observed for irradiations performed at about one hour after the end of deposition; the initial oedema evolved into erythema and eschar (slough), with full skin reepithelization within about 10 days. Photosensitization studies of keratinocytes with ZnODPc analogues showed **(a)** no mutagenic effect, **(b)** a strong dependency of the photo-efficiency on the chemical structure of the phthalocyanines.

(iii) Herbal Supplements

Photosensitivity is caused directly by photodynamic agents, such as hypericin from St. John's Wart (*Hypericum perforatum*) (Goatweed) which is a photosensitizing agent, found in wet meadows, shorelines and marshy areas; may be more common in high country areas. It is considered unpalatable to livestock. Hypericin absorbed and then reacts with light at the skin's surface.

Secondary photosensitization is caused by **phylloerythrin**, a metabolite of chlorophyll, which is normally excreted in the bile. Agents such as alkaloids causing liver damage, result in phylloerythrin

entering the general circulation and causing skin lesions on reaction with ultraviolet light.

Symptoms

The white or light coloured areas of the animal become sunburned with skin lesions, photophobia death is often caused by starvation or infection of skin lesions. The cow will often not let the calf suckle.

Causative agents

Buckwheat from a green manure crop where both the seeds and forage icterus (jaundice like yellow color) can cause photosensitization.

Alsike clover poisoning is usually seen in horses and the unknown agent acts on the liver causing its failure. Other symptoms include icterus, depression, stupor and "head pushing" from elevated blood ammonia and copper levels and neurological involvement.

Kochia scoparia (kochia weed) toxicity includes signs of icterus and photosensitivity with progressive central nervous system involvement, cirrhosis, gastro-Intestinal (GI) tract inflammation and polioencephalomalacia from a thiaminase or liver toxin causing impaired thiamine utilization. Kochia is usually found in arid and saline soils and is most toxic at seed and in drought periods.

Lupinosis arises from several varieties of **lupines**, which are found in meadows, wooded and submountainous areas. Sheeps, late pregnant or recently calved cows are more susceptible.

Mouldy straw : The Cattle fed on mouldy straw show liver damage and even when off straw for some time and placed on lush spring pasture will show photosensitivity (phylloerythrin reaction).

Pyrrolizidine alkaloids give similar symptoms as alsike clover poisoning. Tansy ragwort (Senecio family - ragwort/groundsel) is well documented to cause the necessary liver damage.

Ranunculin from buttercups in the fresh state (not in dried) generally growing in wet soils and marshy areas, cause blistering of the lips and irritation to the mouth and GI tract. It is not a major problem maker.

Sporidesmin in ryegrass pastures is caused by spores of a fungus (*Pithomyces chartarum*), which grows in the dead litter of ryegrass pastures. Action is through liver damage as spore numbers increase dramatically with warm weather. Facial eczema and lesions of the udder and leg areas predominate.

Lady's thumb and Water Smartweed (*Polygonum* spp.) found in shallow water and slough and meadow margins can also cause photosensitivity when eaten green.

Another photosensitizer is **fall rye** when grazed during flowering. Problems, possibly an allergic reaction seems to be related to the occurrence of pollens.

Solution is to remove cattle from the source of problem. If the problem arises from primary photosensitization, symptoms should disappear within a few days. However, liver damage has occurred, the phylloerythrin reaction may continue for some time.

Most of the cases arise when cattle eat something that they don't eat normally as in overgrazed situations. Some plants may grow in abnormal or unexpected areas. Most troublemakers are unpalatable and cause problems in few animals only. If photosensitization is throughout the herd, it is not usually an abnormal plant consumption problem, but an abnormal plant physiology problem.

Producers are advised to work closely with their veterinarians if photosensitivity reactions occur in their animals. Photosensitization may be an indicator of larger problems related to liver damage and production losses and deaths may be the outcome.

PHOTOSENSITIZING AGENTS IN THERAPY (Fig. 10.1)

The photosensitizing compounds are used in the treatment of **vitiligo disease**, in which **melanin** formation is deficient (hypomelanosis). **Melanin**

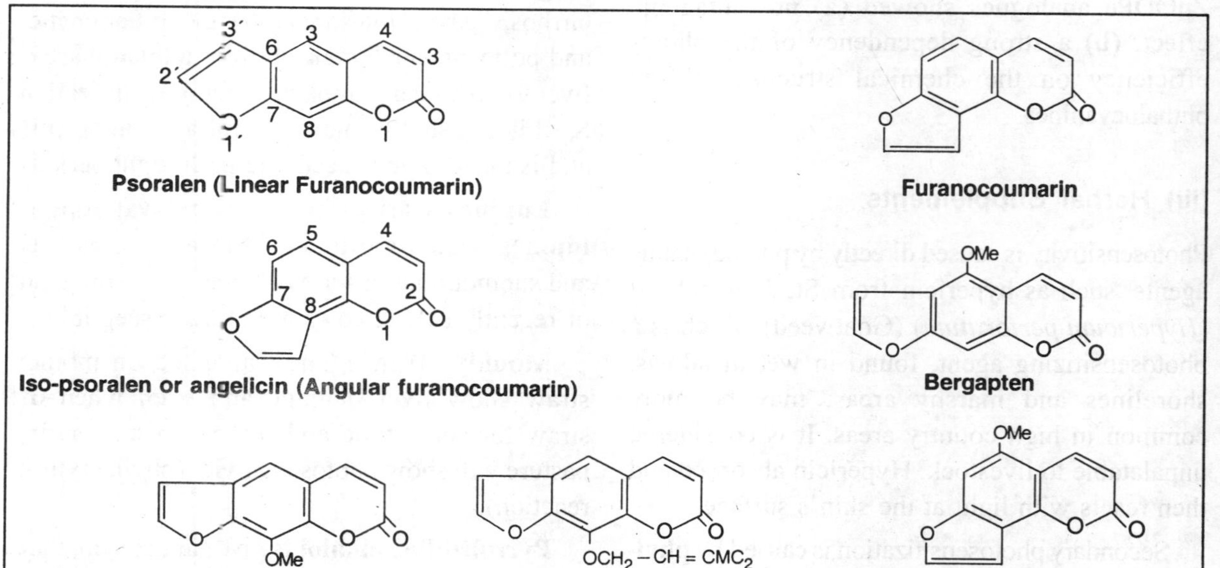

Fig. 10.1. Photosensitizing Agents in Therapy.

is the main pigment in mammalian skin, hair and eyes. It is a complex heterogenous polymer (containing both **eumelanin and pheomelanin** in varying proportions), derived from tyrosine (hydroxy phenylalanine). Tyrosine is oxidized to dihydroxy phenylalanine or DOPA and then further oxidized to dihydroxy indole, which is converted to melanin in melanocytes under the stimulation of sunlight and possibly under the control of melanin-stimulating hormone (MSH) of hypophysis (Fig. 10.2).

There are certain plant extracts and juices e.g. an extract of *Ammi majus* L (Apiaceae) or juice of the fruits of *Psoralea corylifolia,* that have long been used in treatment of vitiligo, a disease characterized by the presence of white spots on the skin (hypomelanosis). The fruit extract of *Ammi majus* is either given orally or painted on the unpigmented spot of the patient. The patient is then exposed to sunlight for 1-2 hours. After 7-12 hours, reddening, and sometimes blisters, appears on the irradiated parts of the skin, and is followed by the development of a strong brown colour after 2 days. The enhanced tanning cannot be obtained by the use of plant extract alone without subsequent irradiation also the exposure to sun alone has only slight therapeutic effect. This form of the therapy, based on the joint action of medicine and irradiation, is called **photochemotherapy** (PUVA).

The photodynamic sensitizing properties of **psoralen, bergapten, xanthotoxin**, isopimpinelin and **isoperatorin** are applied during PUVA treatment or photochemotherapy of psoriasis and other dermatological disorders. The therapy consists of the administration, generally by the oral route, of the **furanocoumarin** (0.6 mg/kg of **xanthotoxin** or 1.2 mg/kg of **bergapten**), 2 or 3 hours latter, followed by exposure to UV radiation of long wavelength (320-380 nm or UVA). The exposure must be brief initially (1-3 J/cm2) and lengthened progressively to 6-8 J/cm2, generally in three weekly sessions. The results for severe psoriasis

are generally obtained in about 20 sessions. Localized treatment is also possible (e.g. in case of hepatic insufficiency) but must be conducted with the greatest caution. PUVA treatment is contraindicated for pregnant women & children, in cases of cutaneous disorders (aggravated by sunlight), and in cases of renal or cardiac insufficiency. Side effects of therapy: gastrointestinal disorder (xanthotoxin), dry skin, photosensitization (pruritis, burns, hence the need to avoid over exposure with protective clothing, sun screens), and latter on, accelerated aging of the crystalline lens of the eye (sunglasses during treatment), aging of the skin, and pigmentation problems. Even the chances of cancer formation occur on the prolonged use of therapy. However, PUVA treatment is useful especially for extensive psoriasis, because it improves the quality of life of the patient.

The natural products such as bergamot oil are used as photodynamic sensitizer in cosmetic products (sun lotions). They increase the number of melanocytes, as well as their melanin production; thus they provide extra protection against UV radiation.

PHOTODYNAMIC THERAPY

Photodynamic therapy (PDT) is based on the discovery that certain chemicals can kill one celled in the presence of light. Recently it has been reported that some of these substances have a tendency to collect in cancer cells.

Photodynamic therapy (PDT) is as a bi-component therapy method: photosensitizing agent (medicine dye which enhance tissue sensitivity to light) serves as one component, and low energy laser irradiation with certain wavelength is another component. Photosensitizing agent interacting with light of certain wavelength causes intense singlet oxygen flow. All this causes phototoxic effect leading to damage and elimination of the cells absorbing photosensitizing agents.

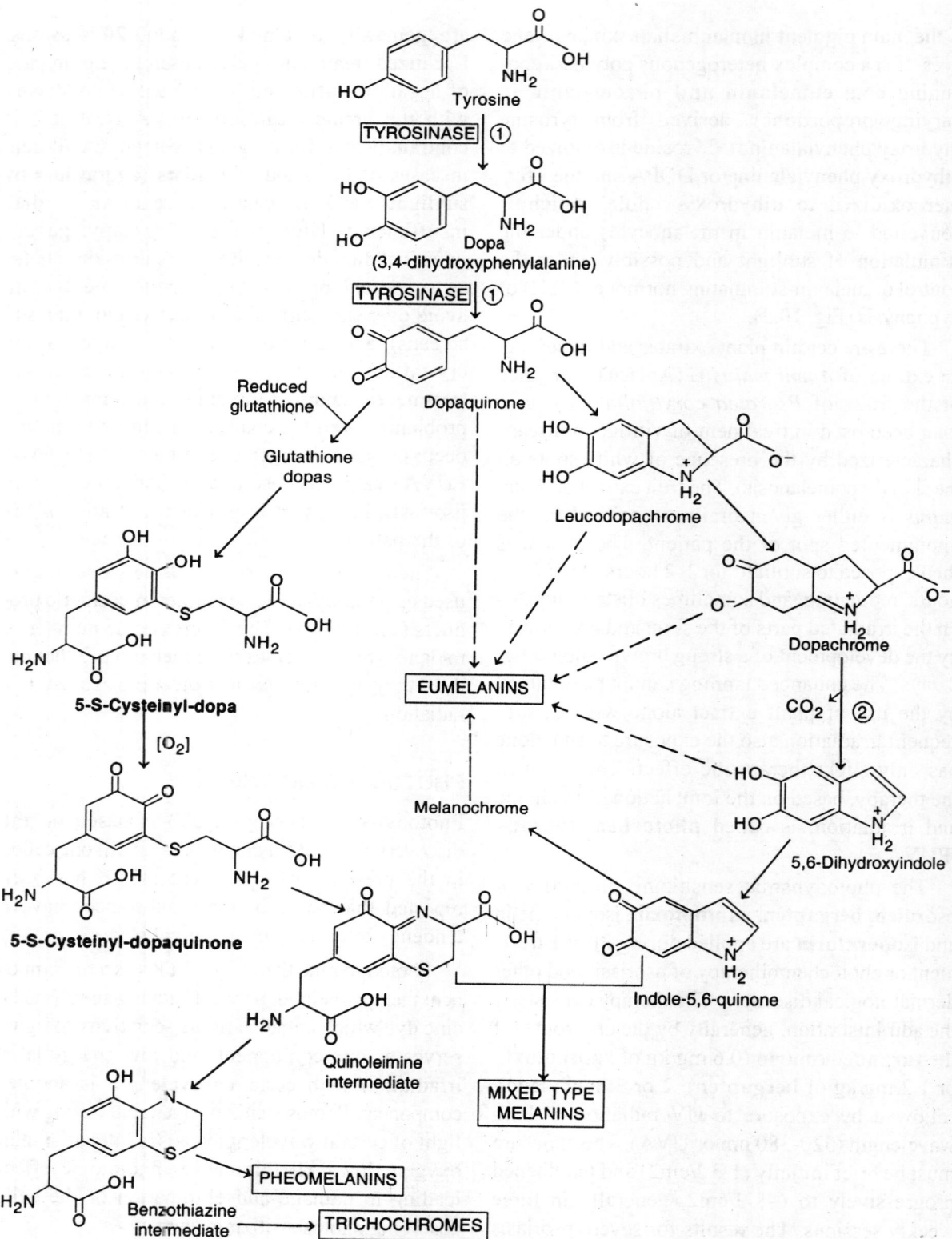

Fig. 10.2. Biosynthesis of Melanin Polymers.

In Russia, National Scientific Research Center "NIOPIC" in collaboration with a number of leading research centers in Physics (CENI IOPh RAS, JSC "BIOSPEK") and medicine (Hertzen Institute (MHRF), RAMS Oncology Center (Sechenov Medicine Academy) developed and introduced PDT method for treatment of tumor diseases using original domestic photosensitizing agents (PS) based on aluminimum phthalocyanine sulfuratted derivatives (Photosensitizers) and 5-aminolevulenic acid (Alasense). Selectivity of PDT effect on malignant tissues is ensured primarily through accumulation of photosensitizing agents and pro-sensitizer in tumor tissues (as compared to healthy tissues) due to more intensive blood supply of tumors.

Cancer Treatment

The photosensitizing agent injected into the body is absorbed by all cells. The agent remains in or around tumor cells for a longer time than it does in normal tissue. When treated cancer cells are exposed to red light from a laser, the light is absorbed by the photosensitizing agent. This light absorption causes a chemical reaction that destroys the tumor cells. Light exposure must be carefully timed to coincide with the period when most of the agent has left healthy cells but still remains in cancer cells. There are several promising features of PDT:

(1) Cancer cells can be selectively destroyed while most normal cells are spared,

(2) The damaging effect of the photosensitizing agent occurs only when the substance is exposed to light and are relatively mild.

Skin Aging Process

Many photosensitizing agents are known to generate reactive oxygen species, singlet oxygen ($1O_2$), superoxide anion (O_2) and •OH radicals which affect in following ways:

(i) The UV generated reactive oxygen species cause cross-linking of proteins (e.g. collagen), oxidation of sulfydryl groups causing disulfide cross-links, oxidative inactivation of certain enzymes causing functional impairment of cells (fibroblasts, keratinocytes, melanocytes, Langerhans cells) and liberation of proteases, collagenase and elastase. The skin-damaging effects of UVA appear to result from type II, oxygen-mediated photodynamic reactions in which UVA or near-UV radiation in the presence of certain photosensitizing chromophores (e.g., riboflavin, porphyrins, nicotinamide adenine dinucleotide phosphate (NADPH), etc.) leads to the formation of reactive oxygen species ($1O_2$, O_2, •OH).

(ii) The formation of protein cross-links in collagen, catalase and superoxide dismutase by $1O_2$ and O_2 (•OH) and the resulting denaturation of proteins and enzyme activities as a function UVA exposure dose.

(iii) The protective role of selective quenchers of $1O_2$ and O_2 (e.g. alpha-tocopherol acetate beta-carotene, sodium azide, ascorbic acid, etc.) is against the photoinactivation of enzymes and the prevention of the protein cross-linking reaction.

NATURAL SOURCE OF FURANOCOUMARINS

Furanocoumarins are natural products in which furan ring is fused with benzene ring of coumarin. These compounds are widely distributed in plants, but are particularly abundant in Umbelliferae/Apiaceae and Rutaceae family. Furanocoumarins are synthesized in plants by prenylation of the benzene ring by dimethyl-pyrophosphate (DMPP) in 6 or 8 position of a 7-hydroxy coumarins. Prenylation at C-6 yields 'Linear' furanocoumarins psoralen whilst at C-8 that of the 'angular' homologs isopsoralen.

Some common furanacoumarins are psoralen, bergapten, xanthotoxin, isopimpinelin and imperatorin. Plants containing psoralens have been used internally and externally to promote skin pigmentation and suntanning (Fig. 10.1). Examples of plants containing furanacoumarins are :

(i) Bergamot oil, (ii) *Ammi majus*, (iii) Babchi, (iv) Heracleum species, (v) *Ligusticum elatum*, (vi) Selinum species, (vii) *Pimpinella diversifolia*, (viii) *Prangos pabularia*, & (ix) *Seseli sibiricum*

(i) Bergamot Oil

Bergamot oil is obtained by cold expression of the peels of unripe fruits *Citrus bergamia* Risso (syn. *C. aurantium* L. Sub species *bergamia wright* and Arn) Family Rutaceae.

Characteristic of oil : The oil is clear mobile, yellowish green liquid with a sweet fragrance and fruity odour. The main constituents are d-limonene, dipentene, l-linalyl acetate, l-linalool, nerol, geraniol aldehyde, terpenes; sesquiterpenes and about 5% furanocoumarin (bergapten).

Use

As flavouring agent in aromatherapy and perfumery. The oil also contain furanocoumarin bergapten (up to 0.5%) and may cause severe photosensitization.

(ii) Ammi majus

Greater Ammi or Bishop's weed indigenous to Egypt and widely distributed in Mediterranean region, Abyssinia, Europe and West Africa.

In India, the plant was first introduced from Egypt at Forest Research Institute, Dehradun in 1955. Now it is cultivated in Jammu, Palampur and Baijnath (H.P.).

It is an erect branching herb, up to 1.5 to 2 m in height, leaves broad, ternate or pinnate, leaflets lanceolate, flowers white in loose compound umbels, fruit oblong, 1.5–2.0 mm long and 1 mm or less broad.

Cultivation

Seed propagation : The fine seeds 2.5 kg per hectare are mixed with fine soil or sand before sowing in furrow 90 cm apart. The soil is ploughed twice and brought to the fine filth. After sowing the seeds are covered with fine layer of soil. The seeds can be sown from 1st October to middle of November.

Fertilizer

Superphosphate 2.5 kg/hectare mixed with liberal quantity of farmyard manure in the furrow before sowing the seeds. Within a week after sowing liberal irrigation is required, the seeds start germinating within fortnight and takes about month to complete the germination. When seed develop true leaves (8-10 cm in height) thinning is done (60-90 cm apart). Irrigation is done after a week or ten days in dry seasons.

Harvesting

Best stage of harvesting is when the fruits are immature green in colour having maximum contents of xanthotoxin.

The flowering starts in the beginning of March and fruiting by end of April. The primary Umbel fruit are first hand picked towards the end of April or early May, when majority of remaining umbels (Secondary and tertiary) are about to mature, the crop is harvested, cut at middle level and stacked in loose bundles till the fruits dry up. The fruits are separated by thrashing and winnowing. A yield of over 1375 kg/ha is reported.

Chemical constituent

The chief active constituent in the fruit is xanthotoxin (ammoidin), the furanocoumarin marked under the trade name **"oxsoralen"**, other furanocoumarin present were ammidin (imperatorin), majudin (bergapten), marmesinine, isopimpinelin, majurin, ammajin (marmesinin) isoimperatorin, ammirin and 8-isopropenyl-8, 9, dihydro-angelicin.

The leaves contain xanthotoxin and isopimpinellin.

Use

Xanthotoxin in the dose of 50 mg three times a day is given orally or applied externally as one percent liniment followed by exposure of affected areas to sunlight or ultraviolet light for 2-4 hours.

(iii) Babchi

Synonyms : Psoralea; Malaya tea, Bawchang seed

Biological source : The drug consist of dried ripe fruits of *Psoralea corylifolia* L. (Leguminosae).

The plant is available as a common weed throughout India in waste land.

It is an annual errect herb having 60-100 cm

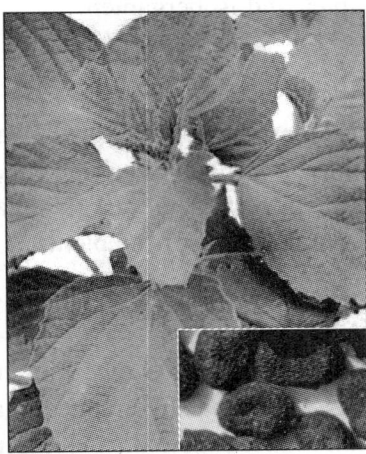

BABCHI (PSORALEA)
(*P. corylifolia*)
(for colour, see Plate 3, Fig. 3)

height. The stem and branches are grooved with glands and white trichomes. It flowers (purple coloured) in the month of August to October. The fruits are one-seeded indehiscent pods, dark brown to black in colour, odourless but on chewing, they produce pungent odour and bitter acrid taste.

Chemical constituent

The fruit contains fixed oil (10-12%), essential oil (0.1 to 0.25%), flavonoids and furanocoumarins. Psoralen and its isomer isopsoralen is the most important furanocoumarin present in this fruit.

Use

Seeds of *Psoralea corylifolia* (Babchi) are used in India in treatment of leucoderma and other skin disease. The curative action of *Psoralea* in leucoderma is due to the presence of Psoralen and Isopsoralen.

(iv) Heracleum candicans (Wall)

A potential source of xanthotoxin the genus Heracleum was reported to contain furanocoumarins, which are convertible to xanthotoxin. This plant is distributed mainly in north temperate region and some tropical mountains. According to estimate every year 150 tonnes of fresh roots of *H. candicans* are extracted from N.W. Himalayan region. During 1990-95 about 1000 tonnes of fresh roots have been extracted from wild sources in Kashmir Himalayas.

Cultivation

Seed propagation : The seeds are planted at a distance of 75 cm × 50 cm to obtain optimum yield. About 25 tonnes of farmyard manure per hectare gives the optimum yield of roots. The roots are harvested after a period of two years (425 kg/ha). The roots from cultivated plants yield **xanthotoxin** up to 1.5%. *H. candicans* can be brought under cultivation without much difficulty. This will greatly ensure a constant supply of quality raw material to the industry.

Vegetative propagation : Vegetative propagation is done from the roots (pretreated with Seridex 'B') arising from the root mass and planted in moist soil. This method of propagation is adopted for clonal multiplication of high xanthotoxin yielding strains.

(a) *H. candicans* : The root yields mixture of twelve furanocoumarins, both of linear and angular type major one is xanthotoxin (1.5% yield). Dealkylation of the total coumarins followed by purification of the product yields crude xanthotoxol, methylation of which with dimethyl sulphate in basic medium form xanthotoxin. The plant grow wild in the North-Western Himalayas and is in great demand by the pharmaceutical industry.

(b) *H. nepalense* : Plant grow wild in Nepal and Bhutan at 2000-4000 m. About 2% yield of furanocoumarin has been reported from the roots of the plant. The coumarins on chromatographic separation gave bergapten, isobergapten, sphondin and isopimpinellin.

(c) *H. wallichi* : The plant is natural habitat of Sikkim and Nepal. Grow wildly throughout the North-Western Himalayan region (2000-2600 m) in Jammu and Kashmir, Himachal Pradesh and U.P. The root contains nearly 2% yield of furanocoumarins viz. bergapten, isobergapten, sphondin, isopimpinallin, columbianetin, marmesin and vaginidiol.

(d) *H. conescens* : Grow wildly in Jammu and Kashmir, Himachal Pradesh and Uttar Pradesh (2000-2600 m).

The roots of the plant are rich source for commercial production of xanthotoxin (light petroleum ether extraction yield about 9% of coumarins). Coumarins and furanocoumarin isolated from roots of these plants are xanthotoxin

(0.005%), Imperatorin (1.5%), 8 geranoxy-psoralen (0.05%), heraclenin (3.0%), heraclenol (0.006%), bergaptin (0.01%) and isopimpinellin (0.01%).

(e) *H. cachemiricum* : The chief habitat are the forest of North-Western Himalayas at 2000-3000 m height.

The coumarin content of the roots is about 7%. The roots of the plant are used for the manufacture of xanthotoxin, giving about 1.5% yield.

(f) *H. thomsoni* : The plant grows wild in Ladakh.

Angelicin, psoralen, bergapten, imperatorin, (furanocoumarin) and their derivatives along with coumarin are obtained from plant root.

(g) *H. obtusifolium* : Grows wild in Sikkim, Nepal and Bhutan (4000 m) Isoimperatorin (furanocoumarin) is obtained from the roots.

(h) *H. sublineare* : Plant grows in Sikkim (3000-4000 m). Bergapten, isobergapten and isopimpinellin (furanocoumarin) are obtained from the roots of the plant.

(i) *H. rigens* : It grows wild in Nilgiris. Furanocoumarins isolated from the roots of the plant are heraclenin, isopimpinellin, imperatorin, bergapten and isobergapten.

(v) Ligusticum elatum

It is source for bergapten (0.001%) and three pyranocoumarins viz. selindin (1.005%), pteryxin (1.6%) and epoxypteryxin (0.1%) have been reported from the roots of the plants.

(vi) Selinum spp.

(a) *S. papyraceum* : Grows wild in Himalayas. Three linear furanocoumarins viz. knidilin, xanthotoxin and isopimpinellin are obtained.

(b) *S. tenuifolium* : Grows in Himalayas at altitude of 2000-4000m. The roots of the plant are source for isoimperatorin and imperatorin.

(vii) Pimpinella diversifolia

This herb grows in the North Western Himalayan region. The plant is a source for Ammirin, isoangenomalin, and oxypeucedanin furanocoumarin.

(viii) Prangos pabularia

It grows abundantly in Kashmir at altitude of 2000-3000 m. Source for isoimpinellin, xanthotoxin alongwith other coumarins.

(ix) Seseli sibiricum

It grows in Jammu and Kashmir. It is source of furanocoumarins viz. isobergapten, bergapten, phellopterin, sibiricin, coumurrain, osthenol and meranzin hydrate.

EXTRACTION PROCEDURE FOR FURANOCOUMARINS

Coumarins in free state are soluble in alcohols and in organic solvents such as ether, petroleum ether and chlorinated solvents, with which they can be extracted. Their glycosides are more or less soluble in water. The process for the production of xanthotoxin from *Ammi majus* is based on the fact that the total coumarins, consisting of xanthotoxin, imperatorin and bergaptin, are isolated of which imperatorin undergoes ready dealkylation to xanthotoxol on treatment with acetic acid-sulphuric acid leaving behind xanthotoxin and bergapten unaffected. Xanthotoxins and bergapten may be separated from hydrolyzed mixture with organic solvents. Removal of solvent and fractional crystallisation of the residue gives xanthotoxin . Xanthotoxol obtained from the hydrolysis of imperatorin, on methylation with dimethyl sulphate in the basic medium gives xanthotoxin. The total yield of xanthotoxin is around 0.6% of the weight of the seed.

Heracleum candicans yields coumarins, majority of which are esters of xanthotoxol (8-hydroxypsoralen). The total coumarins are then dealkylated with polyphosphoric acid. This is then washed with organic solvents to remove the soluble impurities and the purified xanthotoxol on methylation with dimethyl sulphate in alkaline medium gives xanthotoxin.

MECHANISM OF ACTION OF FURANOCOUMARIN IN PHOTOSENSITIZATION

The exact mechanism of action of photosensitization by furanocoumarins is not known. However it is reported that furanocoumarin photoreact with DNA upon irradiation at 366 nm and form complex with DNA which is the preliminary requirement before the initiation of photoreaction, thus they interfere with DNA by forming cross-links between base pairs. It has been reported that the active furanocoumarin are first activated by the UV irradiation and its double bonds at C-3, C-4 and at C-4', C-5' undergo cycloadditions with the 5, 6-double bond of the pyrimidine base in the DNA base-pair (thymine, uracil, cytosine) (Fig. 10.3).

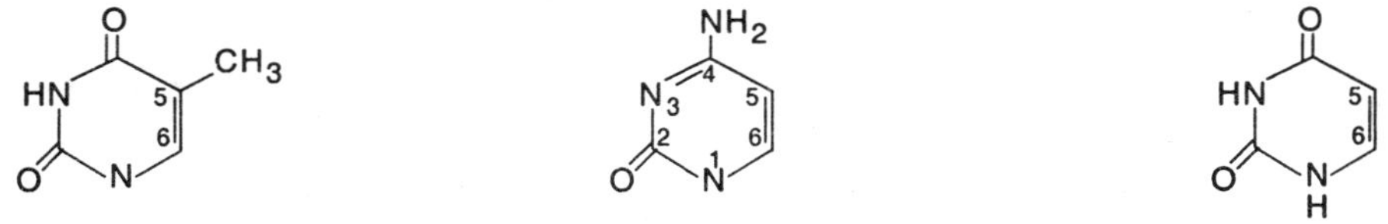

Thymine (2, 4-dioxy-5-methyl pyrimidine)   Cytosine (2-oxy-4-amino pyrimidine)   Uracil (2, 4-dioxypyrimidine)

Fig. 10.3. DNA Base-Pairs for Photo Reaction.

This cross-linking inhibits the replication and transcription of DNA and consequently, the synthesis of RNA, proteins and the occurrence of cell division.

Thus the inhibition of DNA synthesis by the xanthotoxin (active furanocoumarin) is considered to be the major factor in the treatment of vitiligo (psoriasis) (Fig. 10.4).

It is possible that these properties have also something to do with phototoxicity, the mechanism of which remains to be elucidated: they mainly explain the mutagenic and carcinogenic properties.

The efficiency of the ultra violet energy in producing tanning is dependent on the wavelength of the irradiation. shorter wavelength irradiation cause erythema.

Structure Activity Relationship

- Photosensitizing activity is a property of furanocoumarin molecule only.

- Linear structure of furanocoumarin (Psoralen) is more active than angular (Angelicin).
- Methylation of the furanocoumarin molecule in 5-8 position enhances the activity, whereas at 4 or 3' position causes a decrease. A methyl group in 3 position is strongly negative.
- Introduction of –OH group in the molecule of psoralen removes the activity (xanthotoxol, bergaptol) whereas the activity is restored on methylation of –OH group (xanthotoxin, bergapten). Lengthening of the alkyl chain gradually reduces the activity to zero.

Introduction of nitro amino and acetylamine group cancel the activity of parent molecule.

PHOTOBIOLOGICAL EFFECTS OF FURANOCOUMARINS

When irradiated at 365 nm furanocoumarins may produce some interesting photobiological effects. These are:

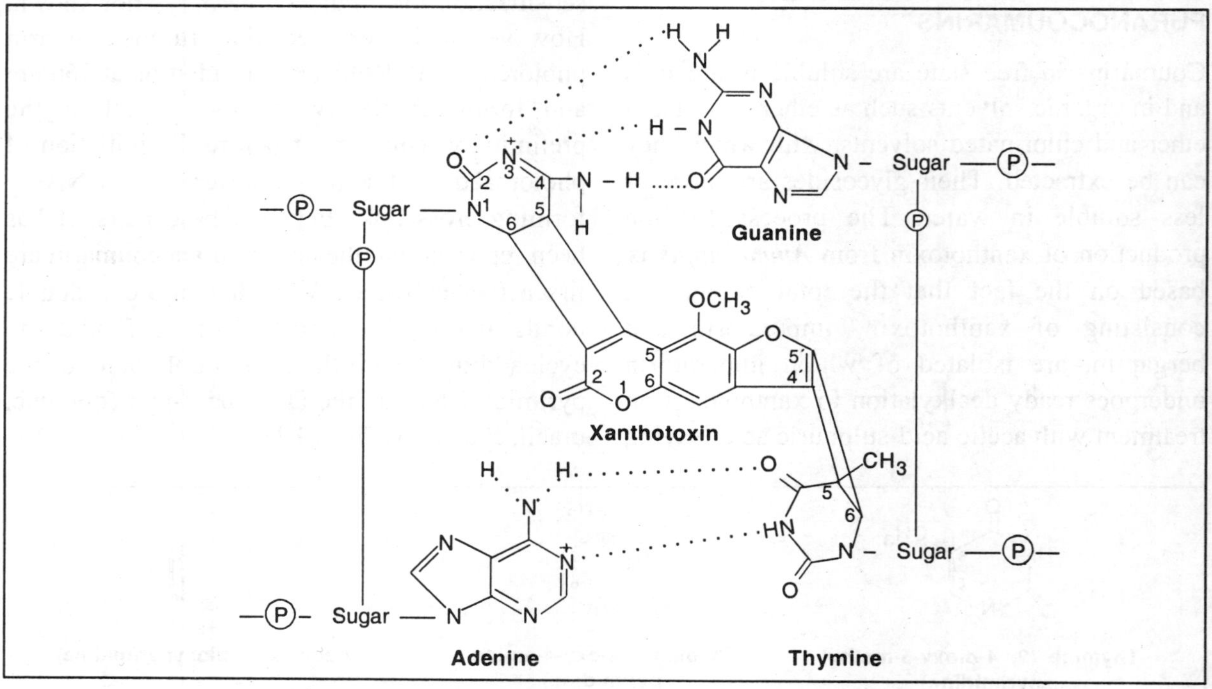

Fig. 10.4. Mechanism of Photosensitization by Furanocoumarin.

(a) **Killing of bacteria -** Irradiation with dermal photosensitizing furanocoumarins can also kill bacteria.

(b) **Formation of mutants -** Mutagenic effect of xanthotoxin were observed on *Escherichia coli, Sarcina lutea*. Psoralen also produces mutagenic effect on Drosophila melanogaster.

(c) **Formation of giant cells -** This effect was noticed on irradiation of mammalian cells (adapted to *in vitro* growth) in the presence of psoralen. The formation of polynuclear cells in sea urchin eggs with sperms irradiated in the presence of psoralen has also been reported.

(d) **Inactivation of viruses -** It has been reported that viruses were completely inactivated when irradiated in the presence of psoralen whilst some RNA viruses proved more resistant.

ANNEXURE I
PRIMARY CLASS OF MEDICATIONS RESPONSIBLE FOR PHOTOSENSITIZING REACTIONS

Antihistamines

Astemizole
Azatacline
Brompheniramine
Buclizine
Carbinoxamine
Chlorpheniramine
Clemastine
Cyclizine
Cyproheptadine
Dexchlorpheniramine
Dimenhydrinae
Diphenhydramine
Diphenylpyralline
Doxylamine
Hydroxyzine
Meclizine
Methapyrilene
Methdilazine
Orphenadrine
Pheniramine
Promethazine
Pyrilamine
Terfenadine
Trimeprazine
Tripelennamine
Triproilidine

Coal Tar and Derivatives
(Examples by brand names)

Alphosyl

Aquatar
Denorex Medicated Shampoo
DHS Tar Gel Shampoo
DOAK Shampoo
Estar
Ionil T Plus
LAVATAR
Medotar
T/Derm
Tar Emollient
Tegrin Shampoo
T/Gel
Therapeutic Shampoo
Zetar Shampoo

Contraceptives, Oral and Estrogens
(Birth control pills, female sex hormones)

Estrogens
Chlorotrianisene
Diethyestilbestrol
Estradiol
Estrogens, conjugated Estrogens,
Esterfled
Estropipate

Progestogens

Ethinyl estradiol
Medroxyprogesterone
Megestrol
Norethindrone
Norgestrel
Quinestrol

(cont'd)

NSAID: Non-Steroidal Anti-inflammatory Drugs (Antiarthritics)

Diclofenac
Diflunisal
Fenoprofen
Flurbiprofen
Ibuprofen
Indomethacin
Ketoprofen
Meclofenamate
Naproxen
Phenylbutazone
Piroxicam
Sulindac
Suprofen
Tolmetin

Phenothiazines (Major transquilizers, anti-emetics)

Acetophenazine
Butaperazine
Carphenazine
Chlorpromazine
Ethopropazine
Fluphenazine
Mesoridazine
Methdilazine
Methotrimeprazine
Perphenazine
Piperacetazine
Prochloroperazine
Promazine
Promethazine
Propiomazine
Thiethylperazine
Thioridazine
Trifluoperazine
Triflupromazine
Trimeprazine

Psoralens

Methoxsalen
Trixsalen

Sulfonamides ('Sulfa' drugs, antimicrobials, anti-infectives)

Acetazolamide

Sulfacytine
Sulfadiazine
Sulfadoxine
Sulfamethizole
Sulfamethoxazole
Sulfapyridine
Sulfasalazine
Sulfinpyrazine
Sulfazoxazole

Sulfonylureas (Oral anti-diabetics, hypoglycemics)

Acetohexamide
Chlorpropamide
Glipizide
Glyburide
Tolazamide
Tolbutamide

Thiazide Diuretics ('water pills')

Bendroflumethiazide
Benzthiazide
Chlorthiazide
Chlorthalidone
Cyclothiazide
Hydrochlorothiazide
Hydroflumethiazide
Methyclothizide
Polythiazide
Trichlormethiazide

Tetracyclines (Antibiotics, anti-infectives)

Chlortetracycline
Demeclocycline
Doxycycline
Methacycline
Oxytetracycline
Tetracycline

Tricyclic Antidepressants

Amitriptyline
Amoxapine
Desipramine
Doxepin
Imipramine
Nortriptylin
Protriptyline
Trimipramine

ANNEXURE-II
OTHER PHOTOSENSITIZING AGENTS RESPONSIBLE FOR PHOTOSENSITIVE REACTION

Classification or Use	Agents
Antifungals	Fentichlor/Jadit/Multifungin
Antimicrobials,	Bithionol/Chlorhexidine
Antiseptics	Hexachlorophene
Artificial sweetners	Calcium cyclamate/cyclamates, Sodium cyclohexylsulfamate
Coal tar and coal tar derivatives for psoriasis and chronic eczema and in hair shampoos	Anthracene/Many phenolic agents Naphtholene/ Phenanthrene/Pitch/Thiophene
Cosmetics and dyes	Acridine/Eosin/Erythrocine, Fluorescein/Methylene Blue, Methyl violet/Orange red/Paraphenylenediamine/Rose bengal, Toluidine blue/Trypaflavin/Trypan blue
Deodorant and bacteriostatic agents in soaps	Halogenated carbanilides, Halogenated phenols/ Halogenated salicylanilides
Fluorescent brigtening agent for cellulose, nylon or wool fibers	Blankophor
Melanogenics (furanocoumarins)	Methoxypsoralens, Petroleum products, Psoralen
Perfumes and toilet articles (essential oils)	Ethereal oils, Msk ambrette, Oil of Bergamot, Oil of Cedar, Oil of **Citron**, Oil of Lavendar, Oil of Lemon, Oil of Lime, Oil of Rosemary, Oil of Sandalwood
Flavoring and spices	Rutaceae and Umbelliferae plants
Tatoos	Cadmium sulfide

Chapter

11

Herbs and Health Food

INTRODUCTION

Herbs are used by the mankind since its origin on the earth; to alleviate human illness and for the maintenance of general health. The products of natural origin for general improvement of the health are referred to as **"health food"** but not as drug or medicinal agent. Hence the health foods may be defined as the food supplemented with herbal ingredients, vitamins, minerals and the nutrients or ingredients isolated from the conventional food. In recent years there is growing interest of the public in the health benefits of dietary food and personal care products, with the results, more attention is being paid by the Pharma Industry towards health food (nutraceutical), herbal cosmetics and personal care products. In west, the fast growing segments of health food products industry look like a revolution. This is because of the increased awareness of the consumers for health benefits of these products and growing desire for the alternative to conventional pharmaceutical products.

The increasing interest and popularity of the health food products in Asia, Latin America, Africa and Middle East countries has opened a new era of international trade in alternative system of medicine (medical care).

Health foods are termed by different names throughout the world i.e. functional foods in oriental and nutraceuticals in the western region, thus the nutraceuticals and functional foods are synonyms for health food products.

Nutraceuticals

Nutraceutical is any substance that can be considered as a food or its part which, in addition to its normal nutritional value, provides health benefits including prevention of disease or promotion of health.

The nutraceuticals are associated with the prevention or treatment of four major diseases like heart disease, cancer, hypertension and diabetes. The other diseases related to role of nutraceuticals are osteoporosis, arthritis and neural tube defects.

The food products used as nutraceuticals contain **antioxidants, prebiotics, probiotics, omega 3 fatty acids and certain dietary fibres.** Except probiotics, all these components are present in fruits, vegetables and different types of herbal foods.

Antioxidants

Antioxidants or inhibitors of oxidation are the

compounds, which retard or prevent the oxidation and in general prolong the life of the oxidizable matter. The reactive oxygen species (ROS) in the body, include superoxide anion, singlet oxygen, hydroxyl radical and hydrogen peroxide. The oxidative damage initiated by them is propagated by lipid peroxidation, which may cause further damage to DNA. The body defence system against the oxidative damage consists of enzymes such as superoxide dismutase, glutathione peroxidase, catalase and the reducing agents such as glutathione, ascorbic acid and iron.

Mechanism of action of antioxidants

In general, reactive oxygen molecules circulating in the body, tend to react with electrons of other molecules of the body and the various enzyme systems; with the result, the molecules as well as the enzyme system of the body is damaged, which may further contribute to conditions such as **cancer, ischemia, aging, adult respiratory distress syndrome and rheumatoid arthritis** etc.

It has also been observed that the presence of free radicals cause cytotoxicity, alteration of enzymes & nucleic acids and peroxidation of the lipids, as a result there is a loss of cell membrane integrity, which initiates the aging process before time.

Naturally occurring antioxidants

Naturally occurring antioxidants which could be of therapeutic use include **superoxide dismutase (isolated or recombinant), tocopherols, ascorbic acid, adenosine transferrin, lactoferrin, glutathione and its precursors, carotenoids and other plant pigments, like defroxamine.**

The natural antioxidants are present in some fixed oils, fruits, vegetables and fishes. The antioxidants present in such fruits/vegetables prevent either the formation of oxygen free radicals or trap them.

Antioxidant like **tocopherols (vitamin E)** lower the susceptibility of LDL oxidation (LDL oxidation increases the chances of atherosclerosis), it also reduce platelet's role in thrombus formation. Examples of natural food rich in vitamin E are **corn oil, wheat germ oil**. Other fruits like **amla, myrobalan and lemon** contain antioxidant in the form of ascorbic acid. It acts by vengering oxygen free radicals as well as prevent their formation.

Beta carotene and vitamin A help to enhance immunity and thus act as antioxidants.

Probiotics

Probiotics are the **living microorganisms,** which improve the intestinal microbial balance. Example: Bifidobacterium and Lactobacilli species such as *L. acidophillus*.

Prebiotics

Prebiotics are the substances, which reach to colon in intact form, i.e. without getting depleted by the gastric pH and digestive acids. These **prebiotics** also selectively promote the growth of colonic probiotic bacteria, hence they act as fertilizers for these symbiotic bacteria. Example **Inulin,** which is a polyfructose obtained from raw chicory (roots of *Cichorium intybus*) or Jeruslem artichoke. Chicory is rich in fibrous polysaccharide inulin, which is soluble dietary fibre and resistant to digestive enzymes, thus reaches to large intestine or colon essentially intact, where it is fermented by resident bacteria, **Lactobacilli and Bifidobacteria** digest inulin and feed themselves on it. The dairy products like sour milk and A/B culture yoghurt contain these prebiotics.

Polyunsaturated fatty acids (PUFA)

The natural vegetable oils and marine animal oils containing polyunsaturated fatty acids (PUFA) belonging to Linoleic group (Omega-6-type and Omega-3-type), help to reduce cholesterol formation/deposition and prevent thromboxane formation and thus useful as preventive measure for atherosclerosis. Example **safflower oil, corn oil, soybeen oil, mustard oil and marine fishes**.

Omega-3-Fatty acids

Omega-3 fatty acids are **eicosapentaenoic acid (EPA)** and doco-sa-hexaenoic acid (DHA). They are polyunsaturated essential fatty acids mainly of marine origin (Fig. 11.1).

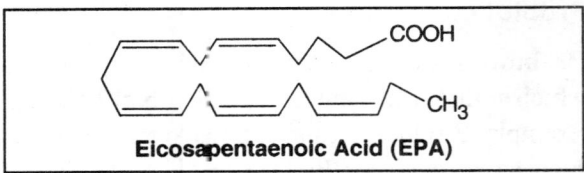

Eicosapentaenoic Acid (EPA)

Fig. 11.1. Eicosapentaenoic Acid (EPA).

Omega-3 fatty acids have been found to be useful for following activities:

- Increase the physiochemical stability and functional integrity of the cell wall.
- Suppression of smooth muscle cell proliferation and migration.
- Reduction of LDL and VLDL levels.
- Reduction in thromboxane formation and increased fibrinolysis.

They are present in cold-water fishes like Cod, Salmon, Tuna, Sardines, Blue fish, Mackerel and Herring. Cold weather bean oil plants like flax seed and canola.

Walnut, soybean and freshly ground wheat germ also contain omega-3-fatty acids.

Dietary Fibres

Dietary fibres are used in Health food products for the normalization of intestinal transit. They have dual effect on intestinal transit. First effect is on the bulk of faeces, which is often increased in substantial proportions (127% after ingestion of

20 g of wheat bran), this action take place with insoluble fibres. The other effect of the dietary fibres is upon the duration of the transit, which get normalized around 48 hours. Long transit gets shortened; short transit gets lengthened. This activity is also due to the insoluble fibre contents (bran, cellulose). It is reported that the bulk-forming effect is enhanced by the presence of short chain aliphatic acids (e.g. propionate, butyrate), released upon bacterial degradation of the water-soluble portion of the fibres. The acids causes phasic contraction. Dietary fibre present in various parts of the plant i.e. leaves, stem and seeds are not digested or absorbed by human body, however, their high intake benefits human body in various ways.

Dietary fibres are generally categorised into two groups:

- Water soluble and
- Water Insolube fibres

Soluble fibres dissolve in water and form a gel that binds the stool and inhibit the non-propulsive colon contractions.

Soluble fibres are present in **Oats, dried beans, legumes, chicory** etc.

Water insoluble fibre mainly helps in bulking of stool and their quick passage through digestive tract.

Insoluble fibres are present in **brown rice, bananas, cassavas, vegetables and whole grain cereals, like wheat, oat, barley and sorghum.**

The regular consumption of soluble fibres (pectin 6-40 g , dried beans 100-150 g, psyllium or guar 10-30 g) or insoluble fibre (bran 25-100 g) in diet, decreases cholesterol (-10%) and LDL-cholesterol (-10 to -14% depending on the initial cholesterolemia).

It is also hypothesized that diet high in fibres and low in animal protein and lipids, causes a lower frequency of colorectal cancer.

Although fibres decrease protein digestibility.

this effect is negligible being that diets are (far) rich in proteins in industrialised countries.

Source of Dietary Fibres

Fresh fruits (**apple, orange, apricot, plum, pineapple**) with fibre 18–30%; vegetables (**cabbage, carrot, lettuce, onion, tomato**) 9–12% total fibres and dried beans peas with 20% total fibres.

To supplement food intake with insoluble fibre one has to consume products like wheat bran (>40% mostly insoluble fibres) and products derived from Oat, brown rice and chicory.

Carotenoids : The **carotenoids** of the vegetable, fruits or other herbal products, on ingestion, are degraded at the level of human intestinal mucosa into **retinol** (vitamin A) and exerts a preventive action against degenerative disorders e.g. vegetable and fruits (**carrots, spinach, mangos, tomatos, citrus and melons**), **animal products (Egg, liver and fish**) and Palm oil. Margarine 1,600,000 IU/g of vitamin A corresponds to 0.3 µg of retinol and 0.6 µg of β-carotene.

Carotenoids also interfere with the photo-oxidation process and are of use in the prevention and treatment of photosensitization linked to porphyrin and dermatitis of phototoxic origin.

Moreover, the carotenoids are useful as natural, efficacious non-toxic food colorant, either natural extracts e.g. **Annatto extract** or carotene extracted from natural origin e.g. carrot (carotene), tomato skin (lycopene), *Tagetes erecta* and **alfalfa** (xanthophylls)

Chief carotenoids containing herbal drugs used as health food and food products are **Alfalfa, Annanto, capsicum, saffron and Palm oil.**

HERBS AS FOOD OR MEDICINE

When the herbal material has been previously licensed as a medicine, is on the Medical Control Agency's (MCA) general sale list and has a long history of use, with proper scientific literature and, if no claims are to be made on the product then the herb may be considered as a food supplement rather than a medicine.

The following are the herbs which are used as health food in the formulation of various health products or as dietary supplements:

Oat bran, Psyllium, Soya. Inulin, Kiwi extracts, *Garcinia cambogia* (fat burners), flax seed, Valerian, Passion flower, chamomile, St. John's wort, *Serenoa repens*, *Echinaceae purpurea*, *Panax gingeng*, *Ginkgo biloba*, *Hypericum perfoatum*, *Allium sativum*, *Hydrastits canadensis* (golden seal), *Matricaria chamomila*, *Silybum marianum*, *Trigonella foenum* (fenugreek), *Tanacetum parthenium*, *Ephedra sinica* and *Cimicifuga racemosa.*

Traditional herbs like ginger, peppermint, fennel, papaya, liquorice, aloe & others and the plants containing isoflavones, lycopene, oligosaccharides, anthocyanins, Lutein, Zea xanthin, phytoestrogens Omega-3-fatty acid and vitamins products are also used as health products.

REGULATION REGARDING THE HERBS AS FOOD

Dietary supplements are regulated under food law, but with certain provisions that apply only to dietary supplements. Thus dietary supplements are eligible for Food and Drug Administration (FDA) authorized health claims under the Nutrition and Labelling Education Act (NLEA). In 1994 when Dietary Supplement, Health and Education Act (DSHEA) was passed, it expanded and clarified the definition of dietary supplements, specified additional requirements for safety provided for four types to support claims of nutritional value. These include:

- Prevention of classic nutritional deficiencies
- Structure or function (S/F) effects
- Mechanism for S/F effects
- General well being

The Office of Dietary Supplement (ODS) was established at National Institute of Health (NIH) by Congress through the Dietary Supplement Health and Education Act (DSHEA) of 1994. The aim of the ODS was to strengthen knowledge and understanding of dietary supplements.

The provision of DSHEA define dietary supplements and dietary ingredients, establish a new framework for assuring safety, guidelines for displayed of literature where supplements are sold, provide for use of claims and nutritional support statements, require ingredient & nutrition labeling and grant FDA authority to establish Good Manufacturing Practice (GMP) regulations.

The DSHEA established a formal definition of dietary supplement i.e. A dietary supplement is a product (other than narcotic) that is intended to supplement the diet that bears or contains one or more of the following dietary ingredients : vitamin, mineral, an herb or other botanical, amino acid, dietary substance for use by man to supplement the diet by increasing the total daily intake, or a concentrate, metabolite constituents, extracts or combinations of these ingredients.

NATURAL HERBS/INGREDIENTS AND HEALTH FOOD

ACACIA
(*Acacia senegal*)

Synonym - Gum arabic.

Gum acacia is the dried, gummy exudate from the stems and branches of *Acacia senegal* (Linn.) wild or of other related Arabian species of acacia (Leguminosae).

Chemical Constituents

Gum acacia consists principally of arabin, which is a complex mixture of calcium, magnesium and potassium salts of arabic acid. The arabic acid is a branched polysaccharide that on hydrolysis yields L-arabinose, D-galactose, D-glucuronic acid and L-rhamnose. 1,3-linked D-galactopyranose units form backbone chain of the molecule and the terminal residues of the 1-6 linked side chains are primarily uronic acids.

Gum acacia also contains 12-15% water and several occluded enzymes (oxidase, peroxidases and pectinases), which get destroyed on heating at 100°C.

Gum acacia is water-soluble gum; one part of the gum can dissolve in two parts of water, forming a weakly acidic solution with pH 4.5-5.5.

Health Food

Gum acacia has been in use as general tonic since ancient times. Currently, its major uses in food are as a suspending or emulsifying agent, stabilizer, adhesive and flavour fixative and to prevent crystallisation of sugar. It is used in practically all categories of processed foods, including candy, snack food, alcoholic and non-alcoholic beverages, baked good and frozen dairy desserts.

Gum acacia along with other polysaccharides, is a potential hypocholesterolemic agent.

Ghati Gum or Indian Gum

It is a product, sometimes used as a substitute for acacia. It is an exudate from *Anogeissus latifolia* (Comberetaceae), a tree indigenous to India and Sri Lanka.

ACEROLA
(*Malpighia glabra*)

Synonym - Barbados cherry; Puerto rican cherry, West Indian Cherry (M. punicifolia); huesito (M. glabra).

Acerola is the globose, ovoid or subglobose fruit of *Malpighia glabra* Linn. and *M. punicifolia* Linn. (Malpighiaceae).

M. punicifolia is native to the West Indies and is also found in northern south America, central America, Florida and Texas. Its fruits are the richest source of natural vitamin C in the edible portion of the fruit (vitamin C content is highest in green and lowest in fully ripe fruit).

Chemical Constituents

Other vitamins present include 4,300-12,500 IU/100 g. Vitamin A, thiamine, riboflavin and niacin. Miscellaneous constituents include Calcium, Iron and Phosphorus in comparable concentrations to those of apple.

Health Food

It is used as a source of natural vitamin C in the form of herbal tea, juice, tablet or capsule.

The fruits have reportedly been used for the treatment of dysentery, diarrhoea and liver disorders.

It is available in the market as fresh fruits, juice and spray dried form, canned juice along with pear, apricot and grape juice (to increase the vitamin C contents of the juices).

ALETRIS
(*Aletris farinosa* Linn.)

Synonyms : Stargrass.

Aletris is the dried rhizome and roots of *Aletris farinosa* Linn. (Liliaceae).

It is the perennial herb with grass like leaves up to 20 cm long, rosette around a slender, with naked flowering stem that grows up to almost 1m high. The plant is native to Florida and west Wisconsin and Texas.

Chemical Constituents

The herbs contain volatile oil, resinous material and saponin glycoside that yield diosgenin on hydrolysis.

Health Food

It is an **estrogenic** plant used in health food in the form of herb teas, crude root, powdered or cut and sifted used in tablets. Capsules, tinctures often in combinations with other herbs for menstrual disorders and as **bitter digestive tonic**. In the form of tea as antidiarrheal tea, as a sedative and as a diuretic.

ALFALFA
(*Medicago sativa* Linn.)

Alfalfa or Lucerne consists of dried leaves, flowering tops and seeds of *Medicago sativa* Linn. (Leguminosae or Fabaceae).

It is a perennial herb with a deep taproot; leaves resemble those of clover, grows to a height of 1 m with mostly bluish purple flowers. Native to western Asia and east Mediterranean regions, now cultivated throughout the World.

Chemical Constituents

It is a saponin containing plant (medicagenic acid, hederagenin) and is better known as a fodder than as a medicinal plant. It contains flavones and isoflavones, coumarin derivatives (medicagol, sativol trifoliol and daphnoretin) and pectin methylesterase. It also contains phenolics (coumestrol) as well as L-canavanine, which is specially concentrated in the seeds (0.8-1.5%) compared to 0.1% in the leaves.

Alkaloids (trigonelline, which is in seeds only; stachydrine and homostachydrine), plant acids, (pantothenic acid; biotin, folic acid etc.), vitamins (A, B, B_6, B_{12}, C, E and K_1, niacin), amino acids (valine, lysine, arginine leucine, methionine and threonine) and plant pigments (chlorophyll, xanthophyll, β-carotene, anthocyanins).

Health Food

Alfalfa sprouts are favorite salad ingredient among health food enthusiasts.

Dried leaves used in tablets, capsules, teas, tinctures are reported as a source of chlorophyll, vitamins, minerals and protein, with unsubstantiated benefit in conditions such as rheumatoid arthritis, to prevent absorption of cholesterol, treating diabetes, stimulating appetite and as a **general tonic to increase vitality and weight in humans;** also as a diuretic, galactogogue and to increase peristaltic action of the stomach and bowels, resulting in increased appetite.

Commercial preparations

Crude and extracts.

ALLSPICE
(Pimentia dioica)

Synonym - *P. officinalis* Lindl.; Eugenia pimentia DC.

Allspice is the berry fully grown but unripe fruits and leaves obtained from 8-20 m high tree of *Pimentia dioica* (L) Merr. (Syn. *P. officinalis* Lindl.; *Eugenia pimentia* DC) (Myrtaceae) native to the West Indies, Central America and Mexico.

The West Indian allspice berries are smaller than Central America and Mexico berries, but they are more aromatic.

Chemical Constituents

The major component of the drugs is volatile oil (eugenol 60-80%). Other constituents are quercetin glycosides, catechins, proanthocyanidins, vitamins (A, C, thiamine, riboflavin, nicacin) and minerals.

Health Food

Allspice, its oil and oleoresin are currently used in many food products including alcoholic and non-alcoholic beverages, frozen dairy desserts, candies baked goods, gelatins, pudding and meat products.

It is considered to be an **appetite stimulant, antioxidant, antimitotic** and inhibits the synthesis of prostaglandin in human colic mucosa.

ANGELICA
(Angelica archangelica)

Angelica is dried fruit, dried rhizome and root of *Angelica archangelica* Linn. (Umbelliferae) containing 0.5% of volatile oil obtained from stout biennial or perennial herb up to 2 m high, with a large rhizome; the fruit with thick corky wings is native to northern and eastern Europe to Netherlands, cultivated in Belgium Hungary, Germany and other countries.

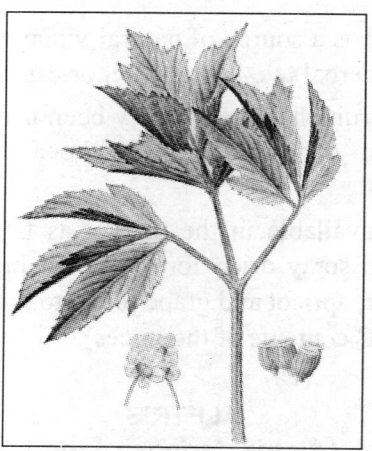

ANGELICA (A. archangelica)
(for colour, see Plate 3, Fig. 4)

Chemical Constituents

Angilica is rich in coumarins, which occurs throughout the plant.

The root and rhizome contains 0.5 to 1% volatile oil, composed mainly of α-phellandrene, α-pinene, limonene, β-caryophyllene, linalool and lactones.

It also contain acids like caffeic, chlorogenic, quinic, linoleic, linolenic, petroselinic and behenic acid.

Health Food

Crude root at a daily dose of 4-5 g and galenical preparations are indicated internally for **appetite loss and digestive ailments including** mild GI tract spasms and flatulence.

Both dried seeds and powdered roots are occasionally used as tea flavourant; aromatic stimulant, bronchial tonic, carminative, diaphoretic, diuretic, emmenagogue and in the treatment of rheumatism and for menstrual regulations.

Roots and seeds were both formerly official in USP and N.F.

ANISEED
(*Pimpinella anisum* Linn.)

Anise or Aniseed is the dried, ripe fruit of *Pimpinella anisum* Linn. (Apiaceae/Umbelliferae) Pimpinella is Latin word meaning two wings.

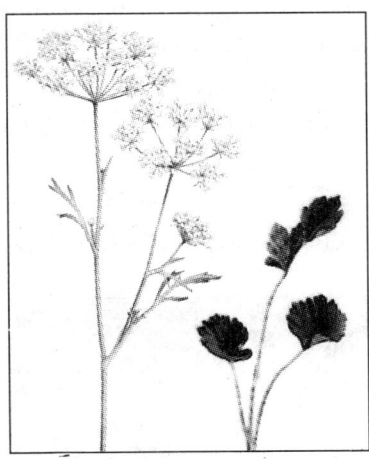

ANISEED PLANT *(Pimpinella anisum Linn.)*
(for colour, see Plate 3, Fig. 5)

The plant is an annual herb indigenous to Asia Minor, Egypt, Greece and also cultivated in South America, Germany, Italy and Southern Russia. Anise grows wild in the near east and widely cultivated, along other places on the Mediterranean rim (Spain, Turkey, North Africa and Asia).

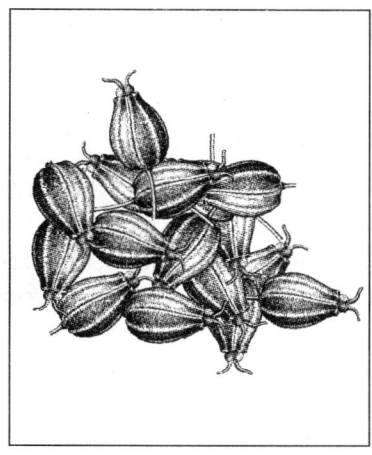

ANISEED
(for colour, see Plate 3, Fig. 6)

Chemical Constituents

The aniseed fruit contains polysaccharides, lipids (15-20%), flavonoids, a glucoside of p-hydroxy-benzoic acid and 2-3% of essential oil. The latter contains 80-90% anethole, estragol and anisaldehyde. Other derivatives (anisic acid, anisyl alcohol and ketone) may be found in partially oxidised essential oils.

Health Food

Aniseed is reputed to be estrogenic, considered to be **galactogogue**, expectorant and carminative, traditionally used for symptomatic treatment of gastrointestinal disturbance.

The fruits are used **as spice in the health food** products, because of their carminative properties.

ANNATO TREE
(*Bixa orellana* Linn.)

Annanto tree (*Bixa orellana* Linn. family Bixaceae) grows wildly in the tropical area of America and is cultivated in tropical area of India, eastern Africa and also widely cultivated in Brazil and Peru.

Its fruit contain 15-20 seeds embedded in a **gooey** bright red pulp.

Chemical Constituents

The main constituent present in the fruit is 9'-cis-bixin, which is lipid-soluble methyl ester of a C-24 dicarboxylic acid 9'-cis-norbixin; cis-bixin occurs along with small quantities of trans bixin and cis-norbixins.

Health Food

The crude product is used to prepare oily extracts, water-soluble extracts or sprays containing 0.2-0.3% bixin, which are used for coloring the food products. Major food categories in which annatto colour is used include alcoholic and non alcoholic beverages, frozen dairy desserts, baked goods, meat and meat products, condiments, fats and oils (salad oil, popcorn oil, margarine and sausages).

APRICOT PITS
(Prunus armeniaca)

Apricot pits is the kernel of varieties of *Prunus armeniaca* Linn. (Rosaceae). Commonly referred to as apricot pits they are sold in "health food" stores throughout USA as a source for amygdalin or laetrile 3%. Fatty acid composition of the oil obtained from the kernel chiefly consists of C_{16}:4-9%, C_{18}:<9%; C_{13}:1:,58-80; C_{18}:2:10-32; C_{18}:3:<0.1.

The fruits are used as spice in the health food products because of carminative properties.

ARNICA
(Arnica montana)

Arnica is commonly known as **Leopard's Bane**. It is a very widely used remedy for the treatment of bruising and contusions and in cases of mental and physical shock. It comes under the category of **homoeopathic natural product**.

Chemical Constituents

Arnica consists of dried flowering heads of *Arnica montana* Linn. and related Arnica species (Compositae). Its alcoholic extract or tincture has been used widely as a counter irritant. Small amount of the extract have also been used to treat inflammation of gums and as a gargle/mouth wash for sore throats.

The chemical constituents responsible for topical action are arnidiol and faradiol (isomeric dihydric alcohols). Arnica extract can be toxic if taken orally in large doses; hence its continuous use should be avoided.

ASTRAGALUS
(Astragalus membranaceus)

Astragalus is the dried roots from 4-7 year old plants of *Astragalus membranaceus* (Fisch) Bge (Syn. *A. propinguus* B. schischk) *A. mongholicus* Var. Mongholicus (Bge.) Hsiao and other Chinese *Astragalus* spp. (Leguminosae or Fabaceae).

Perennial herb native to northern China and some to high regions such as in Sichuan Yunnan and Tibet.

The most commonly used forms are raw (dried root) and cured (honey treated) astragalus.

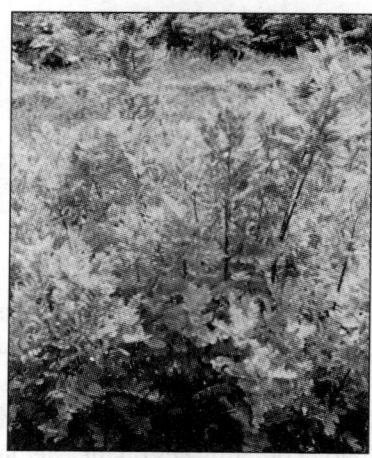

ASTRAGALUS *(A. membranaceus)*
(for colour, see Plate 3, Fig. 7)

Honey treated roots

Sliced roots are fried with honey (25-30 parts to 100 parts of roots) over medium heat until no longer sticky to touch.

Chemical Constituents

The roots contain polysaccharides, saponins, flavonoids, coumarins, folic acid, nicotinic acid, choline, betaine, phenolic acids (ferulic, isoferulic, caffeic and chlorogenic acids etc.), linoleic & linolenic acids, free amino acids and trace of minerals.

Health Food

Astragalus root is a highly valued **Chinese herbal tonic like ginseng**. It is one of the major Chinese (energy) tonic with recorded use history of 2000 years. It is used in the form of crude powder, slices, tea bags, soup mix packets or extracts (decoction or alcoholic extract); singly or in combination with other powdered crude extract (decoction and alcoholic extracts) of herbs in capsule, tablet or liquid (syrup or drink) form primarily as a general tonic or to improve body resistance (immunity), promote suppuration (drain pus) and regenerate tissue or promote muscle growth. Astragalus has antibacterial, antiviral and antiinflammatory powers. It fights flu, colds, fever and bronchitis. It also fights cancer by boosting immunity. It balances the energy of internal organs and improves digestion.

BALM LEMON
(*Melissa officinalis*)

Synonyms : Melissa, Common balm, bee balm and balm

Balm Lemon is the dried leaves with flowering tops; and an essential oil obtained from an aromatic (Lemony) perennial herb, *Melissa officinalis* Linn. (Labiatae or Lamiaceae) growing in the Mediterranean region, Western Asia and widely cultivated widely.

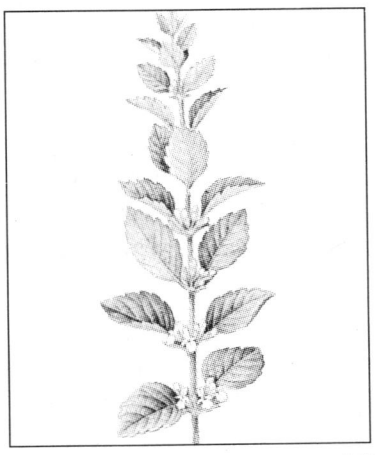

BALM LEMON *(Melissa officinalis)*
(for colour, see Plate 3, Fig. 8)

Chemical Constituents

It contains about 0.1-0.2% volatile oil composed mainly of oxygenated compounds such as citral, α and β-caryophyllene, citronelal, eugenol acetate and geraniol plus smaller amount of terpene hydrocarbons including trans and cis-β-ocimene, polyphenols (Caffeic acid, protocatechnic acid) flavonoid, rosmarinic acid, triterpenoids and glucosides of geraniol, nerol and eugenol.

Use

Hot water extract of the herb have strong antiviral properties against **new-castle** disease, mumps, *Herpes simplex* and other viruses.

Freeze dried aqueous extract of balm has antithyrotropic and antigonadotropic activity.

Balm oil has been reported to have antibacterial activities especially against *Mycobacterium phlei* and *Streptococcus hemolytica* as well as antifungal activities.

Health Food

Balm extract and oil are used in major categories of food products such as alcoholic (bitters) and non-alcoholic beverages, frozen dairy desserts, candy baked goods etc.

Cut and sifted herb, powdered herb, liquid and dried extracts (infusions), tinctures etc. are used as mild sleep aid as well as a stomachic and in neurological disorders. Dried leaves used for tea in doses of 1.5-4.5 g of herb, in infusion used alone and in combination with other herbs.

BASIL SWEET
(TULSI)
(Ocimum basilicum)

Synonyms : Basil and Common Basil

Basil Sweet is an fresh herb as well as essential oil (steam distilled) of *Ocimum basilicum* Linn. (Labiatae or Lamiaceae).

It is an annual herb, 0.5 m high, thought to be native to Africa and Tropical Asia and cultivated worldwide (e.g. Europe, India and the United states). There are many varieties with different flavouring characteristics.

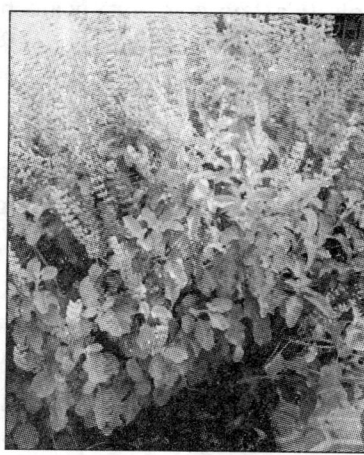

TULSI *(Ocimum basilicum)*
(for colour, see Plate 3, Fig. 9)

Chemical Constituents

The volatile oil contains d-linalool (55-70%) and methyl chavicol (estragole) as the major components. Other components include methyl cinnamate (28%), 1,8 cincole, eugenol, borneol, ocimene, camphor and safrole.

Sweet basil also contains protein (14%), carbohydrates (61%) and relatively high percentage of vitamin A and C, rosmarinic acid (an antioxidant), thymol and xanthomicrol (flavone).

Health Food

Fresh herb now widely available throughout India and United States are considered to be **general tonic, as an appetite stimulant, carminative and immuno-stimulant** and as a source of vitamin C.

The oil and oleoresin are extensively used as a flavour ingredient in all major food products.

It is also recommended for use before and after parturition to promote blood circulation.

BEE POLLEN

Bee pollen refers to pollens collected by bee that in turn harvested for commercial distribution.

Commercial bee pollen is collected by means of net like pollen traps, set up next to the beehives that remove some of the pollen from the hind legs of worker bees as they return to their hives.

The collected pollen is manually rid of impurities (dirt, floral parts, insect fragments etc.) and dried.

The major bee pollen producing countries include China and Spain. The known species that yield commercial bee pollen include buckwheat, maize and pine among others, also Typha pollen (puhuang) collected from Typha species (*T. angustata* Boxy, *T. angustifolia* Linn. and *T. latifolia* Linn.) and pollen collected from numerous Pinus species.

Chemical Constituents

Pollen is very **rich in nutrients** and contain 3-16% water, 5.9-28.3% crude protein; 14.5-21.9% amino acids, sugar, carbohydrates, flavonoids, vitamins (A, B, B_2, C, D_2, E, K, K_3, folic acid, nicotinic acid etc.), trace elements and sterols.

Health Food

Bee pollens are used extensively as a food supplement in tablet, capsule or liquid (drink or Syrup) form.

Used for centuries by different cultures as a nutrient. In China Typha pollen (puhuang) was first described about 2000 years ago as sweet tasting, neutral and having diuretic, hemostatic and stasis dispersing properties.

Pine pollen (songhuafen) also has a long history of use dating back to the 7th century A.D. Traditionally regarded as sweet tasting, warming benefiting vital energy, removing wetness, astringent, hemostatic and to treat rheumatism.

BILBERRY (BLUEBERRY)
(*Vaccinium myrtillus*)

Synonyms : Whortleberry, Huckleberry Dwarf bilberry.

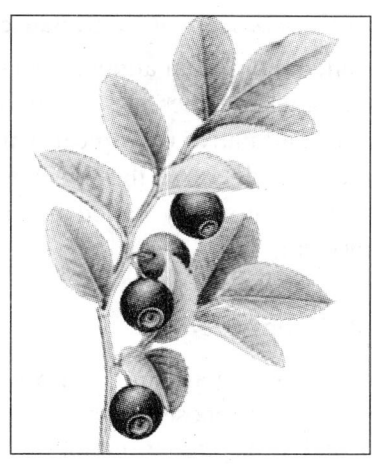

BILBERRY *(Vaccinum myrtillus)*
(for colour, see Plate 4, Fig. 1)

Bilberry is the fruits and leaves of *Vaccinium myrtillus* Linn. (Ericaceae); a deciduous leafy branched subshrub up to about 35-60 cm high arising from a creeping rhizome found in the mountains of southern Europe and subalpine Western Northern America. Shrub has coriaceous leaves bearing bell-shaped flowers grow solitary or in pairs at the base of the leaves. The fruit is multiseeded, tetra or pentaocular globose berry with a fleshy mesocarp on the flattened top.

The bilberry (Blueberry) is well known for its globose edible fruits, used by the pharmaceutical industry for extraction of anthocyanin, a natural pigment. They are also inhibitors of cAMP phosphodiesterase and are free radical scavengers (Antioxidants).

Chemical Constituents

Fruits and fruit juice contain at least 3% anthocyanosides, phenolic acids including caffeic, chlorogenic, p-coumaric, ferulic, gallic, proto-catechuic acids, vitamin C, quinolizidine alkaloids myritine and epimyritine in aerial parts.

The official drug must contain not more than 2% leaves and twigs and the dried extract must contain not less than 9% anthocyanin.

Health Food

The fruit has **nutritive** value, used in various food products e.g. alcoholic and non-alcoholic beverages, pastries and syrup; for **improved vision** (night and day time vision), cataracts, muscular degeneration, glaucoma, retinitis pigmentosa and diabetic retinopathy.

BLESSED THISTLE
(*Cnicus benedictus*)

Synonym : Holy thistle

Blessed Thistle is the flowering top of *Cnicus benedictus* Linn. (Compositae or Asteraceae) indigenous to waste places and fields of Mediterranean region, wildly distributed in Central and South Eastern Europe; casually established as weed in Eastern United States and in Asia.

Chemical Constituents

Leaves contain lignins; 2-acetylnortracheloside, arctigenin, nortracheloside, trachelogenin and arctiin fruit have sesquiterpene lactone, cnicin, lithospermic acid, tannins, mucilage, potassium and manganese salts.

Health Food

Leaf capsules, tablets, tea, extracts & tincture forms as bitter digestive (**bitter tonic**), antiflatulent and in gallbladder disease & a folklore medicine for anorexia, dyspepsia, cold fever and externally for boils and wounds.

BURDOCK
(*Arctinum lappa*)

(See under Cosmetics)

Health Food

Burdock has high concentration of minerals including iron, hence it is very **good blood tonic** and a good blood purifier. The oil of burdock help to expel toxic matter from sweat glands.

CAJEPUT OIL
(*Melaleuca leucadendra*)

Synonyms : Cajuput, Punk tree and Paper bark tree oils; Tea tree oil (M. alternifolia).

Cajeput oil is obtained by steam distillation of the fresh leaves and twigs of *Melaleuca leucadendra* (L'); *M. quinquenervia* S.T. Blake and *M. alternifolia* species.

The plant is 30 m high, evergreen tree and with whitish spongy bark, native to Australia and Southeastern Asia.

Chemical Constituents

The oil contains 14-65% cineole or terpinen-4-ol (upto 47%) as major components. Oil having high percentage of 1-terpinen-4-ol and low in cineole is considered best for predictable clinical results.

Health Food

The oil is used in numerous product forms, either singly or with other ingredients with a broad range of health claims including treatment for burns, sunburn, pimples, boils, stings, ring worm, sore throat, oral infections and bronchial congestion.

It is used as **flavor component** in alcoholic and non-alcoholic beverage, frozen dairy desserts, candy, backed foods, meat and meat products.

CAPSICUM
(*Capsicum frutescens*)

Synonym : Red pepper.

Capsicum consist of dried ripe fruits of *Capsicum frutescens* Linn., *C. annum* Linn. and its varieties *C. chinese* Jacq. *C. baccatum* Linn. Var. pendulum (wild) *C. pubescens* Ruiz (Solanaceae).

Capsicum annum is an annual herb up to 1 m high, while others species are usually perennial woody shrubs, all native to tropical America and now cultivated widely. All the five species yield pungent fruits commonly called red pepper or simply capsicum.

Chemical Constituents

Capsicum fruits contain up to 1.5% pungent principles, mainly composed of capsaicin, dihydrocapsaicin and other constituents like **carotenoids (Capsanthins, Capsorubin** (Fig. 11.2),

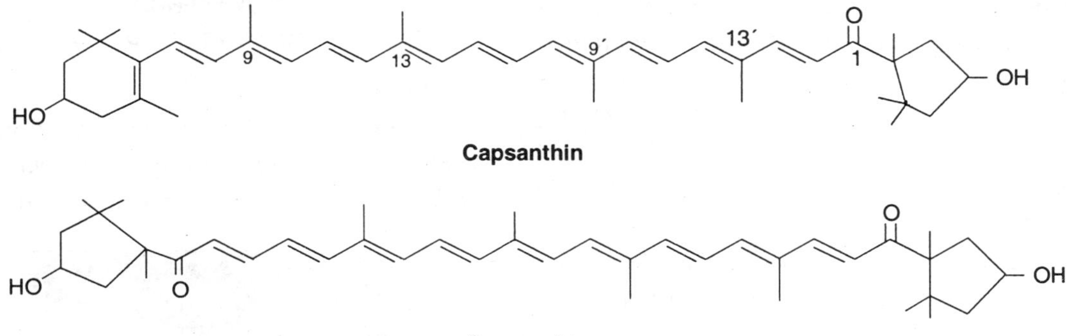

Capsanthin

Capsorubin

Fig. 11.2.

Carotene, lutein etc.), fats, proteins, vitamins A & C and small amount of volatile oil.

The pungent flavour of hot and extra hot peppers is due to amides found in a wide range of concentration namely as capsaicinoids.

Health Food

Capsicums are widely consumed in food preparation as **health food supplement** and **antioxidant** as they are rich in **ascorbic acid**. It is also used as a synergistic ingredient in various herbal formulas, including general tonics, laxatives, sedatives and hay fever remedies.

Capsicum, in whole and ground forms is widely used as spice. Paprika and its oleoresin are primarily used as a colorant in food products to impart yellow to orange color to the food.

Topically capsicum is traditionally used for the symptomatic treatment of minor pain in the joints of neurological origin.

CARAWAY
(*Carum carvi*)

Caraway consists of dried, ripe cremocarp fruit of *Carum carvi* (Umbelliferae). It is biennial herb about 1 m high.

It occurs both wild and cultivated in Central and Northern Europe and in Egypt, Morocco, Australia, China and India.

Caraway fruits were known to the Arbian physicians and introduced into Europe by thirteenth century.

Chemical Constituents

Caraway fruit contains 3-7% of volatile oils, 8-20% of fixed oil, proteins and flavonoids (quercetin, 3-glucuronide isoquercitrin etc.).

The essential oil mainly composed of carvone (50-55%) and limonene (35-45%) and small quantity of dihydrocarvone, thujone, pinene, phellandrene, α-thujene and β-fenchene.

Health Food

Caraway is widely used in domestic spice as food supplements. It is also used in commercial food products; particularly baked goods, meat and meat products, having carminative and flavouring properties help in digestion of the food. It is also used in relieving menstrual discomforts, promoting milk secretion and carminative.

CARRAGEENAN

Synonyms : Carrageenan, Carrageenin, Chondrus extract and Irish moss extract.

Carrageenan is a term referring to closely related hydrocolloids (sea weed gum) that are obtained from various Rhodophyceae seaweeds; *Chondrus crispus* (Linn.), *Eucheuma* and *Gigartina mamilosa*, Agardh (Gigartinaceae) are the major sources of Carrageenan; these algae are commonly known as **chondrus or Irish moss**.

These plants commonly grow along the Atlantic coast of Europe and North America.

Chemical Constituents

Carrageenan is a sulfated, straight chain galactan composed of residues of D-galactose and 3, 6-anhydro-D-galactose with a molecular weight usually 10,000-5,00,000, physically resemble agar, chemically differ from agar because they have higher sulfate ester content.

Carrageenan generally contains two major fractions, a gelling fraction called K-carrageenan and non-gelling fraction called λ-carrageenan. The K-carrageenan contains D-galactose, 3, 6-anhydro-D-galactose and ester sulphate group. While λ-carrageenan contains D-galactose and its monosulfate and disulfate ester.

λ-carrageenan is readily soluble in cold water to form a viscous solution regardless of the cation present where as K-carrageenan is precipitated by potassium ions.

Health Food

Carrageenan is used in various weight loss formulations; also in drinks, especially aloe vera, fruit juice and herbal drinks.

It is extensively used in milk products such as chocolate milk, ice cream, sherbats, cottage cheese, cream cheese, evaporated milk, milk desserts pudding yogurts and infant formulas. It is also reported that seaweed decoction is a demulcent, a nutrient and is recommended to be used in tuberculosis, coughs, bronchitis and in intestinal problems.

CHAMOMILE
(*Matricaria recutita*)

Chamomile is the dried flower heads of :

German : *Matricaria recutita* Linn. (Syn. *Matricaria Chamomilla* Linn., *Chamomilla recutita* (Linn.) Rauschert) (Compositae/Asteraceae).

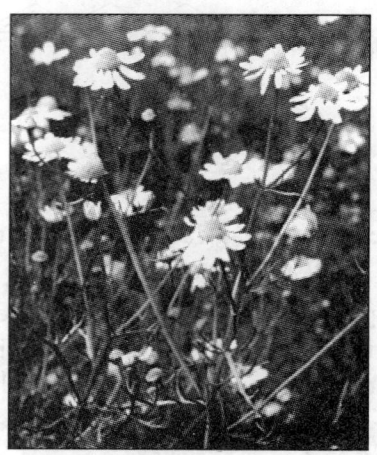

CHAMOMILE *(Matricaria recutita)*
(for colour, see Plate 4, Fig. 2)

Roman : *Chamaemelum nobile* (Linn.) All. (Syn. Anthemis nobilis Linn.) (Compositae).

The herb is native to Europe, Northern and Western Asia but now cultivated extensively in Hungery, Romania, Bulgaria, Greece and Argentina.

Roman herb is a strongly fragrant, hairy, half spreading and much branched perennial herb with flower heads about 2.5 cm. diameter, up to about 0.3 m high, native to Southern and Western Europe, cultivated in England, Belgium and United States.

Blue essential oil is obtained from expanded flowerheads by steam distillation.

Chemical Constituents

The volatile oil of the chamomile contains sesquiterpene lactones, flavonoids including apigenin, rutin, luteolin and quercimeritrin (quercetin-7-D-glucosides) and coumarins.

Health Food

German chamomile and to a lesser extent Roman chamomile crude flowers or extracts are one of the most widely used herbal tea ingredients, singly or in combination with other ingredients. Used internally for gastrointestinal spasms and inflammatory diseases of the GI tract, externally for skin mucous membrane inflammation and bacterial skin disease.

Tinctures and extracts are used as mild sleep aids, antispasmodics and **digestive aids** and antioxidant food supplements.

CHICORY ROOTS
(*Cichorium intybus*)

Synonym : Succory, Blue sailor, Wild chicory and Common chicory root.

Chicory is the dried roots and dried above ground part of *Cichorium intybus* Linn. family Compositae/Asteraceae.

The herb *Cichorium intybus* Linn. is native of Europe and Asia. It is common along roadsides and in vacant lots, it is easy to identify by its terminal and auxiliary capitulums of ligulate lovely blue flowers. It is biennial or perennial herb with spindle shaped taproot and cauline hairy leaves upto 2 m high.

Chemical Constituents

The roots contain high concentration (upto 60% of the dry drug) of **inulin** content; sesquiterpene lactone (bitter principles); tannins, sugars, pectin, fixed oils and choline.

Steam distillable fraction of roasted roots contain pyrazines, benzothiazoles, aldehydes, aromatic hydrocarbons, furans, phenols, organic acids and acetophenone in addition to aromatic compounds, the small amount of two indole alkaloids (β-carboline derivative), harmane and harmine are also reported from roasted roots.

Health Food

Chicory roots are used in food products as a flavour; bitter tonic to increase appetite and to treat digestive problem (prebiotic) usually in the form of herbal tea and juice. The roots are also used in diuretic and digestive formulations for the treatment of gallstone, liver ailments and cancer.

Ground roasted powdered roots are mixed with coffee to impart "richer" flavour and to decrease the caffeine content of the coffee formulation.

CODONOPSIS
(Poor man's ginseng)

Synonym : Radix codonopsis, Bonnet bell flower, Bastard ginseng and Dangshen.

Codonopsis is herbaceous perennials strongly scented thick fleshy cylindrical to slightly spindle-shaped roots of *Codonopsis pilosula* (French) Nannf var modesta (Nannf), *C. tangshen* oliv, *C. tubulosa* Kom. and many other codonopsis species (Campanulaceae).

The plant is native to Asia; distributed throughout China, now extensively cultivated, also as ornamental in the United States.

Chemical Constituents

It contain polysaccharides, sugars (e.g. Inulin, starch, glucose, sucrose and fructose), saponins (tangshenosides I, II, III and IV), amino acids, β-carboline alkaloids (perlolyrine), triterpenes (e.g. taraxeryl acetate, taraxerol friedelin), sterols and their glycosides. Volatile oil is composed of 50% acidic compounds with palmitic acid and methyl palmitate as major component.

Health Food

Powdered herb and extracts are used **in tonic formulas** (in tablets, capsule or liquid form) often as oriental ginseng substitute for boosting one's **immune system and replenishing vital energy**.

Cut or teabag and cut herb is used in tea or soup preparations.

CORIANDER
(*Coriandrum sativum*)

Coriander is the dried or nearly dried ripe fruits of *Coriandrum sativum* (Umbelliferae/Apiaceae), consisting of straw yellow colored, whole cremocarps, about 2.3–4.25 mm in diameter; each consisting of two hemispherical mericarps united by their margins. Indian variety is oval, but the more widely distributed spherical varieties vary in size from Ukrainian 2.4-3.8 mm to Moroccan 4.0 to 4.5 mm bearing two divergent stylopod.

Chemical Constituents

The fruits contain up to 1.8% volatile oil with Linalool as the major constituent (65-78% in ripe fruits) along with camphor (4-6%), geranyl acetate (1.5-3.5%) and the minor component are α-pinene, γ-terpinene, limonene and p-cymene.

The fruits also contain flavonoids, coumarins, isocoumarins, phthalides and phenolic acids.

In addition to volatile oil the fruits contain high content of fats (16-25%) and proteins (11-17%). The unripe fruit has unpleasant content (n-decanol) present in the vittae.

Health Food

It is most highly priced spice (curries, bakery products and liquors etc.) in food preparation because of its antispasmodic, carminative and flavouring properties as well as antioxidant properties due to the presence of flavonoids and phenolic compounds.

CORN OIL
(*Zea mays*)

Corn oil is the refined oil obtained from embryo of *Zea mays* Linn. (Gramineae).

The steeped grains are separated from the germ prior to fine milling; the germs are recovered and may contain up to 20% lipids (dried germs), Pharmacopoeia specifies that the oil is obtained from Caryopsis.

Chemical Constituents

The corn oil contain fatty acids the major one are stearic, oleic, linoleic, linolenic, arachidic and behenic.

The unsaponifiable matter (0.8-2%) contains β-sitosterol and campesterol (63-70%) and 16-21% of the total sterols respectively, as well as γ and α-tocopherol (68-69%) and 8-22% of total tocopherol respectively.

Health Food

This oil is used as **dietary supplement** because of the presence of glycerides with component acids of the linolenic acid (50%), oleic acid (37%), palmitic (10%) and stearic (3%).

It is an edible oil and as such is used in salad and in the preparation of food.

An emulsion containing 67% of corn oil is employed as high caloric dietary supplement, having natural antioxidant (tocopherol).

DEVIL'S CLAW (HERBAL TEA)
[*Harpagophytum procumbens* DC]

Synonyms : Grapple fruit and wood spider.

Devil's claw is the dried tubers of *Harpagophytum procumbens.* Decandelle (Pedaliaceae), is south African plant widely sold in both Europe and United States **under the name of Devil's Claw.**

Plant grows wildly in steppes on red sand in South tropical Africa, especially in the Kalahari desert and in the Namobian steppes plus Madagascar.

It is herbaceous trailing perennial, bearing red

flowers in the axils, fruits with pointed and barbed woody grapples 1.5 to 2.5 cm long. Tuber is about 6 cm in diameter and 20 cm long.

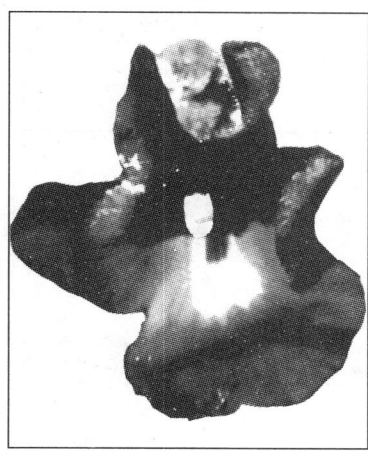

DEVIL'S CLAW *(Herpagophytum procumbens)*
(for colour, see Plate 4, Fig. 3)

Chemical Constituents

The plant contains iridoid glycosides - including harpagoside (0.1-3%) in the tubers, phytosterols, triterpenes, flavonoids including kaempferol and luteolin glycosides.

Health Food

Oral dosage forms including extracts, tablets and capsules are sold in natural food or health food stores; primarily for relief of arthritic symptoms. It is also used in Europe and African countries as **bitter tonic** and blood purifier and as anti hyper-cholestremic as well as folk remedy for cancer. A smaller dose of 1.15 grams of dried root powder is recommended for loss of appetite.

ECHINACEA
(*Echinacea* species)

Synonyms : Purple cone flower, Common purple cone flower (*E. purpurea*) and Pale purple cone flower (*E. pallida*)

Echinacea are *Echinacea angustifolia* DC; *Echinacea pallida* (Nutt) and *Echinacea purpurea* Linn. (Compositae/Asteraceae).

Echinacea angustifolia is herbaceous perennial, about 60 cm high, leaves lanceolate; flowers violet long ray florets. It grows wildly in Minnesota to Texas.

E. pallida is about 120 cm high, leaves lanceolate, purple ray flowers 9 cm long, grow wildly in eastern texas to Iowa, cultivated in United States and Europe.

E. purpurea is about 90 cm high, leaves ovate, coarsely toothed, basal one often cordate, fibrous root grow wildly in mideastern United states. Cultivated in Europe, North America and Australia.

Chemical Constituents

Leaves contain essential oils and flavonoids.

Essential oil components common to the aerial parts of *E. pallida*, *E. purpurea* and *E. angustifolia* include borneol, bornylacetate, pentadeca-8-en-2-one, germacrene, α-caryophyllene, caryophyllene epoxide and palmitic acid.

Rutoside is the major leaf flavonoid of all the three species of Echinacea.

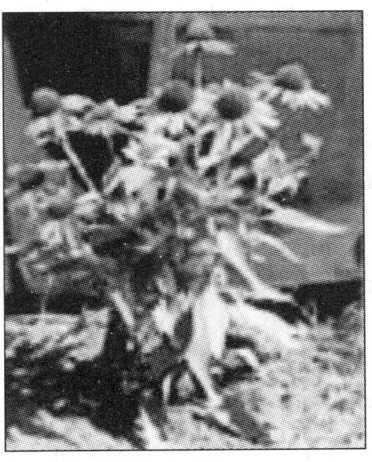

ECHINACEAE *(E. angustifolia)*
(for colour, see Plate 4, Fig. 4)

Polysaccharide includes inulin (5.9%), fructans and other constituents include a resin yielding oleic, linoleic, cerotic and palmitic acid on hydrolysis.

Alkaloids include glycine betaine in *E. purpurea*. The pyrrolizidine alkaloids tussilagine (0.006%) and isotussilagine have been identified from dried roots of *E. angustifolia* and *E. purpurea*.

Health Food

Numerous oral dosage products are available in food stores of Germany and USA as food supplement. Echinacea species has immuno-stimulant properties and is used as prophylactic at the onset of cold and flu symptoms and for the treatment of *Candida albicans* infections, chronic respiratory infections and in rheumatoid arthritis.

In Europe the entire fresh, flowering plant is employed medicinally. The plant Echinacea was introduced into American medicine in 1885.

The wound healing property of the drug has been reported to be attributed to a polysaccharides, (inulin and fructans), echirachin B, which forms complex with hyaluronic acid that is resistant to attack by hyaluronidase.

EPHEDRA
(Ephedra sinica)

Synonyms : Mahuang, Herba Ephedrae, Cao mahuang (Chinese ephedra) Zhong mahuang (Intermediate ephedra) and Muzei mahuang (Mongolian ephedra).

Ephedra is the dried stems and roots separated from Chinese ephedra *Ephedra sinica* stapf and other Ephedra spp. (Ephedraceae).

Chemical Constituents

Stems contains 1-2% alkaloids composed mainly of l-ephedrine and d-pseudoephedrine.

Other compounds present include glycans (ephedrans A, B, C, D and E), catechin, gallic acid and condensed tannins, flavonoid glycosides, inulin, dextrin, starch, pectin and other common plant constituents, including plant acids (citric, malic, oxalic etc.).

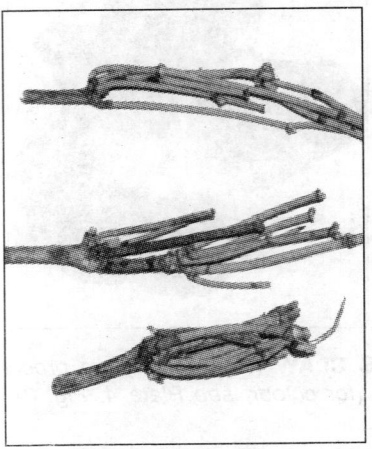

EPHEDRA *(E. sinica)*
(for colour, see Plate 4, Fig. 5)

Health Food

Used in diet formulas for its appetite suppressive effect and in "energy" formulas for its Central nervous system stimulant action; also used in cold and flu remedies. Usually in tablet, capsule and tea forms.

EVENING PRIMROSE
(Oenothera biennis)

Evening primrose is annual or biennial *Oenothera biennis* Linn. (Onagraceae).

Chemical Constituents

Seeds of the plant contain about 14% fixed oil (Evening primrose oil) with 50-70% cis linolenic acid and 7-10% cis-γ-linolenic acid with small amount of oleic, palmitic & stearic acid, steroids campesterol and β-sitosterol.

Health Food

Capsulated seed oil products widely available as dietary supplements for the addition of essential fatty acids to diet.

FENUGREEK (METHI)
(*Trigonella foenum-graecum*)

Synonyms : Fenugreek and Greek hay.

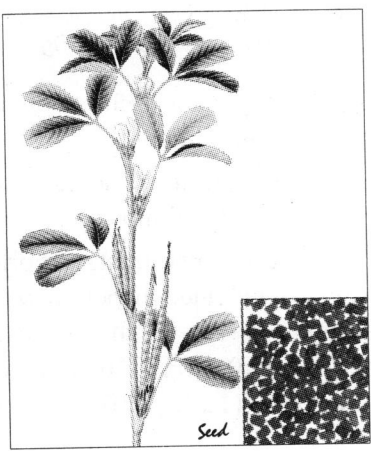

FENUGREEK (*Trigonella foenum-graceum*)
(for colour, see Plate 4, Fig. 6)

Fenugreek is an annual herb (*Trigonella foenum-graecum* family *Leguminosae*) with alternate leaves on a long petiole, each consisting of three ovate leaflets up to 0.6 m high. The flowers, solitary or in pairs, have a creamy white corolla with a posterior triangular petal. The fruit is an elongated arched pod, containing 10–20 very hard seeds with light brown tegument marked with slanted groove, some what flattened, resembling triangle.

The plant grows wildly and is cultivated especially in India, both as a spice and as a forage crop. This plant is also cultivated for the production of steroid in temperate countries.

Chemical Constituents

The seeds contain saponins, which on hydrolysis yield 1-2% of sapogenin (diosgenin and trigafoenosides, foenugraecin) and trigonellin.

The seeds contain volatile oil with main constituents having sesquiterpenes hydrocarbons, alkanes and lactones. Rich in proteins (30%), lipids (7%) C-flavonoids and many sterols, abundant carbohydrates, fibres (cellulose, hemicellulose), mucilage and soluble galactomannan.

Health Food

Used as an ingredient of curry powder and many spice blends and other food products, which include alcoholic and non-alcoholic beverages frozen dairy desserts, candy baked goods, gelatin and puddings, meat and meat products throughout the world.

As herb health food to facilitate weight gain, in France as well as in Germany and as spice in India. It is also used as a demulcent, emollient and in treatment of indigestion, diabetes and hypercholesterimia.

FENNEL
(*Foeniculum vulgare*)

Commonly fennel is of the two types:
- Bitter fennel
- Sweet fennel

Bitter fennel consists of the dried ripe fruits of *Foeniculum vulgare*, subsp. *vulgare*, var. *vulgare* (Umbelliferae). It is cultivated in Europe and much is imported from India, China and Egypt.

Sweet fennel is derived from *F. vulgare* subs. *vulgare* var. *dulce* and is also included in the 1994 BP addendum.

Chemical Constituents

Fruit contain 1-4% volatile oil, the principal constituents are the phenolic ether *trans*-anethole (60%)

and ketone (fenchone 10-30%). Minor constituents are hydrocarbons (monoterpene like limonene), anisaldehyde and estragole.

Sweet fennel contains more than 80% of *trans*-anethole, (10%) methylchavicol (Estragole) and less than 5% (+)-fenchone and also contain furancoumarin, including imperatorin, bergaptin and xanthotoxol.

Health Food

Fennel fruit is used in spice, as health food, because of its carminative and flavouring properties (traditionally used for symptomatic treatment of gastro-intestinal disturbance such as epigastric bloating, impaired digestion, eructation flatulence etc.).

Crushed or ground fruit in teas, tinctures, and sweet fennel oil are widely used in most major food products, including alcoholic and non-alcoholic beverages, frozen dairy desserts, candy, baked goods, gelatins and puddings.

FO-TI (Raw and cured)

Raw fo-ti are freshly collected tubers of *Polygonum multiflorum* Thumb, (Polygonaceae), washed with water, cut in half or sliced and dried in oven or sun.

Cured FO-TI

The raw fo-ti slices are first stirred in to black soybean broth in a non-iron container, sealed and cooked in water or steam bath until all liquid is absorbed and fo-ti slices turn dark brown to reddish brown, then dried in oven.

It is native to China; now distributed mainly along coastal provinces, from Guangxi to Hebei and extending inland to Sichuan and Yunnan.

Chemical Constituents

Both raw and cured fo-ti contains anthraquinone,

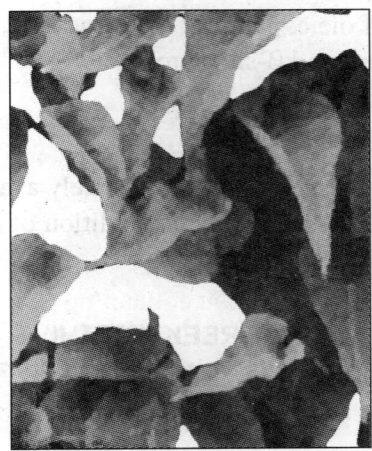

FO-TI *(Polygonum multiflorum)*
(for colour, see Plate 4, Fig. 7)

including chrysophanol, chrysophanic acid anthrone, emodin and rhein.

It also contain lecithins. The cured fo-ti contains more quantity of lecithin.

Other chemical constituents reported to be present in raw fo-ti include rhapontin, α-sitosterol, catechins and relatively high concentration of calcium (222.5 ppm), iron (350 ppm), zinc (24.5 ppm), manganese (18.5 ppm) and other trace minerals.

Health Food

Powdered and occasionally extracts are used in tonic formulation in America (anti-aging, immuno-suppressive, antiartherosclerotic, liver protectant and anti-mutagenic effect). It is also used in sliced form in soup mix packets.

Cosmetic Use

Extract of the cured fo-ti is a popular ingredient in hair-care products (shampoos and tonics) especially in China and Hong Kong for its alleged hair darkening and growth promoting properties also used in skin care products (e.g. Creams and lotions) for its traditional detoxicant (antiallergic) and nourishing properties.

FEVERFEW
(Tanacetum parthenium)

Feverfew is the leaves and stems of strongly aromatic perennial herb *Tanacetum parthenium* (L) *Schultz Bip* (Syn. *Chrysanthemum parthenium* (L) Bernh; *Leucanthemum parthenium* (L) Gren. et .Godron, *Pyrethrum parthenium* L Sm.) (Compositae or Asteraceae).

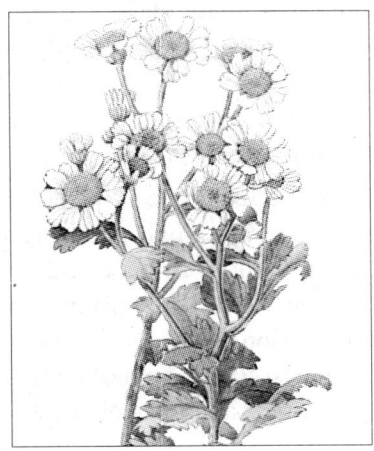

FEVERFEW *(Tanacetum parthenium)*
(for colour, see Plate 4, Fig. 8)

It is indigenous to rocky mountain scrub of Balkana peninsula and cultivated throughout Europe.

Chemical Constituents

It contains sesquiterpene and lactones (parathenolides costunolide, reynosin, canin and artecanin).

Health Food

Feverfew extracts standardized to contain 0.1-0.2% parthenolide (leaf only; Canada) are used for the prophylactic treatment of migraine, asthma, rheumatism, gynaecological problems etc. The herb is also used in the form of tea, capsules and tablets for stimulant tonic and for vermifuge activity.

GANODERMA
(Ganoderma lucidum)

Synonym : Holy mushroom Reishi lingzhi

Ganoderma is the fruiting body of *Ganoderma lucidum* (Leyss ex Fr.), Karst (Syn. *Polyporus Japonicus* Fr.) and *G. Japonicum* (Fr.) Lloyd (Polyporaceae).

G. Japonicum (purple lingzhi) resemble closely to that of *G. lucidum* (red lingzhi) with cap sizes ranging from 2 × 1.4 cm to 20 × 20 cm. Both ganodermas are widely distributed in China, growing at stumps and decaying logs of oak and other broad leaf trees as well as on decaying conifers, especially *Tsuga Chinensis* (Franch) Pritz which is parasitized by *G. lucidum*. The later can also be found as hardwoods in North America as well as in Japan and Korea.

The mushrooms are collected in autumn, washed to rid of dirt and dried under the sun. Although now commercially cultivated in China, much of ganoderma are still gathered wild. In America mainly red Lingzhi (*G. lucidum*) is cultivated and imported. It is also cultivated in China Taiwan, Japan and Korea.

Other species of polypores, which are occasionally used as substitutes of Lingzhi including *Ganoderma applanatum* (Pers. ex. Gray), *Ganoderma lobatum* (Schw.), Atk *Ganoderma eapense* (Lloyd), Teng. *Fomes pinicola* Cke, *Trametes diekinsii* Berk *Polyporus montanus* (Quel), Freey. *P. grammocephalus* Berk and *Polysticus vernicipes* (Berk) Cke.

Chemical Constituents

Chemical constituents include ergosterol (0.3-0.4%), β-sitosterol, 24 methylcholesta, 7, 22-dien-3-β-ol and other sterols, fungal lysozyme, acid protease and other enzymes (Lactase endopolygalacturonase, cellulase, amylase etc.). Also water soluble protein, polypeptide, amino acids, trehalose and other sugars, mannitol; betaine; adenosine and fatty acids (tetracosanoic, stearic, palmitic non-decanoic and behenic acids).

Polysaccharides present include water-soluble branched **arabinoxyloglucan**.

Triterpenes are mainly of lanostane type (lucidenic acids and lucidones)

Health Food

Powdered form or extracts are used singly or in combination with other herbs in capsule, tablet, or liquid (syrup or drink) form as a **general tonic to improve energy, stamina and resistance to stress** and diseases; hydroalcoholic extracts are also used to flavour instant soup mixes and herbal drinks because of their mushroom aroma.

GARLIC
(Allium sativum)

Garlic is a fresh or dried bulb of *Allium sativum* Linn. (Liliaceae). Garlic oil is obtained by steam distillation of crushed fresh bulb of *Allium sativum*. Powdered garlic is derived from the dried bulb.

It is cultivated on a large scale in India & other Asian countries and to a lesser extent in Europe, America and Africa.

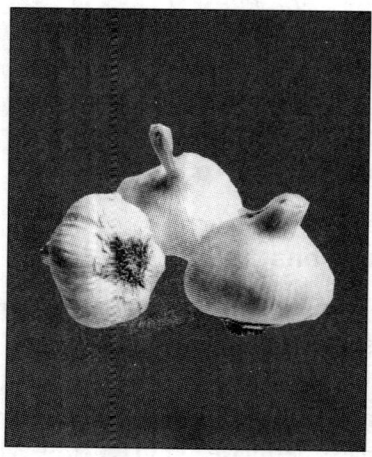

GARLIC (Allium sativum)
(for colour, see Plate 4, Fig. 9)

It is strong scented perennial herb with long flat and firm leaves (0.8–1.6 cm wide) flowering stem upto 1.1 m high, bulb with several bulblets (cloves) enclosed in membranous skin.

Chemical Constituents

It contains 0.2-0.3% volatile oil, allin (S-allyl-L-cysteine sulfoxide) S-methyl-L-cysteine sulfoxide, enzymes (alliinase, peroxidase and myrosinase), ajoenes (E-Z-ajoene, E-Z-methylajoene and dimethylajoene), protein (16.8% dry weight basis), minerals, vitamins (thiamine, riboflavine, niacin etc.), lipids, amino acids and others.

The strong smelling juice of the bulbs contains a mixture of aliphatic mono and polysulphides. The chief constituent is allicin and diallyldisulphide oxide. The latter result from spontaneous enzymatic reduction of allicin and 5-allylcystine sulphamide, thioglycoside, amino acids, fatty acids, flavonoids, vitamins and trace elements.

Prostaglandins A_2 and F_1 are recently isolated from fresh homogenized garlic extract.

Health Food

Fresh garlic and dried powdered garlic are widely used as herb health **food supplement** and as domestic spice. In these days garlic preparations are the best selling over the counter drug in **Germany** and in **Asian countries**. It has been used for thousand of years in treating cough, cold, bronchitis, hypertension, arteriosclerosis, also used extensively in cancer, generally as juice, cold infusion or tincture. In addition, fresh cloves, garlic tea, syrup and other preparations have been used as aphrodisiac, to treat fever, gout, rheumatism, antihyperglycemic and in pulmonary tuberculosis.

Garlic has antibacterial and antifungal activity against many common pathogenic organisms i.e. *Staphylococcus aureus*, *Escherichia coli*, *Candida albicans*, *Shigella sonnei* and *Salmonella typhi*. There are several reports showing the hypoglycemic activity of garlic and allicin in animals.

Fried and raw garlic use has shown an increase in fibrinolytic activity in ischemic heart disease patient. It also has cholesterol and triglyceride lowering effect in animals as well as in human being.

Safety : Normal use of garlic as a food has not reported any toxic effects, but prolonged chronic feeding of large amounts of garlic powder (350 mg/kg) reported to have severe testicular lesions after 70 days and arrest in spermatogenesis i.e. 20 g (Freeze dried, garlic powder in a 60 kg body weight man). Its asthmatic allergic reaction has been reported in some sensitive person.

Formulations and Dosage:

Rasonadivati tablet   – 2-3 b.i.d.

Lashoonadi taila   – 1-2 drops in ear

Pearls of garlic oil   – 2-4 b.i.d.

Lashoonadi ghrita   – 1-2 teaspoonful b.i.d.

GENTIAN
(*Gentiana lutea*)

Gentian or Gentian root is dried root and rhizome of *Gentiana lutea* Linn. (Gentianaceae), plant

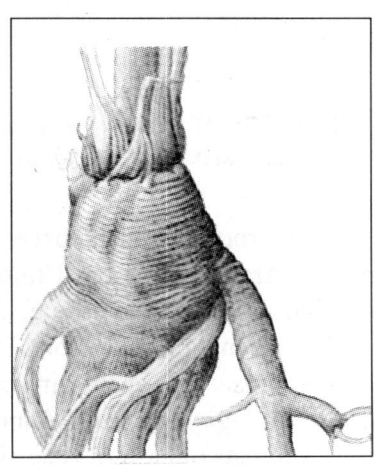

GENTIAN (*G. lutea*)
(for colour, see Plate 5, Fig. 1)

indigenous to Central and Southern Europe. A tall and hardy herb (1-1.5 m), with simple erect stem, large oval leaves and yellow color flowers.

The drug consists of simple or branched, cyclindrical pieces upto 20-25 cms long and 1.5 to 3.0 cms diameter, covered with yellowish brown cork. The rhizomes are larger in diameter than the roots and are wrinkled transversely, whereas the roots wrinkle longitudinally, **fracture** is brittle when perfectly dried. It has characteristic **odour,** sweet taste which latter becomes bitter.

Stemless gentian (*G. acaulis*) is a small perennial herb, with basal rosettes; leaves lance shaped; up to 10 cm high, native to Europe whole herb is used in health food.

Chemical Constituents

The drug contains 2-3% secoiridoids, gentiopicroside, amarogentin and other esters of sweroside and swertiamarin, which are responsible for the bitter taste of the drug. Presence of xanthone (gentisin, isogentisin gentin) gives yellow color to the drug. It is rich in sugas (gentionose, gentiobiose and sucrose).

Health Food

Traditionally the drug is used as health food, because of its property to **stimulate the appetite** and is used in liquor industry. The bitter substance present in the drug stimulate salivary and gastric secretions via reflex activity and thus this tonic is used for gastrointestinal pain and lack of appetite, the enzymatic hydrolysis of gentiopicrin take place at the time of improper drying and yields a darker reddish brown product that is inferior for use as a medicinal bitter.

GINGER
(*Zingiber officinalis*)

Ginger is the fresh and dried root and rhizome of *Zingiber officinale* Roscoe (Zingiberaceae) as well as ginger oil obtained from freshly ground, unpeeled dried ginger by steam distillation.

It is native to Southern Asia, extensively cultivated in the tropics (e.g. India, China, Jamaica, Haiti and Nigeria).

It is an erect perennial herb with thick tuberous rhizomes, sympocially branched pieces known as hands. The branches arise obliquely from rhizomes, (1-3 cm long) terminating in depressed scars or in undeveloped buds. The outer surface is buff colored and longitudinally striated.

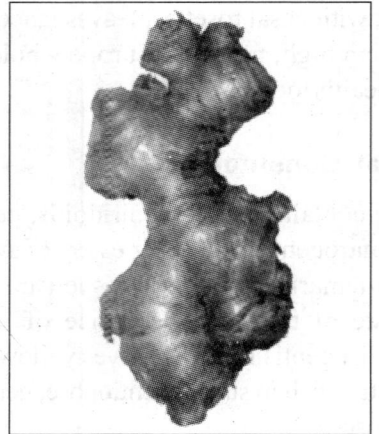

GINGER *(Zingiber officinalis)*
(for colour, see Plate 5, Fig. 2)

Chemical Constituents

Ginger oil contains sesquiterpene, hydrocarbons zingiberene and bisabolene.

Ginger has been reported to contain 0.25-3.3% (usually 1-3%) volatile oil, pungent principle (gingerols and shogaols) about 6-8% lipids composed of triglycerides, phosphatidic acid, lecithin, free fatty acid (lauric, palmitic, stearic, oleic, linoleic) and protein (9%), starch (upto 50%), vitamins (especially niacin and A), minerals, amino acids and resin.

Health Food

Ginger is used as domestic spice. It is used

commercially in many foods, including non-alcoholic beverage, baked goods, gelatin, pudding meat and meat products as a digestive aid, anti-nauseant and potential source of food antioxidant. It is also used to treat flu and cold, rheumatism and as a **general stimulant**.

Ginger oil oleo-resin and extract are widely used in soft-drinks and frozen dairy desserts. The highest average maximum use level reported to be about 0.004% for oil in baked goods and food products to about 0.525%.

GINSENG

Synonyms : Chinese ginseng; Korean ginseng and Japanese ginseng (*P. ginseng*); Western ginseng, (*P. quinquefolium*) seng and sang.

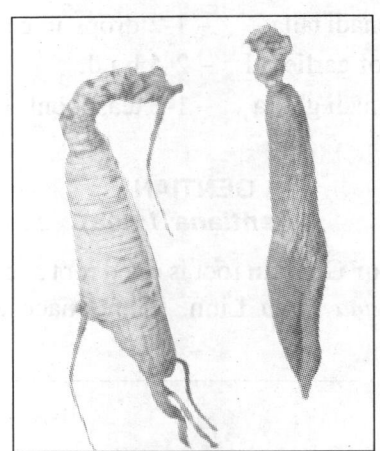

GINSENG ROOT *(Panax ginseng)*
(for colour, see Plate 5, Fig. 3)

Ginseng is dried root of the herbaceous plant Panax ginseng (Araliaceae) from China, Korea and Russia and related species e.g. *P. quinquefolium* (American ginseng) from USA and Canada, *P. notoginseng* (Sanchi-ginseng) from China and *P. pseudoginseng wallich* indigenous to mountainous forests of eastern Asia. The roots are carefully gathered from 3-6 years old plants and carefully cleaned and dried.

White ginseng is the dried and usually peeled roots, where as red ginseng is obtained by steaming the roots, this process reputedly enhancing biological activity.

Both are perennial herbs with simple single stems bearing at flowering a whorl of three to six long petioled compound leaves at the top. The most expensive one that derived from Korean ginseng root. The plant is about 50 cm tall with a crown of dark green verticillate leaves and small green flowers, giving rise to clusters of bright red berries. Flowers appear in 3 years old plant.

Chemical Constituents

It contains large number of triterpenoid saponins known as ginsenosides or panaxosides. These are derivatives of two main aglycones, protopanaxadiol and protopanaxatriol. About 30 ginsenosides have been characterized from different varieties of ginseng; these panaxoside saponin glycosides are apparently responsible for all these functions.

The benefits of ginseng treatment are yet to be confirmed at the pharmacological level, though CNS-stimulating, CNS-sedative, tranquillising, antifatigue, hypotensive and hypertensive activities have all been demonstrated.

Health Food

Because of the relatively high cost of the drug and almost totally lack of quality control in the "health food" industry consequently most of the preparations have shown great variations in the panaxosides glycoside content. It is reported that about 60% of the products in one sampling were found worthless and about 25% of those sampled contained no ginseng at all.

Recently, western interest in the ginseng drug has vastly increased and it has become widely available in "health food" outlets. It is reported that at present ginseng is the top selling herb among first time herbal users, in US health food stores. Approximately 6–10 million people use this herb in the United State alone.

Both American and Asian ginseng are available in a wide variety of product forms, the powdered root or leaves alone or in combination in the form of teas, capsules, tablet, liquid extracts and instant tea (upto 5% extract on fructose, carrier). The standardized preparations contain 4-7% ginsenoside.

Ginseng is classified as an adaptogen helping the body to adapt to stress, improving stamina and concentration; and normalizing and restorative effect. It is also widely promoted as an aphrodisiac.

Ginseng is favourite remedy in Chinese medicine and considered to have tonic, stimulant, diuretic and carminative properties. It is also reported to have hypoglycemic properties as it acts favourably on metabolism, central nervous system and the endocrine secretion. It is employed in the treatment of anaemia, diabetes insomnia, neuralgia, gastritis and especially sexual impotence.

Note : The FDA found no evidence of enhanced sexual experience or potency resulting from its use.

GINKGO
(*Ginkgo biloba*)

Synonyms : Maiden hair tree.

Ginkgo or the maiden hair tree, also called in French the forty-coin tree, is a small tree, primitive member of the gymnosperms and the only survivor of the family Ginkgoaceae, all other species being found only as fossils. It is native to China, but widely planted as an ornamental and cultivated for drug with leaves used in Korea, France and United States.

It is deciduous tree 40 m high, leaves alternate or borne on spurs in clusters of 3-5; parallel veined, broad fan shaped upto 12 cm, notch at the apex, forming two distinct lobes hence the

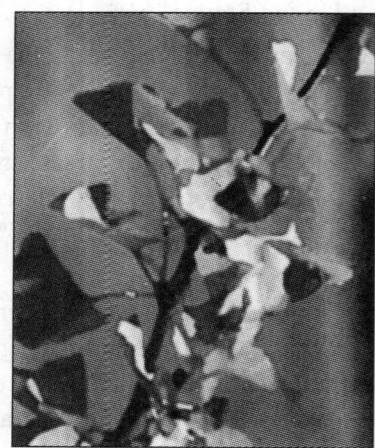

GINKGO *(G. biloba)*
(for colour, see Plate 5, Fig. 4)

species named "biloba". Flowers dioecious, male flowers with numerous loosely arranged anthers in stalked pairs on a slender axis; female flowers in pairs on long footstalks. The drupelike fruits have an arid, foul smelling pulp.

Chemical Constituents

The active constituents have been characterized as mixture of terpenoids and flavonoids (flavonol glycosides). The dried leaves contain 0.1-0.25% terpene trilactones comprising five ginkgolides (A, B, C, J and M) and bilobalide.

Use

Biological properties of ginkgo leaf or extract have been reported to have efficacy to improve peripheral and cerebrovascular circulation and thus have beneficial effect to correct the symptoms of senile cerebral insufficiency in the elderly (difficulties in concentrating, memory loss, confusion, mood problems, lack of energy, headaches) and assist with other symptoms such as vertigo, tinnitus and hearing loss.

Ginkgo may be combined with ginseng in the treatment of geriatric disorders. Extracts of ginkgo for herbal drug use are standardized to contain flavonoid glycosides and terpenes lactones in a ratio of 24 : 6% or 27 : 7%.

For the above mentioned indications, ginkgo extract is more efficacious than merely adopting a healthy lifestyle and diet supplement.

Health Food

In U.S., various ginkgo leaf preparations or crude leaf are sold as dietary supplements in the form of tablets, capsules, tincture and standardized extracts and tea.

The leaves are used in prescriptions for arteriosclerosis, anginapectoris, high serum cholesterol levels, dysentery and filariasis.

LIQUORICE
(*Glycyrrhiza glabra*)

Synonyms : Indian liquorice (*G. glabra* var. typica) Turkish liquorice (*G. glabra* var. violaceae, glycyrrhiza and sweet wood)

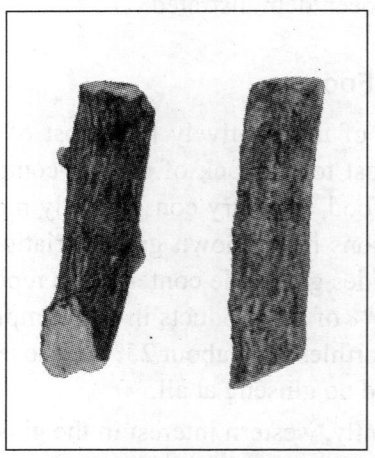

LIQUORICE ROOT *(G. glabra)*
(for colour, see Plate 5, Fig. 5)

Glycyrrhiza or Liquorice has long history of folk-loric use for a wide variety of purposes.

Liquorice is the dried unpeeled rhizome and root of the perennial herb *Glycyrrhiza glabra* (Leguminosae/Fabaceae). Different varieties of liquorice are cultivated commercially, including *G. glabra* var. typica (Persian liquorice) in Spain, Italy and France.

G. glabra var glandulifera (Russian liquorice) in Russia (Generally peeled drug). *Glycyrrhiza uralensis* (Manchurian liquorice) from China.

Chemical Constituents

It contains starch, glucose & surcrose, coumarins, triterpenoids, flavonoids & flavanones (liquiritin, isoliquiritin and glabrone), isoflavanols, isoflavenes, coumestanes and saponins (glycyrrhizin).

Health Food

Most of the liquorice produced are used in confectionary and for flavouring, including tobacco, beer and stouts. The drug is used in the orient for its sweetening power. It contains glycyrrhizin, which is reported to be 50-150 times as sweet as sucrose and drug has thus long been used in Pharmacy to mask the taste of bitter drugs. Greek recommended the use of drug for ulcers and Arab physicians to treat the cough and to relieve the side effects of laxative, being its demulcent property.

Phytopharmaceuticals based on liquorice claim the following indications; Traditionally used to treat the symptoms of digestive ailments such as epigastric bloating, **impaired digestion**, eructation and flatulence and soothing in cough.

It is widely used in the food technology industry for its **sweetening properties** and for its role as flavour enhancer. It is an ingredient of beverages including anise-flavoured cocktails with or without alcohols.

HONEY
(*Apis melifera*)

Honey is a saccharine secretion deposited in the cells of honeycomb by the hive bee, *Apis melifera* (Apidae) and other species of Apis.

Purified honey BP is prepared from the crude honey, by melting it at moderate temperature, skimming of any impurities by decantation and diluting with water to a weight of 1.35-1.36 g/ml at 20°C.

Honey when freshly prepared is a clear, syrupy liquid of pale yellow or reddish-brown color. On keeping, it crystallize and becomes opaque in appearance.

Chemical Constituents

Dextrose and fructose in equimolar quantities are the major constituents of honey. Some sucrose, small quantities of other carbohydrates, volatile oil, pigments and pollen grains are also present

Health Food

Honey is a useful **nutrient and sweetner**. It is used as a demulcent in cough preparation and for many special claims to cure folklore ailment and remedies, for which no scientific evidence to support the claim is yet available. It **improves digestion**, facilitate wound healing and had sedative, antiarthritic and antibacterial effects. In pharmacy honey is used as a component of linctuses for cough mixtures.

HOPS
(*Humulus lupulus*)

Hops consist of the dried pistillate inflorescence of *Humulus lupulus* Linn. (Moraceae/Cannabaceae) a tall dioecious perennial herb, with trio to pentalobate leaves, with pistillate flowers gathered in recemes commonly referred to as hop, hop cones (strobiles). It grows wild in the hedges and wood skirts of Europe and North America but also widely cultivated in British isles.

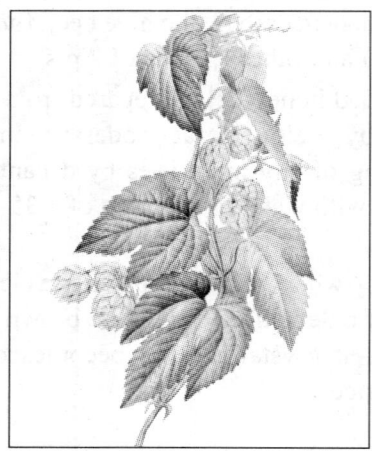

HOPS *(Humulus lupulus)*
(for colour, see Plate 5, Fig. 6)

Chemical Constituents

The drug contains flavonoids, rutin, quercetin, astragalin, chalcones, flavanones, xanthohumol and isoxanthohumol.

Steam distillate produce 0.3 to 1% essential oil, chief constituents of which are mono and sesquiterpenoid hydrocarbons (β-myrcene, humulene, caryophyllene), esters of myrcenol, linalool and numerous minor constituents and 30% is a resinous fraction. Chemically unstable phloroglucinol derivatives such as humulone and lupulone are found in resinous fraction. The later components isomerize to produce bitter principles, whose bitter taste and bacteriostatic properties account for the use of hop in the brewing process.

Health Food

Hops are marketed in "Health food" stores in the United States, not only for the preparation of sedative tea but also as a legal intoxicant, because the plant is closely related to marijuana; it produces mild sensation of euphoria when smoked but prolonged use produce dizziness, intoxication and jaundice.

It is also used as **appetite stimulant** in powdered and dried extract powder form for tea, tincture, capsules and tablet dosage form. Extracts and oil are also used as flavour component in nonalcoholic beverages, frozen dairy desserts, candy and baked goods as sedative. Also used in "dream pillow" to promote sleep.

LEMON OIL
(*Citrus limon* LINN.)

Synonyms : Expressed lemon oil; Cedar oil (terpene less)

Lemon oil is volatile oil obtained from the fresh peel of fruit of *Citrus limon* Linn. (Rutaceae); by expression in cold.

Citrus limon plant is indigenous to northern India but cultivated in subtropical regions such as southern Italy, Sicily, southern California, Florida, Jamaica and Australia. In India cultivation is done in U.P., M.P., Karnataka, Maharashtra and Punjab.

Lemon oil is pale yellow colour liquid with characteristic odour.

Lemon oil is volatile oil obtained by expression, without the aid of heat, from the fresh peel of the fruit of *Citrus limon* (Linn.) Burmann filius (Rutaceae) with or without the previous separation of pulp.

A small evergreen tree upto 6 m high, with fragrant flowers and stiff thorns.

It is indigenous to northern India but is cultivated in Spain, Italy and Sicily.

Chemical Constituents

Lemon oil contains about 90% of terpenes consisting chiefly of (+) limonene (monoterpene hydrocarbons) present in the range of 70–80%, other monoterpene hydrocarbons are β-pinene and γ-terpinene, approximately 8–10% each. The presence of aliphatic aldehyde (0.2-0.5%) including nonanol, octanol and monoterpenoid aldehyde (2-3% including neral, geranial and citronellal; together called citral). Some lemon oil contain up to 13% citral but the optimum range for citral is 2 to 4%.

Health Food

Lemon oil is used as **flavour for food products**. It has power to give strength to the body's defence mechanism and also has stimulant, carminative and stomachic properties.

Lemon oil is also employed in cosmetics and liquid cleansers.

Note : All the essential oils containing terpenes, carotenoids, limonoids, flavonoids (Isoflavones) are used in health food products because they have disease prevention property.

MUSTARD OIL
(*Brassica nigra*)

Mustard oil is obtained from the black or brown mustard dried ripe seeds of *Brassica nigra* or *Brassica juncea* (Brassicaceae/Cruciferae). The plants are annual herbs, slender erect stem with yellow flowers. They are cultivated in Europe and USA while *B. juncea* is naturalized and cultivated in India and former USSR.

Chemical Constituents

The mustard seeds contain both fixed oil (25-27%) and volatile oil (0.5-1.3%). The seeds also contain proteins (30%) and mucilage (20%). The volatile oil is obtained by hydrodistillation and fixed oil is obtained by expression.

The volatile oil fraction contains about 90% allyl isothiocyanate (mustard oil) obtained from sinigrin (glycoside) by hydrolysis with the enzyme (myrosinase) present in the seeds.

The fixed oil contain lipids (erucic, oleic and linoleic acids).

Health Food

Mustard seed is used as condiments and as **food supplements**. Mustard family vegetables are reported to have anticarcinogenic properties.

Mustard oil is also used externally as rubefacients and counter irritants.

Mustard (especially white) is extensively used in prepared mustard form, where it is commonly used with vinegar and other spices. Other food products in which mustard is used include baked goods, meat and meat products, processed vegetable, fats and oils, snacks foods etc. Highest maximum average use level are about 12.4%.

NUTMEG (MACE)
(*Myristica fragrans*)

Nutmeg are the dried kernels of the seeds of *Myristica fragrans* (Myristicae). The trees are indigenous to the Molucca and neighboring islands but also cultivated in tropical regions including Ceylon and the West Indies.

The nutmeg tree is an evergreen tree with spreading branches and dense foliage up to about 20 m high. The fruits are fleshy like an apricot (about 6 cm long) on ripening splits in half, exposing a bright red net like aril wrapped around a dark reddish brown and brittle shell within which lies a single seed. The net like aril is known as **mace**.

Chemical Constituents

Nutmeg was introduced in Europe by Arabs in the middle of the twelfth century.

Nutmeg contains fixed oils (25-40%) which are solid at ordinary temperature, known as nutmeg butter. It also contain volatile oil (8–15%), proteins and starch.

The volatile oil (myristica oil) is obtained from the kernels by steam distillation. The oil is colourless or pale yellow liquid with characteristic odour and taste of nutmeg.

Health Food

Myristica is used in food products as flavour and condiments having carminative properties.

ONION
(Allium cepa)

Allium cepa Linn family Liliaceae is the common onion plant available into two varieties depending upon whether the external part of the bulb is white or colored. The shape and size of the bulb differ with each variety (from 2–20 cm; flattened spherical or pear shaped).

Chemical Constituents

A fresh onion bulb contains fructans with a low degree of polymerization, flavonoids and sulphur containing compound, (also contain prostaglandins), trans (+)-S-(1-propenyl)-L-cysteine sulfoxide and other cysteine derivatives.

Health Food

It is being used as herb health food and medicine in India, China, Pakistan Middle East for the last more than 1000 years and still employed as daily **food supplements**. It has variety of physiologic effects, including stimulation of bile production, lowering of blood sugar and blood lipids, reduction of hypertension, acceleration of wound healing and curing of common cold. It has been clinically proved that diet having consumption of onion and garlic more than 600 g and 50 g respectively per week, significantly lowers triglycerides and beta-lipoproteins.

Its juice is known for its diuretic properties (true diuretic or stimulant of water elimination), is an antimicrobial agent *in vitro* and experiment in animals demonstrate its hypoglycemic activity. As in garlic it also has an activity against platelet aggregation and fibrinolytic activity.

Currently onion is marketed as a soft extract presented as "pulvic decongestant". In folklore medicine, onion is being used for boils, anthrax or whitlow. It is also frequently used in homoeopathy medicine.

Garlic and Onion : Antithrombic, hypolipidaemic, hypoglycaemic, hypotensive, diaphoretic, expectorant and antibiotic properties. The hypoglycaemic action derives from disulphide such as allicin (diallyldisulphide oxide) and allylpropyldisulphide.

It has been investigated that by virtue of their thiol groups, these disulphides act as sparing agent, for insulin by competing with it for inactivating compound.

PARSLEY
(Petroselinum crispum)

Synonyms : Common parsley and garden parsley

Parsley, the leaf, root and fruit have been used for centuries in folk medicine. *Petroselinum cris-*

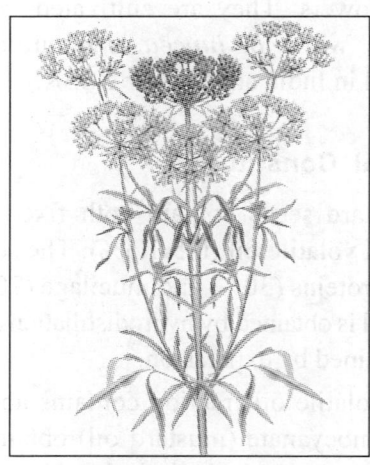

PARSLEY (Petroselinum crispum)
(for colour, see Plate 5, Fig. 7)

pum (Mill) (Syn. *P. sativum* Hoffm; *P. hortense* Hoffm; *Apium petroselinum* L; *Larum petroselinum*, Benth et Hook) family Umbelliferae/ Apiaceae. The leaf of this common garden herb, cultivated throughout the world, is also employed as culinary garnish.

Chemical Constituents

Parsley leaf contains essential oils containing myristicin, p-mentha-1,3,8-triene and hydrocarbons (limonene, β-phellandrene and α-pinene). It also contains flavone glycosides, furanocoumarins (bergapten, heraclenol). Roots contain phthalalides and apiol containing essential oil. Fruit contains mainly apiol, myristicin and tetramethoxybenzene.

Health Food

Parslay (fresh and dehydrated) is widely used in home cooking. Herb, its seed oil and oleoresin are extensively used in flavouring meat sauces, canned meats and spice blends. Herb or its roots are sometimes used as tea ingredients, also in diuretic formulations. It is also used as health food being a rich natural source of carotene, ascorbic acid (**antioxidant**), iron and other minerals.

According to tradition parsley is a diuretic and an emmenagogue.

ROSE HIPS
(*Rosa canina* Linn., *R. gallica* and *R. villosa*)

Rose hips are elongated red pseudofruits containing very hard polyhedral alkenes.

The drug rose hips consist of the ripe and dried receptacle cup as well as alkene from the bushy shrub of *Rosa canina* L (Rosaceae). Must contain not less than 0.2% ascorbic acid. Vitamin content of the commercially available dried fruit is highly dependent on exact botanical source, environment, time of collection and method of drying. Many of the marketed samples no longer contain detectable amount of vitamin C.

Health Food

The drug is used as a health food in the form of tea, jam, soup, or other preparation for oral use. The commercial product such as vitamin tablets that contain rose hip in combination with synthetic ascorbic acid, rarely state the proportion of vitamin derived from the natural source.

Rose hips are used in the treatment and prevention of influenza type infections, infectious disease and **vitamin C deficiencies**, to facilitate digestion, for arthritis, as a diuretic, as an astrigent and so on but none of these use is justified and more synthetic **vitamin C is available** in the market at cheaper rate than the natural vitamin C to be obtained from rose hips, hence, it is not recommended for the therapeutic use. But rose hip can be employed to **enhance the flavour** of herbal tea mixture or in **the food industry**.

SAFFRON
(*Crocus sativus*)

Saffron (*Crocus sativus* Linn. Iridaceae) is a small plant of oriental origin, cultivated from a bulb.

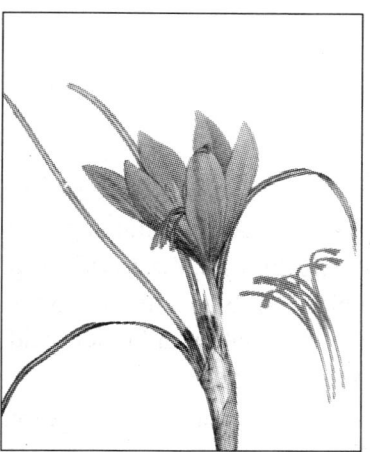

SAFFRON (*Crocus sativus*)
(for colour, see Plate 5, Fig. 8)

It is an perennial herb with large fleshy corm from which leaves and flowers are produced in fall; native to the eastern Mediterranean region; cultivated as an annual or perennial worldwide crop (Spain, France, Italy and India).

Chemical Constituents

The color of the drug is due to carotenoids, chiefly due to crocin (2%), which is diester of crocetin (Fig. 11.3) (8, 8'-diapocarotene-8, 8'-dioic acid) and of gentiobiose. Other constituents are picrocrocin (Fig. 11.4) (4%) (glucoside of 4β-hydroxycyclocitral) and a small amount of essential oil, containing mainly safranal, which is responsible for the characteristic odour and together with picrocrocin for the taste of the saffron.

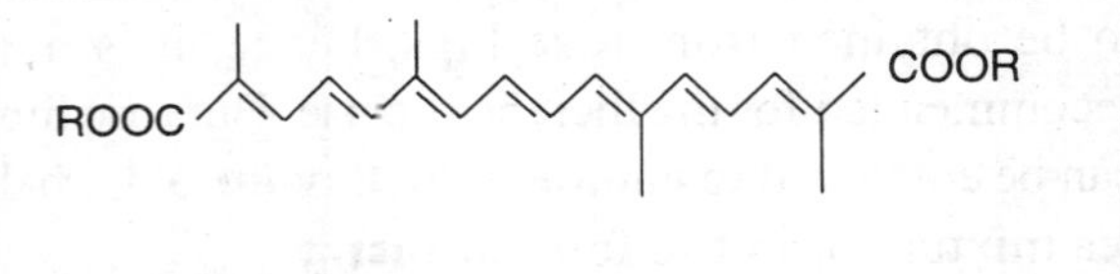

R = H. Crocetin
R = β-D-Glc (1 ⟶ 6) β-D-Glc(1 ⟶ 4) : CROCIN

Fig. 11.3.

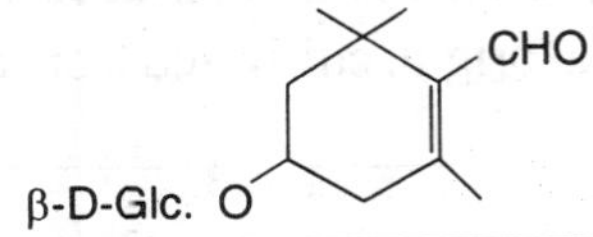

Fig. 11.4. Picrocrocin.

Health Food

The stigma of the flower are used in health food. These stigma have an aromatic odour and slightly bitter and pungent taste. **Antioxidant properties** of saffron claimed to be superior to vitamin E in its inhibition of oxidation of linoleic acid. It is used as **dietary supplement**.

German commission E. monograph describe that saffron stigma is a traditional nervous sedative, but no proof of its activity available hence not recommended for therapeutic use. The dried stigma are used as a spice in health food products.

SAFFLOWER OIL

Safflower oil is fixed oil obtained from the seeds of *Carthamus tinctorius* Linn. family Compositae.

Safflower is a glabrous annual herb, up to about 1 m high, flowering from May to July; extensively cultivated worldwide, especially for its seeds.

Health Food

The oil is used as **dietary supplement** in health food products in the form of margarines and as oil filled capsules. This oil is rich in linoleic acid (75%), oleic acid (18%) and mixture of saturated acids (6%).

SASSAFRAS
(*Sassafras albidum*)

Synonyms : Common Sassafras bark.

Sassafras is the dried root bark obtained from a small tree of *Sassafras albidum* (Nuttall) Nees family Lauraceae indigenous to Eastern North America.

It is a decidious tree with leaves ranging in shape from two lobbed to three lobed, up to 40 m high. The plant is native to Eastern United States.

Safrole-free Sassafras extract is obtained by dilute alcoholic extraction of the bark which is used in health food preparation.

Chemical Constituents

Contains essential oil known as sassafras oil, which contains over 80% safrole, other phenylpropane derivatives and hydrocarbons (α-pinene, phellandrene). In addition, the drug contains isoquinoline alkaloids and lignans.

Health Food

The bark is widely used as a **spring tonic and**

"**blood thinner**". It is still sold by "Health food" outlets and writers of popular accounts of herbs continue to praise its virtues as an unexcelled home remedy.

Both sassafras oil and sassafrole are **presently prohibited by the FDA from use as flavors or food additives,** as it is reported that 0.66 mg/kg dose of safrole prove hazardous to human beings. One cup of tea prepared from 2.5 g of sassafras could yield as much as 200 mg of safrole (equivalent to 3 mg/kg).

SOYBEAN OIL
[*Glycine soja* Sieb and *Glycine max* (L) Merr.]

Soybean oil is a refined fixed oil obtained from the ripe seeds of *Glycine soja* Sieb and *Glycine max* (L) Merr. (Fabaceae). About 10% oil is obtained by expression.

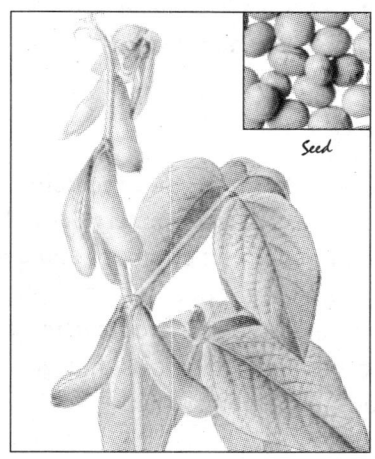

SOYBEAN (Branch & Seed) *(Glycine soja)*
(for colour, see Plate 5, Fig. 9)

Chemical Constituents

The oil contains mixture of fatty acid (Palmitic 9-12%, stearic 2-4%, oleic 27-60% and linoleic acid 25-56%).

The unsaponifiable matter contains sterols;

β-sitosterol (47-59%), stigmasterol (17-19%), campesterol (19-23%), Δ^5-avenasterol (2-4%), Δ^7-sterols (2-4%) as well as tocopherols γ-(44-60%), δ-(30-43%), α(5-10%), β(2-3%).

Health Food

Soybean oil is most important oil crop in the world. In the terms of total production, it is largely dominated by the United States, Brazil, China and Argentina are also the major producer far ahead of India and Canada.

Soybeans are used as a general food for humans and live stocks. The oil is consumed principally as salad oil, shortening and margarine. The main use of the oil is as **dietary supplements**.

In pharmacy the soybean oil is used for parenteral feeding for caloric and essential fatty acid intake. It is administered in the form of (O/W) emulsion containing 10-20% of the oil.

Soybean oil is also a source of **Lecithin**; which is an ingredient in a number of proprietary products that are used in controlling deranged lipids and cholesterol metabolism.

SUNFLOWER OIL
(*Helianthus annuus*)

Sunflower oil is fixed oil obtained from the seeds of cultivated varieties of *Helianthus annuus* Linn. (Asteraceae). Russia ranks first in the production of oil and the Argentina is second in ranking followed by Russia, Ukraine and France.

Chemical Constituents

This oil consist of a mixture of triglycerides which are rich in unsaturated fatty acid, the main fatty acid are Palmitic 3-10%, stearic 1-10%, oleic 14-35%; Linoleic 55-75% and Linolenic <0.3%.

The unsaponifiable matter characterized by many sterols; β-sitosterol (60%), alongside Δ^7-

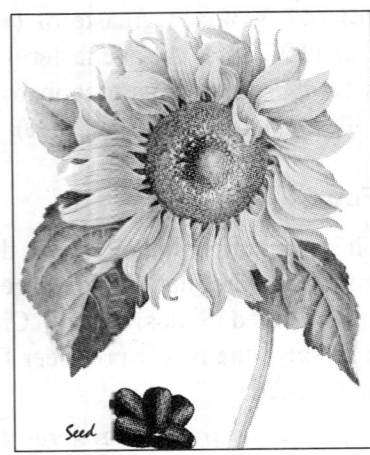

SUNFLOWER *(Helianthus annuus)*
(for colour, see Plate 6, Fig. 1)

stigamasterol (7-14%) and Δ^5-avenasterol (4-6%) are also present.

Tocopherol are mainly represented by α-tocopherol in this oil.

Health Food

It is used as **dietary supplements**. This oil is used as an alternative to corn and Safflower oil for culinar purposes and it is an ingredient of a number of **speciality dietary** supplements.

TAMARIND
(Tamarindus indica)

Tamarind is the partially dried ripe fruit of *Tamarindus indica* Linn. **(Leguminosae/Caesalpinieaceae)**.

It is an evergreen tree with large trunk and dark grey bark, up to 20 m high; native to tropical Asia and Africa. Cultivated worldwide (e.g. China, India, Africa and West Indies).

The fruit is an indehiscent pod with fleshy mericarp, which hold from 4-12 irregular seeds. The drug has been deprived of the outer layer of pericarp and preserved with sugar. The pulp is reddish brown, has a mild sweet taste.

Chemical Constituents

Pulp is rich in pectin and monosaccharide (20-40%). It contains 10-15% organic acids such as tartaric acid, citric acid in the free state but as salt the main component is potassium hydrogen tartarate.

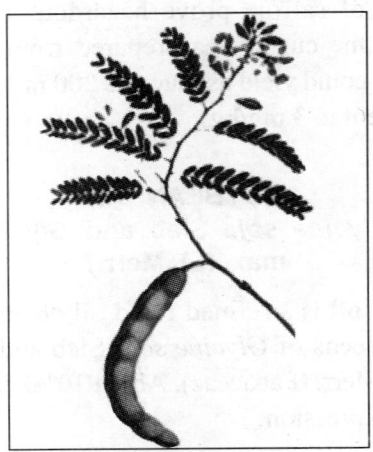

TAMARIND *(Tamarindus indica)*
(for colour, see Plate 6, Fig. 2)

Health Food

Tamarind is used in folklore medicine as health food, as laxative and in dysentery. Widely used in Asia as an ingredient in chutneys and curries and also used in making refreshing drink in tropics. It is also used as flavour ingredient in sauces and other food products, fats, oils and gravies as an health food supplements.

TURMERIC
(Curcuma longa Linn.)

Synonyms : Curcuma.

Turmeric is prepared rhizome of *Curcuma longa* Linn. (Zingiberaceae)

It is perennial herb of ginger family, having thick rhizome; native to Southern Asia; extensively cultivated in India, China Indonesia and other tropical countries.

Rhizome is boiled, cleaned, sun dried (prepared turmeric) and polished. India is the major supplier to the world market.

Chemical Constituents

Turmeric contains 3-7% orange-yellow colored volatile oil which is mainly composed of turmerone (60%), α, β-atlantone and zingiberene (25%) with minor amounts of 1,8 cineole, α-phellandrene, d-sabinene and borneol. Others than above it contains yellow coloring matter including 0.3–5.4%

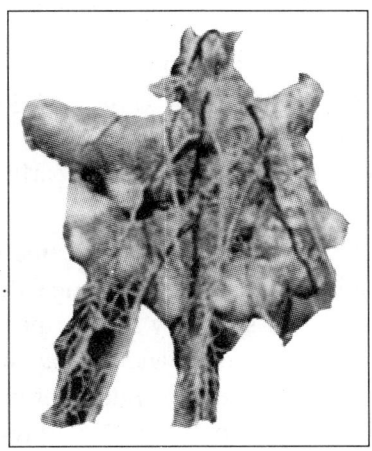

TURMERIC *(Curcuma longa)*
(for colour, see Plate 6, Fig. 3)

Curcumin, sugars (glucose 28%; fructose 12% and arabinose 1%), fixed oil, proteins, minerals (high in potassium) vitamin C and resin.

Turmeric water and alcoholic soluble fraction have been reported to have antioxidant activities (which is due to curcumin).

Health Food

Turmeric is the major ingredient of curry powder (both for flavour and color) to stimulate appetite. It is used as an antioxidant in capsules, tablets and flavoring tea. It is recommended as food supplement to treat numerous conditions like flatulence, liver problems, menstrual difficulties, haemorrhage, chest pain, colic, skin diseases, constipation and also in religious rituals.

Turmeric and turmeric oleoresin are used extensively both for color and flavour in many food products including baked goods, meat and meat products. It is a major ingredient of curry powder and also used in prepared mustard.

Pharmacy uses turmeric rhizomes as a constituent of phytopharmaceuticals with the following indications as a choleretic and cholagoghe for functional dyspepsia attributed to hepatic origin and as an appetite stimulant. It is also used for its broad-spectrum antimicrobial activity. It has also been employed to stimulate biliary secretion and to treat gallstones.

HERBAL PRODUCTS OR HERBS IN COSMETICS

Herbal products in cosmetics or herbs in cosmetics can also be referred as botanical origin products in cosmetics. Personal care products containing ingredients from the plant origin are finding an increasing receptive trend in the domestic as well as world market.

Beginning in the 1990's, cosmetic manufacturers adopted a trend of using the terms cosmeceuticals to describe the OTC skin care products that claim therapeutic benefits by the addition of plant based active ingredients such as alpha hydroxy acids, retinoic acids, ascorbic acid and co-enzyme Q-10 (Ubiquinone, Fig. 7.8) to increase the skin elasticity, delay skin ageing by reducing the wrinkles, antioxidant as protectant against UV radiation by antioxidant property and to check the degradation of the collagen respectively. Thus the **herbal cosmetics are defined as the beauty products, which possess desirable physiological activities, such as skin healing, smoothning, appearance, enhancing and conditioning properties** because of herbal ingredients.

The Herbal cosmetics can be grouped into following major categories:

- For enhancing the appearance of the facial skin
- For hair growth and care
- For skin care, specially in teenager (acne, pimples, sustaining)
- Shampoos, soap, powders and perfumery etc.
- Miscellaneous products

Among the above mentioned categories, the skin care will dominate cosmeceutical demand in the coming years specially for the professional products used for appearance enhancing facial implants, chemical peels and related products. The US demand for cosmeceutical products is projected to increase by 7.6 percent per annum, likely to reach about US$ 5 billion by 2005. On the whole global market for cosmeceuticals has been estimated at about US$ 22 billion. In USA, the market for cosmeceuticals in 1998 was estimated at about US$ 2.5 billion. The key market demand was of the products effective in anti-wrinkle treatment, to increase microcirculation, sun screens, analgesic and promotion of hair growth. In USA alone, the market for herbal cosmetics and toiletries stood at US$ 345 million in 1998, data available is shown in the Table 12.1.

In olden days the herbal products were used for medicinal purposes, both, internally as well as

Table 12.1. Demand of botanical extract in cosmetics and toiletries from 1989–98 in USA

Item	Demand value (Million US $)		
	1989	1993	1998
Aloe extract	38	46	63
Botanical extracts	180	230	345
Others	22	34	67
Plant acids/enzymes	19	37	65
Essential oils	101	113	150
Other natural products	85	115	180
Total	445	575	870

externally. The drugs were used in crude form i.e. either their juice/latex, crushed fresh drugs or dried in fine powder form. In the case of seeds, they were crushed and pressed for the removal of oils, which were applied locally. But with the advancement of phytotechnology, the herbs are available in the forms of their extracts, oils, tinctures and even in more purified forms with the objective to provide improved performance and a reduced risk of skin irritation e.g. the availability of coenzyme Q-10 (polyhydroxy acid) which provides combine (antioxidant and exfoliant) action.

Manufacturers are frequently replacing vitamins with herbal ingredients, such as **aloe gel, ginseng and ginkgo.**

Indena is one of the world's largest botanical extract suppliers with a wide range of extracts with cosmetic potential. **Balsara Herbal Products Ltd.** are also marketing herbal extracts in India under the name of Folicon.

Table 12.2 shows lists few Herbal extracts available in the market for the use as herbal cosmeceutical products.

HERBS AS COSMETICS

The examples of herbs which are commonly used in Cosmetics.

ALKANET
(*Alkanna tinctoria* Linn.)

Synonyms : Alkanna, anchusa, orcanette, dyer's alkanet, and spanish bugloss.

Alkanet is the dried roots of *Alkanna tinctoria* (L) Tausch. (Boraginaceae), found in Hungary, Southern Europe and Turkey.

It is biennial or perennial herb about 0.5 m high with hairy leaves, bearing bluish or purple violet trumpet-shaped flowers.

Chemical Constituents

The roots contain alkannin about 5% (colouring matter), which is known as anchusin, anchusic acid and alkanna red; other constituents include tannin, alkannin isovalerate, alkannin angelate and alkannan, wax, and flavones.

Cosmetic Uses

Alkanna roots are used in cosmetics colouring oils, tars, in lipsticks formulation and in hair dyes.

Commercial Preparation

It is widely available either in crude or extract forms. It was official in USP.

ALOE VERA GEL
(*Aloe barbadensis*)

Aloe vera gel is obtained after eliminating the outer most tissue of the leaf of Aloe barbadensis (liliaceae) (see colour plate 2, Fig. 5), found in South Africa, West Indies and India.

Chemical Constituents

It is rich in water, amino acids, lipids, sterols, enzymes and in polysaccharides (pectin and hemicellulose).

Table 12.2. Selected herbal extracts with their cosmetic potential

Product	Botanical Source	Potential
Amla extract	*Embelica officinalis*	Hair tonic
Amla oil	--do--	Hair care
Aloe gel	*Aloe vera*	Skin bleaching
Bhringraj Aq. extract	*Eclepta alba*	Hair dye
Bhringraj oil	--do--	Hair tonic
Bilberry dry extract	*Vaccinium myritillus*	Antioxidant
Butcher's broom dry extract	*Ruscus aculeatus*	Cream to enhance appearance
Brahmi Aq. extract and Brahmi oil	*Centella asiatica*	Hair care
Chamomile dry extract	*Matricaria Chamomilla*	Soothing effect on irritated skin
Echinaceae dry extract	*Echinacea* spp.	Anti ageing
Ginkgo extract	*Ginkgo biloba*	Microcirculation
Hawthron	*Crataegus* spp.	Antiaging
Henna/Mehandi Aq. extract	*Lawsonia inermis*	Hair dye and Conditioner
Haldi Aq. extract	Turmeric	Skin care
Roselle Aq. ext.	*Hibiscus sabdariffa*	Skin & Hair care
Ivy soft extract	*Rhus toxicodendron*	
Khus Aq. extract	*Vetiveria zizanioides*	Skin and Hair care
Brahmi Leaf extract	*Centella asiatica*	Stimulation of collagen synthesis
Lemon peel Aq. extract	*Citrus limon*	Skin and Hair care
Methi Aq. extract	Fenugreek	Skin and hair care
Melilot dry extract	*Melilotus officinalis*	Microcapillary protection
Marigold dry extract	*Calendula officinalis*	*Emollient*
Neem Aq. extract	*Azadirachta indica*	Skin and Hair care
Neem oil	--do--	--do--
Peruvian bark fluid extract	*Cinchona succirubra*	Stimulation of scalp hair
Pumpkin seed lipophilic extract	*Cucurbita pepo*	Stimulation of sebaceous gland
Rose petal Aq. extract	*Rosa* spp.	Skin and hair care
Shikakai Aq. extract	*Acacia coneinna*	Hair care
Soybean saponin	*Glycine max*	Soothing effect
Sandalwood oil	*Santalum album*	Skin care
Tulsi Aq. extract	*Ocimum* spp.	Skin care

Cosmetic Uses

This gel is widely used in **cosmetology** as a **hydrating ingredient** in liquid or creams: sun lotion, shaving creams, lip balms, healing ointments, face packs and hair conditioner.

Extract of aloe or aloin are also used in sun-cream and other cosmetic preparations as emollient, anti wrinkles and wound healer.

Commercial Preparation

Aloe gel products are available in liquid and solid forms (spray-dried) in different qualities, depending upon the viscosity, based on glucomannan contents. Aloe vera gel is available in a wide range of ladies and gents health and skin care preparations such as aloe vera juice, medicated jelly, medicated cream, heat rub, moisturiser, hand

and body lotion, facial cleansing wash and mini lift mask.

AMLA
(*Emblica officinalis*)

Amla is a fresh and dried fruit of *Emblica officinalis* (Euphorbiaceae), a deciduous tree found in deciduous forests upto 350 m on hills. In India, often cultivated in UP, Gujarat, Rajasthan and Maharashtra.

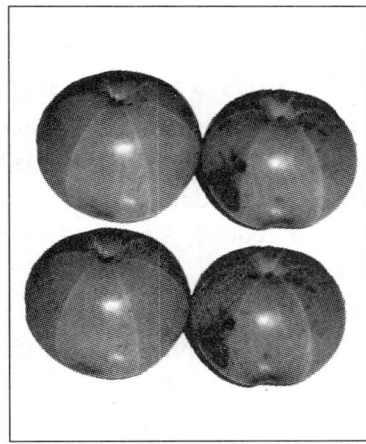

AMLA *(Emblica officinalis)*
(for colour, see Plate 6, Fig. 4)

It is a tricarpellary globose drupe (fruit) with fleshy edible mesocarp and stony endocorp. Its colour is green when unripe but turns yellow on ripening. The surface of fruit is smooth and shiny with six verticle furrows. The taste is sour and astringent.

Chemical Constituents

Amla contains about 5-6% tannins (gallic acid, ellagic acid and phyllembelin). It is a rich source of natural vitamin C, which is about 500-950 mg per 100 gm of fresh pulp. It is destroyed on heating and drying in sun. The fruit is also a rich source of pectin and minerals like phosphorus, iron and calcium.

Cosmetic Uses

Amla has antifungal, antibacterial, antiviral and antioxidant properties. It is used in the herbal **cosmetic preparations, hair dyes and as hair conditioner**. It also checks dandruff.

Amla is used in the form of fresh juice of the pulp, aqueous extract as well as its oil.

Commercial Preparation

Cosmetics, Shampoos and Hair oils.

ALMOND OIL
(*Prunus dulcis* (Miller) D.A.)

Almond oil is the fixed oil obtained by cold expression from ripe seeds of *Prunus dulcis* (Miller) *D.A. Webb var dulcis* or var. amara (DC) Buchheim or a mixture of two varieties (Rosaceae); widely cultivated around mediterranean region, including Greece, Italy, Spain and North Africa.

The fruit is an ablong drupe with light green velvety epicarp. The seed is oval, flattened and has thin, wrinkly and easy to peel off (fresh) tegument.

Chemical Constituents

Both the varieties of almond oil contain 40-55% fixed oil, about 20% proteins, mucilage and emulsion. The only chemical constituent which distinguishs two varieties (amara and dulcis) is the presence of 2.5-4% of the colourless crystalline, cyanogenetic glycoside (amygdalin).

The chief constituents of fixed oil are oleic acid (62-86%), linoleic acid (7-30%) and palmitic acid (4-9%).

Cosmetic Uses

Almond oil is mainly used in cosmetology, dermatology and for many toilet articles. The cosmetic industry also use fraction containing low molecular weight proteins, associated with carbohydrates. This active fraction is reported to relieve skin irritation (after sun lotions, shaves, make up removers and so on). The purified essential oil of almond is used as flavour, chiefly in the agricultural food industry.

Commercial Preparation

Anti wrinkle cream, herbal beauty care, moisturiser, hair lotions and cold creams.

BERGAMOT OIL
(*Citrus aurantium* Linn.)

Bergamot oil is obtained by mechanical processes without heating, from fresh (nearly ripe fruit) pericarp of *Citrus aurantium* Linn. (Rutaceae) a species Bergamia, cultivated in Calabrian coast (Italy).

Its source is a small tree, bearing fruits which ripen to look like miniature oranges.

Chemical Constituents

The oil contains β-pinene (5-9.5%), limonene (33.42%), γ-terpinene (6-10.5%), linalool (7-15%), linalyl acetate, (22-33%) and geraniol (0.5%). The bergapten concentration is between 0.15–0.35%.

Cosmetic Uses

The oil free from bergaptin is used in **perfumery** (colognes) and **cosmetology industry**; the bergamot oil is authorised as photodynamic sensitizer and used for the treatment of psoriasis, vitiligo and mycosis fungoides in cosmetic creams and in sun lotions up to 0.25% and up to 3% concentration in perfumes. It is used in **aromatherapy** for stress related conditions, as an antidepressant and for its antiseptic properties. Combined with *Eucalyptus* and carrier oil it has been used to relieve the symptoms of shingles

and cold sores and to suppress the irritation of chicken pox.

Commercial Preparation

Bergamot oil expressed and rectified.

BRAHMI (INDIAN PENNYWORT)
(*Centella asiatica*)

Synonym : Hydrocotyl asiatica

Brahmi consist of fresh and dried leaves and stem of *Centella asiatica* (Umbelliferae), growing at the edges of river i.e. wet damp and marshy places in India, Srilanka and Pakistan.

Brahmi is a herbaceous creeping herb having prostrate stem with long internodes, small rounded leaves, more or less cordate and adventitious roots at the nodes of reddish stem and umbels with very small flowers.

Herb *Bacopa monniera* (Sym. *Herpestis monniera*), family Scrophulariaceae is confused with Brahmi and is also found in wet places on the river edges throughout India.

Both the herbs differ in the shape of their

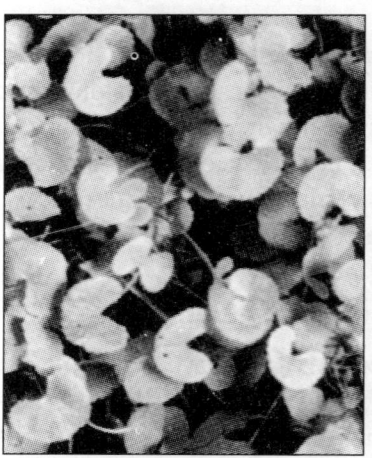

BRAHMI *(Centella asiatica)*
(for colour, see Plate 6, Fig. 5)

leaves. *Centella asiatica* has reniform leaves with sheathing base while *Bacopa monniera* leaves are obovate and entire with broad apex.

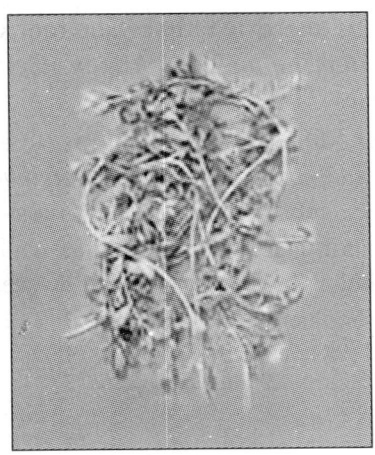

BRAHMI *(Bacopa monniera)*
(for colour, see Plate 6, Fig. 6)

Chemical Constituents

Brahmi contains essential oil, sterols, flavonol glycoside and triterpenoid saponins. They are β-amyrin derivative and known as **asiaticoside and madecassoside**. In these glycosides sugar moietes are attached to –COOH group of asiatic or madecassic acid (brahmic acid), on hydrolysis they yield asiatic acid and madecassic acid respectively along with two glucose and one rhamnose).

Cosmetic Uses

The drug is used since ancient times in India, to treat various forms of **dermatitis** and is thought to accelerate the healing of superficial wounds. Although its use is difficult to evaluate clinically but is linked to asiaticoside and its derivatives. It is also reported to **promote fibroblast proliferation and collagen synthesis**, and to have anti-ulcer activity.

Centella extracts are used topically as the adjunct in the treatment of surgical wounds and minor burns, and as a complementary treatment of leg ulcers of venous origin (at the granulation stage).

Orally, it is indicated to relieve the symptoms of venous and lymphatic vessel insufficiency, and used on atonic wounds, as well as in case of hypertrophic healing.

Alcoholic extract of the whole brahmi plant is reported to have anti-cancer activities.

Commercial Preparation

Brahmi oil and soft extract.

BHRINGRAJ (BHANGRA) (*Eclipta alba* (Linn) Hassk)

Bhringraj is used as an entire fresh or dried weed plant *Eclipta alba* (Linn) Hassk (Compositae or Asteraceae) found in moist places throughout India, ascending up to 600 fts on the hills. It is mostly seen in rainy seasons in dry areas and all the year round in wet and watery places.

It is an annual or perennial, erect or prostrate, branched plant with leaves opposite, flowers white or yellow in capitulum inflorescence.

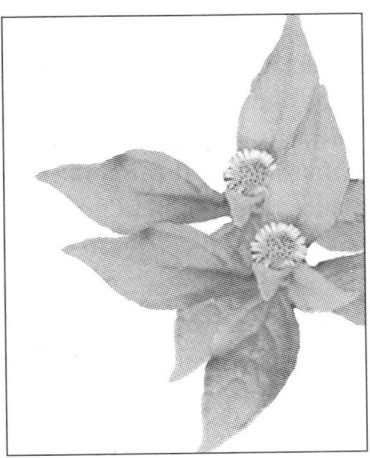

BHRINGRAJ *(Eclipta alba Hassk)*
(for colour, see Plate 6, Fig. 7)

Chemical Constituents

It contains coumestans (wedelolactone and de-methyl wedelolactone); alkaloid (ecliptine), glycosides, (β-amyrin), triterpenic acid, fatty acid, resin and steroids (ecalbasaponins).

The presence of coumestans is reported in fresh herb only.

Cosmetic Uses

Plant is used all over India as a constituent to hair oil for healthy black and long hair. The oil is very **good hair tonic**. Externally, it is used as anti-inflammatory for minor cuts and burns. The fresh leaves juice is considered very effective in stopping bleeding. The leaf juice is also used as a hepatic tonic deobstruent (removing obstruction).

BILBERRY (BLUEBERRY)
(*Vaccinium myritillus*)

Bilberry *Vaccinium myritillus* Linn. (Ericaceae).

Chemical Constituents

See page no. 215

Cosmetic Uses

Extracts obtained from the fruits, enriched in anthocyanins are ingredients of drug designed to treat symptoms of **cutaneous capillary fragility**. The dried extract of the plants used in cosmetic preparation, for having **anti-oxidant properties** as well as **colouring pigment**.

The french market is largely dominated by import of *V. myritillus* (from Poland) and other species (*V. corymbossum*) cultivated in Germany are also used in the agricultural food industry.

Commercial Preparation

Crude drug and aqueous extract containing 36% anthocyanosides.

BURDOCK
(*Arctium lappa* Linn.)

Synonyms : Arctium majus Bernh

Burdock is the dried first year root collected from *Arctium lappa* Linn. Hardy (Compositae/Asteraceae).

Arctium lappa Linn. is hardy, biennial or perennial herb up to 3 m high, is very common in vacant lots and on trail edges almost all over Europe, having large cordate leaves, capitulum of purple tubular flowers surrounded by green bracts ending in hooks.

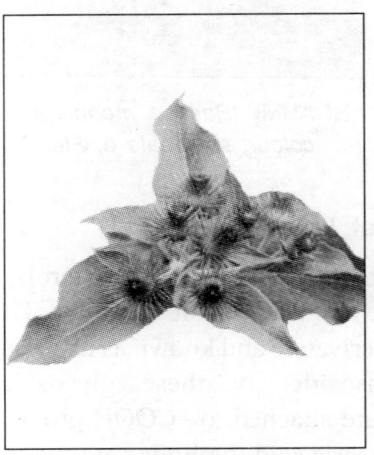

BURDOCK (*Arctium lappa* Linn.)
(for colour, see Plate 6, Fig. 8)

Chemical Constituents

Roots contain inulin (up to 50%) rich in poly-unsaturated compounds, polyalkenes, polyalkynes, volatile acids and non-hydroxy acid (lauric, myristic, stearic and polyphenolic acids (2-3%) (e.g. caffeic and chlorogenic).

Leaves have been reported to contain arctiol, fukinone, β-eudesmol and taraxasterol.

The **dried roots** of the plant are official in French Phamacopoeia and are used for the treatment of dermatosis and furuncuosis. In phytotherapy, it is recommended for the treatment of acne, and pilo-sebaceous infections and psoriasis.

The **leaves** are used locally as an emollient and itch-relieving adjunctive therapy for dermatitis and as topical protective agent for cracks, abrasions, scratches and insect bites.

Commercial Preparation

Crude and extracts of leaves and roots.

Cosmetic Uses

This plant (**roots and leaves**) is used in **herbal cosmetics** due to the presence of polyunsaturated compounds, (Inulin) polyalkenes and polyamines; whose *in vitro* antimicrobial and antifungal properties have been demonstrated. Also used in toiletry preparations for its skin-cleansing and hair tonic (stimulate hair growth) properties and used in chronic skin conditions such as psoriasis.

Traditionally, the plant roots are used orally for the treatment of moderate acne and to improve renal and digestive elimination functions.

Commercial Preparation

Crude form as well as extracts of leaves and roots.

CADE OIL (JUNIPER TAR)
(*Juniperus oxycedrus*)

Cade oil is the lightest fraction obtained after destructive distillation of *Juniperus oxycedrus* Linn. (Cupressaceae) wood. The plant is indigenous to Southern France and other countries bordering the mediterranean area.

Juniper tar (cade oil) is a viscid, clear, dark brown liquid with a tarry odor and a faintly aromatic bitter taste.

Chemical Constituents

The oil contains sesquiterpene, (*S. cadinene*, cadalene, calacorene, α1-murolene) associated with some phenolic (guaiacol cresol) compounds.

Cosmetic Uses

It has been used in creams designed to treat skin disorders (keratosis, eczema and neurodermatitis). It is also used in veterinary medicine and in various hygiene products (shampoos for seborrheic dermatitis of the scalp).

Commercial Preparation

Crude and rectified oil, official in U.S.P.

CASTOR OIL
(*Ricinus communis*)

Castor oil is the fixed oil obtained from the seeds of *Ricinus communis* Linn. (Euophorbiaceae) by cold expression.

The plant is an annual in temperate climate or a tree attaining the height of 15 meters. There are many forms of plant with variations in the

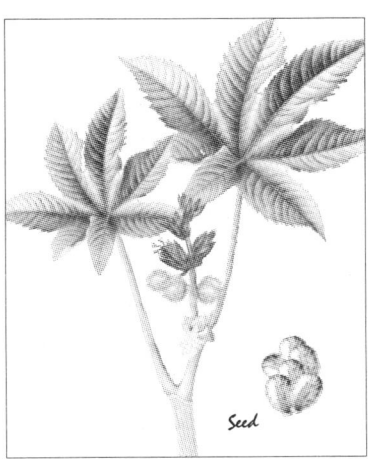

CASTOR OIL PLANT & SEED
(for colour, see Plate 6, Fig. 9)

shape of leaves and colour, size and marking of the seeds.

The fruit is a three-celled spiny capsule, each cell containing albuminous elliptical ovoid, somewhat compressed seeds from 8–18 mm in length and from 4–7.5 mm in thickness. It is mottled grayish and brown, but varies considerably in colour.

Castor oil is a pale yellowish or almost colourless, transparent and viscid liquid. It has a faint, mild odor and a bland characteristic taste.

Chemical Constituents

Castor seeds contain 46–53% fixed oil, which consists of triglycerols containing an unsaturated and hydroxylated C-18, fatty acids (ricinolic acid, isoricinoleic acid, stearic and dihydroxy stearic acids).

Cosmetic Uses

Hydrogenated castor oil (USP/NF) is used as stiffening agent. **Undecylenic acid**, which is prepared from castor oil, is used in fungistatic preparation and is also used as a preservative in cosmetology. Castor oil is employed in the manufacture of soaps.

Commercial Preparation

Two grades oil is available. It is official in IP and USP.

COCONUT OIL
(Cocos nucifera Linn.)

Coconut oil is a fixed oil obtained by expression or extraction from seed kernels of the coconut palm, *Cocos nucifera* Linne (Palmae) grown in Africa and South East Asia.

The tree is tall strait'ly rising to a height of 30 meters; has a tuft of leaves at the top and bears 100 or more fruits (coconut) each year.

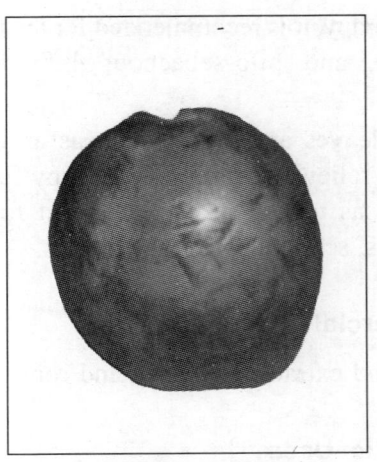

COCONUT FRUIT *(Cocos nucifera)*
(for colour, see Plate 7, Fig. 1)

Chemical Constituents

The oil consists of mixture of glycerides in which 80–85% of the acids are saturated; semisolid at 20°C. Lauric (50%) and myristic (20%) are the major fatty acids. The oil also contains glycerides of caprylic and capric acids.

Cosmetic Uses

It is used in cold creams and in sun tan formulations. The coconut oil yields quality soaps and shampoos because of its high saponification value.

COMMON IVY
(Hedera helix LINN.)

Common Ivy is dried leaves and flowering tops of the *Hedera helix* Linn. (Araliaceae), official in 10th edition of French Pharmacopoeia.

It is a very common plant growing at altitude upto 1,200 m in woods, hedges and cool rocky areas. It is a shade and half-shade loving plant that climb trees and walls. It has creeping and climbing stem, which emit roots and grow hooks. The cauline leaves are divided into 3-5 triangular lobes (8-10 × 10-12 cm). The flowers are gathered in terminal umbels and fruits are globulous blackish berries with circular features near the top.

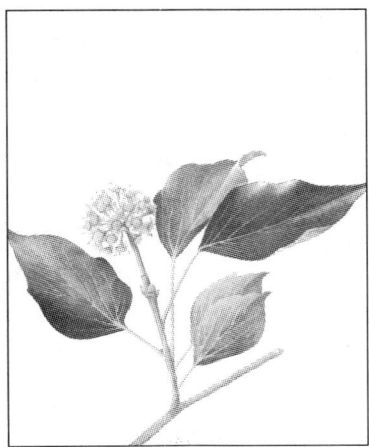

COMMON IVY *(Hedera helix)*
(for colour, see Plate 7, Fig. 2)

Chemical Constitutents

The leaves contain sterols, a small quantity of steam distillable products (germacrene, β elemene), caffeic esters of quinic acids, flavonoids (rutin), polyalkynes and saponins (the three chief saponins are hedera saponin, B and C and saponin K-10).

Cosmetic Uses

The leaf extract (30% ethanol) has antifungal and antibacterial properties. Ivy based preparations are mostly used in cosmetic products, cream lotions, shampoos and anticellulite preparations.

ECHINACEAE (CONE FLOWER)
(*Echinaceae angustifolia*)

Echinaceae, the dried rhizome and roots of *Echinaceae angustifolia* de Candolle (*E. pallida* Nutt) is used in USA.

The plant is perennial herb (Compositae/Asteraceae) and native to the mid-Western states.

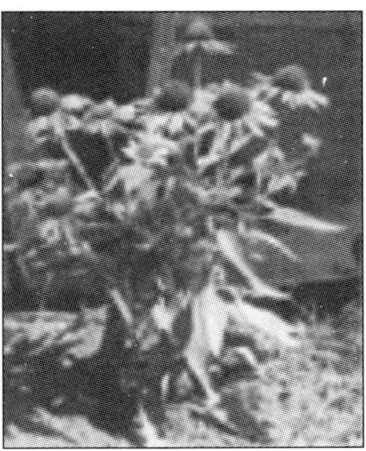

ECHINACEAE *(E. angustifolia)*
(for colour, see Plate 7, Fig. 3)

In Europe, the entire fresh, flowering plant *E. purpurea* (Linne) Moench is used in medicine.

Echinaceae spp. (*E. angustifolia* DC *E. purpurea* (Linn.) Moench and *E. palliada* (Nutt) (Asteraceae) are the hardy plants with oval or lanceolate leaves entire or more or less pinnate (Purpurea). The large size-capitulums comprises of purplish tubular flowers gathered into three spheres.

Chemical Constituents

The drug contains essential oil, pyrrolizidine alkaloids and phenolic compounds derived from caffeic acid.

Cosmetic Uses

The plant is used externally in lotions and cosmetics as wound healing, immunostimulatory and antiageing drug.

EUCALYPTUS OIL
(*Eucalyptus globulus*)

Eucalyptus oil is volatile oil obtained by hydro distillation from the scythe-shaped fresh leaves of

Eucalyptus globulus and from other species of Eucalyptus (Myrtaceae).

This tree is indigenous to eastern Australia, Tasmania and is cultivated in Southern Europe and in Asian countries.

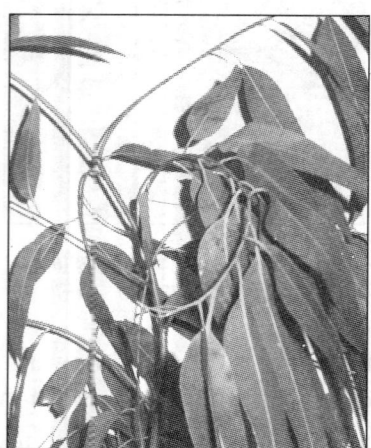

EUCALYPTUS LEAF BRANCH *(E. globulus)*
(for colour, see Plate 7, Fig. 4)

The oil is a colourless or pale yellow liquid that has a characteristic aromatic, somewhat camphoraceous odour and a pungent, spicy and cooling taste.

Chemical Constituents

Eucalyptus oils contain about 70-85% cineole, plus lesser amount of volatile aldehyde, terpenes, sesquiterpenes, aromatic aldehyde, alcohols (geraniol) and phenols.

Cosmetic Uses

The essential oil is used externally to facilitate the transcutaneous absorption of other substances present in the **cosmetic preparation**.

Two eucalyptus ointments are available:
- Compound Resin Ointment B.P.C. and
- Eucalyptus Ointment.

Compound Resin Ointment BPC

	By weight
• Resin	20
• Eucalyptus Oil	15
• Hard paraffin	10
• Soft paraffin	55

Eucalyptus Ointment (Benn's Botanic Doctor's Advisor):

• Elder oil	12.0 ounces;
• White wax	2.0 ounces;
• Spermaceti	1.5 ounces.
• Eucalyptus oil	2.0 drachms;
• Winter green oil	20 drops.

Eucalyptus ointments have antiseptic and healing properties. It produces very satisfactory results in scruf, chapped hands, chafes dandruff, tenderfeet, spot on the chest, arms, back & legs and pain in the joints.

As local application for ulcers and sores, one ounce of oil is added to one pint of lukewarm water and used for washing.

Commercial Preparation

Leaf oil and eucalyptol. It is official in IP, USP and NF.

GINKGO
(*Ginkgo biloba*)

Synonyms : Maidenhair tree.

Ginkgo are dried leaves obtained from the deciduous tree *Ginkgo biloba* (Maidenhair tree) (Ginkgoaceae), native to China and Japan but cultivated ornamentally in many temperate regions.

Chemical Constituents

Ginkgo leaves contain terpenes, trilactones (ginkgolides) flavonol glycosides and biflavonoids (kaempferol).

Cosmetics Uses

Leaf extract has property to increase vasodilation and peripheral blood flow rate in capillary vessels and also has free radical scavengering properties hence the leaf extract is used in cosmetic formulations (shampoos, creams and lotions).

Commercial Preparation

Crude herb, extracts, dried leaves, tinctures and purified ginkgolide.

HAWTHORN
(*Crataegus laevigata* DC)

Synonyms : Northern Chinese hawthorn (*C. pinnatifolia*) or Southern Chinese hawthorn (*C. Cuneata*).

Hawthorn is dried leaves, flowers and false fruits of *Crataegus monogyna* and *Crataegus laevigata* (Rosaceae) and is official in EP, BP and BHP.

Crataegus monogyna is thorny shrub or small deciduous tree with branched twigs bearing red fruits, native to Europe and has a long medicinal and ethanobotanical history.

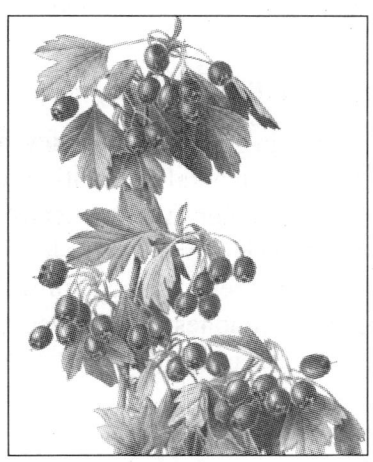

HAWTHORN *(Crataegus laevigata)*
(for colour, see Plate 7, Fig. 5)

Crataegus laevigata is a spiny shrub, leaves mostly smooth obovate, three to five lobed serrulate, flowers white to pink with red anthers, fruit globose and deep red in color.

Plant found in woods from North-West to Central Europe from England to Lativa.

Crataegus pinnatifolia var. major and *Crataegus cuneata* are source plant for the Chinese drug shanzha (dried hawthorn fruit).

Chemical Constitutents

The fruit contains 1-3% oligomeric procynidins, which appears to be partially ascertained together with flavonoids principally heparoside. The leaves contain less heparoside and more vitexin rhamnoside, about 1% pentacyclic triterpenes (0.5-1.4% in fruits), olanolic acid, ursolic acid, acantolic acid, xanthine derivatives, vitamins B_1, B_2 and C, calcium, iron and traces of essential oils.

Cosmetics Uses

Hawthorn extract or decoction is antibacterial against *Shigella flexneri*, *Shigella sonneni*, *Proteus vulgaris* and *Escherichia coli*.

It is also reported that water extract of *Crataegus pinnatifolia* has free radical scavenging activity.

Its extract or decoctions are used in skin formulations for sores, ulcers and antiageing preparations.

Commercial Preparation

Crude and extracts (solid and liquid) and purified form of flavonoids.

HIGH MALLOW
(*Malva sylvestris* (Khubzi) Linn.)

High Mallow is the dried leaf and flowers of *Malva sylvestris* Linn. (Malvaceae), grows wildly in Europe, mainly in the damp area of the atlantic seaboard.

It is a tall perennial herb with lobate and dentate leaves. The flowers are pentamerous and include calyculus with 6-9 divisions fused at the base and shorter than the calyx; the corolla has five pinkish-white petals emarginate at the top. The stamens are numerous and fused by their filaments.

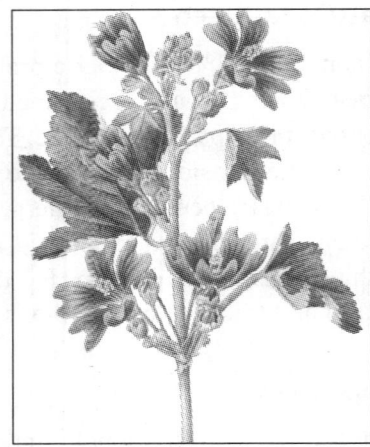

HIGH MALLOW (Malva sylvestris)
(for colour, see Plate 7, Fig. 6)

Chemical Constituents

The leaf and flower contains flavonoids (anthocyanins), phenolic acids, scopoletin and polysaccharides.

Cosmetic Uses

Leaf and flower extracts are used in cosmetic preparations as **adjunctive emollient and for itch relieving treatment** of dermatological conditions, protective trophic in the treatment of cracks, chaps and insect bites. It also has traditional use as local applicant for eye irritation or discomfort due to smoky atmosphere and sea water.

HENNA (MEHNDI) (*Lawsonia inermis*)

Henna consists of dried leaves of *Lawsonia inermis* (Lythraceae). A globous much branched shrub with grayish brown bark, grows wild and is also cultivated as garden plant throughout India, North Africa to Middle East.

Leaves are opposite subsessile, elliptic or broadly lanceolate with acute apex. 2-3 cm long and 1-2 cm wide. Flowers are numerous, small with rose coloured fragrance.

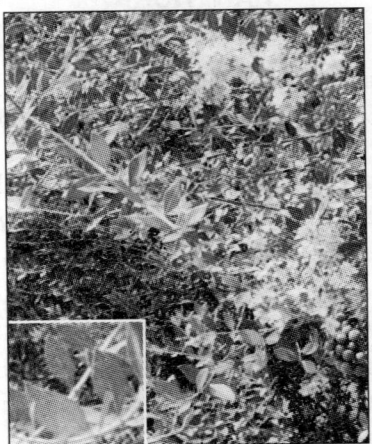

HENNA (Lawsonia inermis)
(for colour, see Plate 7, Fig. 7)

Chemical Constituents

The leaves contain soluble matter **lawsone**. This quinone dissolves in alkaline solution to give an intense orange red color. It is practically nontoxic and fungicide. The lawsone level in the dried drug is about 1%. Henna leaf also contains flavonoids, coumarins and xanthones. The flower owes their fragrance to an essential oil due to ionone.

Cosmetic Uses

It is used in cosmetic preparation in many ways as a colouring and cosmetic ingredient. It has been in use for nearly three millennia as a **hair colour**, nail colour, and in the muslim world for the (traditional) decoration of the soles of the feet and palm of hands. The drug is widely used in **cosmetology** for its dyeing properties due to the strong binding of lawsone to hair, probably due to the reaction of thiol group with keratin. It is also used in the form of **shampoo and hair lotion**.

Henna is used in Ayurvedic preparation for the treatment of skin ailments, burns and wounds.

Commercial Preparation

Mainly the crude powder form.

HIMALAYAN CEDAR
(*Cedrus deodara*)

Himalayan Cedar is a large perennial handsome tree of *Cedrus deodara* (Roxb) (Pinaceae), found at the height of 150-180 feet in Himalayan forest.

The leaves are triangular, acicular 11-12" long single spiral on long branches and in clusters on short branches.

Chemical Constituents

Plant contains volatile oil, sesquiterpene and toxifolin. Wood contains more amount of aromatic oil than the bark. It also contain black coloured tar and brown-yellow coloured oil.

Cosmetic Uses

Oil is used in skin diseases (chronic eczema and itches) and is used aromatically for relief of nervous stress.

Red Cedar oil is obtained from *Cedrala toona* (Mediaceae), used in skin ulcers, burning sensation and leucoderma.

HYSSOP
(*Hyssopus officinalis* Linn.)

Hyssop oil is obtained by steam distillation, of leaves and flowering tops of *Hyssopus officinalis* Linn. (Labiatae/Lamiaceae).

A perennial aromatic subshrub with slender herbaceous stem arising from woody base upto about 0.5 m high; native to Southern Europe and temperate Asia.

Major producing countries include France, Hungary and Holland.

Chemical Constitutents

The essential oil contains mainly pinocamphone, α- and β pinene, camphene and α-terpinene. Other constitutents include cineole, linalool, terpineol bornyl acetate, cis-pinic acid, cis-pinonic acid and myrtenic acid etc.

The leaves also contain volatile oil (0.3-2.0%), tannins (5-8%), flavonoid glycosides, ursolic acid and oleanolic acid.

Cosmetic Uses

Hyssop oil is used as a **fragrance** component in soaps, creams, lotions and **perfumes**, with a maximum use level of 0.4% in perfumes.

Hyssop extracts have been reported to exhibit antiviral activities against *Herpes simplex*. It also

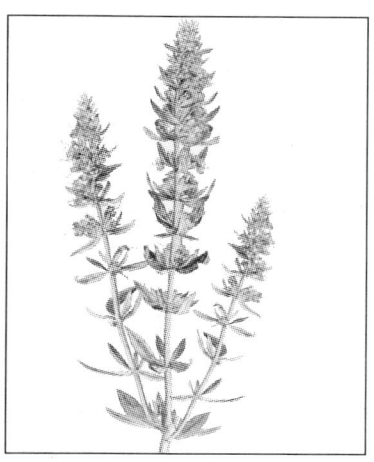

HYSSOP (*H. officinalis*)
(*for colour, see Plate 7, Fig. 8*)

has **antioxidant activity**; which are due to the presence of rosmarinic acid in oil.

Commercial Preparation

Mainly crude and oil.

LAVENDER OIL
(*Lavandula angustifolia* Miller)

Lavender oil is volatile oil obtained by steam distillation from the fresh flowering tops of the dwarf shrub, *Lavandula angustifolia* Miller (*L. officinalis* chaix), (Labiatae); cultivated in France, Bulgaria, Australia and North Africa.

When grown in a fairly high altitude yields best oil (**petite lavande**). The lower altitude '**Lavande moyenna**' yields somewhat less essential oils. '**Grande lavande**' (*Lavandula latifolia* villers) yields a much coarser oil (oil of spike). '**Grosse lavande**' or lavadin is the oil of intermediate characters (hybrids of two species).

The plant is evergreen flower from July to September, the fresh flowering spikes yield about 0.5% of volatile oil; the amount varies with varieties of season and method of distillation.

Chemical Constituents

The genuine continental lavender oil contains over 30% of esters (linalyl acetate). The oil of spike, which is used in cheap perfumery contain less esters but high proportions of free alcohols (about 20-40% calculated as borneol). Linalool, geraniol, cineole and camphor is also present.

Cosmetic Uses

Lavender oil is principally used in perfumery industry in toiletry preparation and occassionally in ointment and lotion formulation to mask the disagreeable odours. Topically the oil is used in creams for rheumatic pain and to treat minor

wounds, sun burns and superficial burns. It is also extensively used in aromatherapy.

Commercial Preparation

Oil, official in N.F.

LEMON OIL
[*Citrus limon* (L.)]

Synonyms : Cedro oil (terpeneless).

Lemon oil is obtained from the lemon peel by cold expression, while lemon petitgrain oil is produced from leaves and twigs.

Cosmetic Uses

Lemon oil is used as a fragrance ingredient in soaps, detergents, creams, lotions and perfumes (e.g. colognes).

Lemon petitgrain oil is used in creams, lotions and perfumes. Lemon peel aqeous extract is used in skin and hair care formulation.

LITHOSPERMUMS
(*Lithospermum officinale*)

Lithospermums consist of dried wood, leaves and seeds of *Lithospermum* officinale (Boraginaceae) native to Japan.

Chemical Constituents

It contain shikonin, a naphthaquinone derivative: scyllitol, a cyclitol; a cyanoglucoside - lithowspermicide, caffeic, chlorogenic and ellagic acid and catechin type of tannins. Shikonin is also produced for the cosmetic and pharmaceutical industry in Japan by cell culture of the plant.

Cosmetic Uses

It is used in the treatment of burns, inflammation, wounds and ulcers.

MARIGOLD
(*Calendule officinalis*)

Marigold (*Calendule officinalis* Linn. Family Asteraceae) is a small perennial herbaceous plant, with hardy and angular stems having sessile leaves. The inflorescences are big capitulums the tubulous disc-flowers and ray-flowers with tridentate ligula, all are orange yellow in colour.

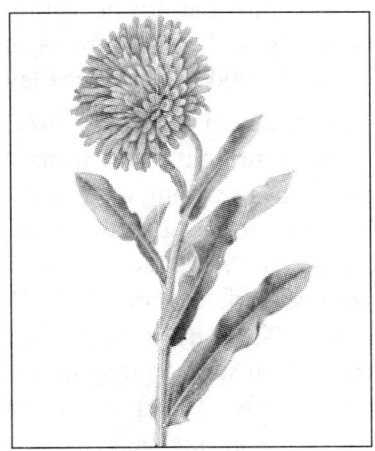

MARIGOLD (*Calendule officinalis*)
(*for colour, see Plate 7, Fig. 9*)

Chemical Constituents

The drug (flower or capitulum) contains flavonoids, (quercetin) carotenes, xanthophyll, and essential oil (containing sesquiterpenoid derivatives; mono, di and trihydroxylated derivatives free or ester form triterpenoids).

Cosmetics Uses

The **ethanolic extract** possesses *in vitro* antibacterial properties. The drug is useful for topical application to treat skin disorders (as an **emollient** and **itch-relieving** agent); as a protective agent for cracks, abrassions, chaps, for sunburns, superficial and limited burns, and diaper rashes. The drug is widely used in cosmetology

as an emollient and hydrating agent in lotion, creams, soaps and after sun lotions.

MATRICARIA FLOWERS
(*Chamomilla recutita*)

Matricaria flowers are the dried capitulums of *Chamomilla recutita* Linn. (*Matricaria chamomilla*) (Asteraceae), listed in French Pharmacopoeia.

A common plant of the neglected fields of Europe particularly abundant in Hungary and in Croatia.

It is an annual herbaceous plant with much ramified stems bearing bipinnatisect leaves. The capitulums (10–17 mm) comprises 12–20 mariginal ligulate florets and numerous central tubular florets. Unlike chamomile flowers, matricaria possesses a hollow receptacle, which is devoid of paleae (membranous inner bract). The capitulum is surrounded by an involucure composed of one to three rows of lanceolate bracts with a scarious brownish grey edge. The drug has a pleasant aromatic odour.

Chemical Constituents

The flower heads contain 0.3–1.5% of blue essential oil, consisting mainly of sesquiterpenes (α-bisabolol, chamazulene and farnesene). The chamazulene is formed from a sesquiterpene lactone (matricin) during steam distillation.

It also contains flavones and coumarins (herniarin), apigenin glucosides, and phenolic acids.

The essential oil of matricaria is an antibacterial and antifungal agent.

Cosmetic Uses

It is used in **Shampoos** (to lighten the hair color) and in suntan lotions. The oil is ingredient of **perfumes and soaps**. The presence of lactones in matricaria based preparation may cause allergic reactions (contact dermatitis) in sensitive persons.

Orally used to treat the symptoms of digestive ailments (epigastric bloating, impaired digestion, eructations, and flatulence), hence it is often used in spices.

NAGKESARA (MESUA FERREA)
(Mesua roxburghii, M. coromandalina)

Nagkesara (Mesua ferrea) (*M. roxburghii, M. coromandalina*) (Guttiferae) is common on the Eastern Himalayas, East Bengal, Assam, Eastern & Western Ghats and up to about 5000 feet in Burma and the Andamans. It is also cultivated in garden.

Chemical Constituents

Young fruits contain oleoresin from which an essential oil is obtained. Seeds contain fixed oils. Hard pericarp contain tannins.

Cosmetic Uses

Fixed oils expressed from the seed is used as an application for cutaneous infections such as sores, scabies, wound etc. **Powdered flowers mixed with clarified butter** (washed hundred times with water) are **used in the form of cream** for the healing touch to the burning of feet.

NEEM
(Azadirachta indica)

Neem [*Azadirachta indica* (Melliaceae)] is a tree indigenous to all plains in Indian subcontinent. It is commonly cultivated for providing shade. It also grows wildly in the sub-Himalayan track at altitude of 700-10,000 m above sea level.

The tree is medium or large in size, 40 to 50 feet tall, with a straight stout trunk and large spreading branches carrying a circular evergreen crown of un-usual leaves glabrous, impairpinnate with serrate margin. Moderately thick, dark brown rough furrowed bark covers the trunk and the older branches. The tiny, five-petalled, whitish flower appear in clusters on long dropping stems from March to May. The fruits are small, oval berries green when unripe, yellow on ripening.

Chemical Constituents

Neem leaves contain flavonoids (kaempferol, quercetin, myricetin, quercetin-3-galactoside

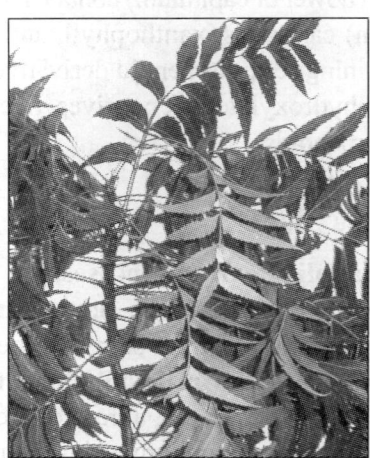

NAGKESARA *(Mesua ferrea)*
(for colour, see Plate 8, Fig. 1)

NEEM LEAVES *(Azadirachta indica)*
(for colour, see Plate 8, Fig. 2)

kaempferol-3-glucoside, myricetin-3-L-arabino-side), oxalic acid, steroids, terpenoids, sterols and Nimbolide.

The seeds and seed oil contains many bitter limonoids (nortriterpenoids) including nimbin, nimbibin, salanin etc. to which most of the pharmacological activities is attributed.

Cosmetic Uses

The leaves and seed oil is widely used in cosmetology in common skin diseases — eczema, ring worm infection, scabies and psoriasis.

Neem oil is used in the manufacture of **shampoos** that control ticks, fleas and lice. In Germany, it is used in **herbal hair oil, hair tonic and nail oil**. In India, neem is becoming popular beauty aid. Few companies are using neem oil and leaves for production of cosmetics like **facial creams**, nail polish, nail oils, **shampoos and conditioners**. All parts of the neem plant has antiseptic, antimicrobial properties and are used in the treatment of various skin infections, septic sores, infected burns and inflammatory diseases. The decoction of the bark and leaves are also used for the above mentioned ailments. The oil in the form of cream and lotion is used for all type of skin infections and inflammation.

OLIVE OIL
(*Olea europoea* Linn.)

Olive oil (salad oil, sweet oil) is a fixed oil, which is obtained by cold expression from the ripe fruits of *Olea europoea* Linn. (Oleaceae).

The olive tree is evergreen tree with a cracked bark, indeciduous leaves and small white tetramerous flowers grouped in recemes. The leaves are opposite, subsessile, entire and coriaceous, have a grayish green upper side and a whitish underside with a fine down (can be easily scraped off.). The tree lives for long ages but never exceed 12 m in height.

Olives (fruits) are ellipsoid drupes (1.3 × 1.5 cm) with thin and smooth epicarp, hard pit and mesocarp rich in oil, green coloured that gradually turns from green to blackish purple during ripening. The var. *Latifolia* bears larger fruits than the var. *Longifolia* but the later is said to produce best quality of oil. The olive is produced in all the mediterranean countries and in California, Italy, Spain, France, Greece, Tunisia and Libya.

Tunisia produce 90% of the world production.

Olive oil is a pale yellow liquid, which some times have greenish tint, with slight odour and bland taste. Olive oils from different source differ somewhat in the composition.

Chemical Constituents

The BP limits of the olive oil are : Oleic acid (56-85%), Linoleic acid (3.5-20.0%), Palmitic (7.5-20%) and Stearic acid (0.5-5%). There is also limit of sterols. It also contains volatile (C_6) alcohol (hexanol, E-2-hexanol, 2-3 hexenol) (C_6), aldehyde and acetylated esters.

Cosmetic Uses

Olive oil is employed in **cosmetology** and pharmaceutical Industry for its **demulcent and emollient properties**. It is also used in the preparation of **soap** and **face creams**.

PRIMROSE
[*Primula veris* Linn. = *P. officinalis* Linn. (Hill)]

Primrose consist of dried flower of *Primula veris* L. (*P. officinalis* (Linn.) Hill) family Primulaceae.

Primrose plant is indigenous to western Europe. It is characterised by almost oval leaves which abruptly narrow into wide petiole, by a floral stalk covered with fluffy hair (down), and by bright yellow flowers with lengthy tubular swollen calyx; obtuse-teeth and small concave corolla with five orange spot at top of the tube.

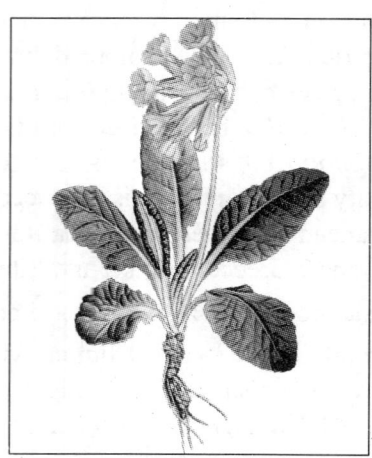

PRIMROSE (Primula veris. L.)
(for colour, see Plate 8, Fig. 3)

Chemical Constituents

The flower contains flavonoids (gossypetin) and about 2% of saponin in calyx. The subterranean part contains 5–10% saponins, represented by primulic acid and oleanolic acid.

Cosmetic Uses

Essential oil of the flowers and the alcoholic extract of primrose root is used locally in mouth washes, and as an adjunct in emollient and itch relieving treatment of skin disease and as a topical protective agent for cracks abrasions, frostbites, chaps and insect bites.

Evening Primrose Oil

The fixed oil from the seeds of Oenothera spp. (Onagraceae) contains substantial amount of esterified γ-linolenic acid (GLA), C_{18} 6,9,12-triene.

The principle species cultivated in the UK are Oenothera biennis, which yield oil containing 7-9% GLA; Oenothera paradoxa (14.41%), Oenothera acerviphilla nova (15.68%).

The oil is widely marketed as a dietary supplement. For cosmetic purpose, it is specifically used in the treatment of atopic eczema.

QUINCE SEEDS
(Cydonia oblonga)

Quince seed is a ripe seed of Cydonia vulgaris Persoon (Rosaceae), a tree cultivated in South Africa, Central Europe and the Middle East. Iran supplies about 75% of the World production.

The seeds are obtained from the apple or pear shaped fruits. They resemble apple pips (hard body seeds) and are frequently adhered together in masses.

The seeds possess a mucilaginous epithelium, which is equivalent to approximately 20% of their weight.

Chemical Constituents

The mucilage is composed of units of arabinose, xylose and uronic acid derivative, 15% of fixed oil and a small quantity of cyanogenetic glycosides and an enzyme which effects the hydrolysis.

Cosmetic Uses

The hydrocolloid forms viscous solutions with

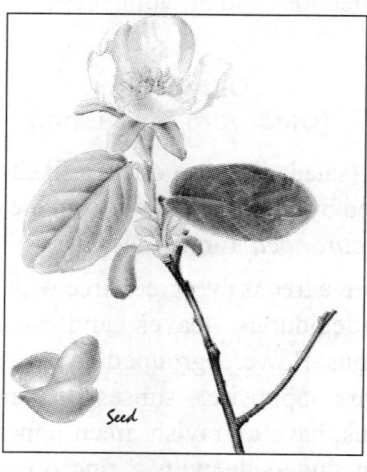

QUINCE SEEDS (Cydonia oblonga)
(for colour, see Plate 8, Fig. 4)

thixotropic properties, and is used as a **demulcent**, as a good **emulsifying agent** and in the preparation of hair-fixing lotions.

ROSEMARY OIL
(*Rosmarinus officinalis*)

Rosemary oil is volatile oil distilled from the flowering tops of leafy twigs of *Rosmarinus officinalis* (Labiatae). The plant is native to Southern Europe and the oil is produced principally in Spain and North Africa.

The plant is a bushy evergreen shrub with rigid opposite sessile, linear and coriaceous leaves about 3.5 cm long and 2--4 mm broad with grey and woolly lower surface; typical labiate glandular hairs contain volatile oil. The two lipped or light lilac flowers with purple spot and grouped in racemes inflorescences common in all the mediterranean basin.

Chemical Constituents

Rosemary oil mainly contains monoterpene hydrocarbons, e.g. α-pinene and camphene, 0.8-6% esters, mainly bornyl acetate, 8-20% alcohols, mainly borneol and cineole and phenolic compounds represented by flavonoids (glycosides of luteolin and methoxylated flavones) and phenolic acids (rose-marinic acid).

Cosmetic Uses

The oil is mainly used in **perfumery industry**, and is frequently used in **aromatherapy**. Rosemary extract is employed in **cosmetology,** because of its **antioxidant activity** it is used to facilitate the tissue damage and restoring the healthy status of the skin.

ROSE OIL
(Otto or Attar of Rose, *Oleum rosae*)

Rose oil is the volatile oil obtained by distillation in copper alembic stills, from the fresh flowers of *Rosa damascena, R. gallica, R. alba* and *R. centifolia* (Rosaceae).

The main producing countries are Bulgaria, Turkey and Morocco and in smaller quantity from India.

Chemical Constituents

The oil is a pale yellow semisolid. The solid (at

ROSEMARY *(Rosmarinus officinalis)*
(for colour, see Plate 8, Fig. 5)

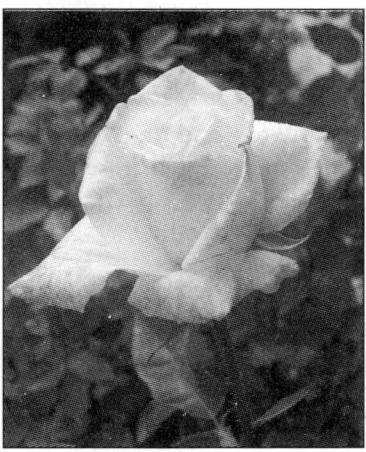

ROSE *(Rosa damascena)*
(for colour, see Plate 8, Fig. 6)

ordinary temperature) portion of the oil (about 15-20%) is odourless mainly consisting of saturated aliphatic hydrocarbon (C_{14} to C_{23} paraffins). The liquid portion forms the clear solution, mainly consisting of alcohols (geraniol, citronellol, nerol and 2-phenylethanol) with smaller quantities of esters. The odour of the oil is modified by the other constituents, such as sulphur containing compounds.

Cosmetic Uses

The oil is chiefly used in **perfumery industry** and aromatherapy. It is also used to prepare **rose water**, which is used in **dermatology**, collutoriums, gargles and in eye drops. The rose oil also has antimicrobial properties, used locally as an adjunctive **emollient** and **itch-relieving** treatment in skin disorders (formulation).

Note: The oil is very expensive and is liable to adultration.

SANDALWOOD OIL
(*Santalum album*)

Sandalwood oil is pale yellow viscous liquid obtained by steam distillation from the heartwood of *Santalum album* (Santalaceae) an evergreen tree 8–12 meter in height, which is widely distributed in India and Malaya's archipelagoes.

More than 90% of the sandalwood oil of commerce is produced by steam distillation of the pulverized heartwood and roots. The volatile oil is contained in all the elements of wood; medullary ray cells, vessels, wood fibres and wood parenchyma.

Chemical Constituents

The oil contains about 90–97% of sesquiterpene alcohol (Santalol). The hydrocarbon fraction contains about nine components. The other ingredients viz. acids, aldehydes, ketones etc. form comparatively minor part.

Cosmetic Uses

Sandalwood oil has a strong antiseptic and soothing action on dry inflamed skin. It is widely used in **cosmetology and perfumery**, in the production of essence and as a food flavour. It is also used in the manufacture of **soap, face cream, toilet powder, attars** etc. Its pale colour enables a good blending with a wide variety of other perfumery raw materials.

SESAME OIL
(TEEL OIL OR GINGELLY OIL)
(*Sesamum indicum*)

Sesame oil is refined, fixed oil obtained by expression or extraction from ripe seeds of *Sesamum indicum* L (Pedaliaceae). The oil is official in the EP and BP.

It is an annual herb of modest size (0.6–1 m). It has flowers with a white or pinkish bilabiate corolla. **Capsular fruit** with four locules containing numerous seeds which escape spontaneously at maturity. Cultivated widely in China, India and Africa.

The seeds are small flattened, oval or ovate, smooth and shiny, and whitish, yellow or reddish brown colour.

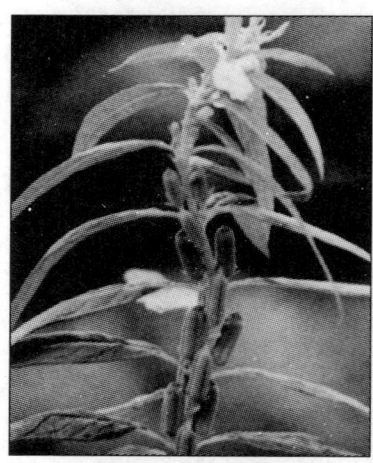

SESAME (*Sesamum indicum* Linn.)
(*for colour, see Plate 8, Fig. 7*)

The oil is a pale-yellow, oily liquid, almost odourless and bland tasting; which on cooling to about 4°C solidifies to a buttery mass; with saponification value same as that of olive oil and with somewhat higher iodine value (104 ± 20).

Chemical Constituents

Sesame seeds contain fixed oil (lipids) (40-50%), carbohydrates (20%) and proteins (20-35%). The unsaponifiable matter contains diaryl-furanofuranic lignans, sesamin and sesamolin which on hydrolysis produce sesamolin and lignan. The unsaponifiable matter also contains sterols campesterol (18-19%), stigmasterol (6-7%), β-sitosterol (59-62%) and tocopherols, γ-tocopherol and δ-tocopherol about 8.3% and 11.0% respectively.

Fatty acid composition of the fixed oil contains : Palmitic (9%), oleic acid (45%), linoleic acid (50%), linolenic, stearic acid (4-5%), arachidic, behenic and gadoleic in the range of 0.5 to 1%.

The stability of the oil is due to the phenolic constituent sesamol, which is produced from the hydrolysis of sesamolin.

Cosmetic Uses

Seed extract enriched in unsaponifiable matter (lignans) used in **cosmetic industry as antioxidant**, radical scavenger and **"regenerating agent"** in the skin preparation and in hair tonic formulation.

Sesame oil is also used as food products being nutritive, laxative, demulcent and having emollient properties.

SENNA (SANA)
(*Cassia acutifolia*)

Senna or Senna leaves consist of dried leaflet of *Cassia acutifolia* Delile known in commerce as **Alexandria Senna** or *Cassia angustifolia* Vahl known as Bombay or **Tinnevelly senna** (Leguminosecae/Fabaceae). Most of the commercial supply of the drug is collected from plants cultivated in southern India (Tinnevelly); some material is also produced in the Jammu Distt. of India and in northwest Pakistan. Medicinal important plant is highly drought resistant and may be suitable for deserts, as the plant requires dry, warm climate & bright sunshine.

The young leaves and 3–5 days old pods contain high percentage of sennosides. The leaves are picked once in 15 or 20 days. Eight to ten pickings can be obtained under very favourable conditions.

The harvested leaflets are dried under shade in thin layers. The leaves dry in 7-10 days, which is indicated by thin yellowish green color. The method of drying affects the percentage of sennosides in leaflets. The commercial drug consists of dried, green leaves and shells of nearly dried and ripe pods.

Chemical Constituents

The leaves, pods and roots contain– rhein, chrysophanol, emodin, several mono and di-glucosides of anthrone are present in the seedlings, leaves and roots. Leaves also contain 8-mono-β-D-glucosides of rhein and aloe emodine and water soluble glycosides. Isorhamnetin, kaempferol, palmidin, tinnevellin glucoside, myricyl alcohol and micilage is also present in leaves.

Cosmetic Uses

The powdered leaves in vinegar are applied to wounds & burns and to remove pimples. The leaves along with those of henna are used to dye the hair black.

TAGETES OIL

Synonyms : African marigold, Aztec marigold and big. marigold (*T. erecta*), French marigold (*T. patula*); Mexican marigold (*T. minuta*); and marigold.

Tagetes oil is obtained by steam distillation of the above ground parts of all three species (especially *T. minuta*).

It is an strong scented annual herb usually 0.3–1 m high. *T. erecta* bears the largest flower heads among the three species; generally considered to be native to mexico (*T. erecta* and *T. patula*) and South America (*T. minuta*). Cultivated or found growing wild worldwide, including Ethopia, Kenya, Nigeria, India and China.

Chemical Constituents

Tagetes oil from *T. minuta* contains tagetones ocimene, β-myrcene, linalool, limonene α- and β-pinene, carvone, cineole, linalyl acetate and α-terpineol.

The petals of Aztec marigold (*T. erecta*) is reported to contain mainly carotenoid.

Cosmetic Uses

It is used as a fragrance component in **perfumes**. In India, the juice of the leaves of *T. erecta* is used in the treatment of eczema.

THYME OIL
(*Thymus vulgaris*)

Thyme oil is volatile oil obtained from dried or partially dried leaves and flowering tops of *Thymus vulgaris* and *T. zygis* (Lamiaceae) by water and steam distillation.

Thyme (*Thymus vulgaris* L) is a much branched subshrub, square erect evergreen with numerous white hairy stems, bearing small white or pink two lipped flowers arranged in whorls and woody fibrous root up to about 45 cm high; native to mediterranean region (Greece, Italy, Spain, etc.) extensively cultivated in France, Spain Portugal, Greece and the United States (California).

Chemical Constituents

Thyme oil, (BP) contains thymol (32-55%),

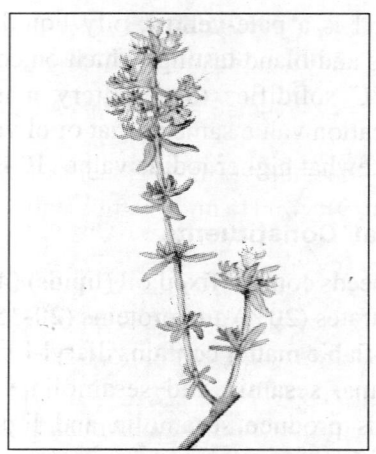

THYMUS VULGARIS (Flowering branch)
(for colour, see Plate 8, Fig. 8)

carvacrol (1-4%), p-cymene (15-28%), γ-terpinene (5-10%), lanalool, β-myrcene and terpinen-4-ol.

Spain supplies about 90% of the world population of thyme oil.

The essential oil content of the drug is rich in phenols and has antibacterial and antifungal properties.

Cosmetic Uses

Both the essential oil and thymol are the ingredients of various proprietary drugs, antiseptic and skin healing ointments and number of herbal remedies for skin disorder.

Thyme oil is also used in **soaps, detergents, creams, lotions and perfumes** with maximum use level of 0.8% v/w.

WALNUT
(*Juglans regia*)

Walnut tree (*Juglans regia* Linn. family Juglandaceae) is originally from the Near-East, cultivated in France to produce walnut. The leaves are imparipinnate, have five or nine entire folioles, ovate lanceolate, acuminate and slightly coriaceous.

The fruit walnut is a drupe with green exocarp, which blacken by oxidation on maturity, the hard, bivalve endocarp surround two "cerebriform and voluminous" cotyledons.

Chemical Constituents

The chief constituent is Juglone (5-hydroxy, 1,4 naphthaquinone), which occurs in the fresh plant (leaf, stain) as 1,4,5-trihydroxy naphthaquinone glycoside (2% in the stain and 0.6% in the leaves) and also in the free state particularly in the epicuticular wax. The leaf and pericarp are rich in hydrolysable tannins.

The leaf also contain essential oil, ascorbic acid and flavonoids. Juglone has antibacterial and fungicidal properties.

Cosmetic Uses

The **leaf extracts** of the plant are used in **cosmetology**, in **dyeing preparations** and in the treatment of sunburns (superficial and limited burns) as well as to treat **scalp itching**, peeling and **dandruff**.

Also as an adjunctive emollient and itch relieving in the treatment of skin disorders.

WINTERGREEN OIL (GAULTHARIA OIL) (*Gaultheria procumbens* Linn.)

Synonyms : Betula oil or Sweet birch oil.

Wintergreen oil is obtained by distilling the dried leaves of *Gaultheria procumbens* Linne. (Ericaceae), but now distilled from the bark of *Betula lenta* (Betulaceae).

Gaultheria oil of the Indian Pharmacopoeia is obtained from the fresh plant of *Gaultheria fragrantissima* and contain not less than 98% of esters calculated as methyl salicylate (teaberry and checkerberry oil).

The plant is a low shrub like perennial with slender creeping or subterranean stems and branches (5 to 15 cm height). The leaves are alternate, evergreen and coriaceous, the upper surface is dark green, shining and the under surface is pale green. Flowers are white & axillary and the fruit is bright red globular, aromatic berry.

Odour is distinct & aromatic, and the taste is aromatic & astringent.

The plant is common in coniferous woods throughout the eastern United States, Canada and India.

Chemical Constituents

Methyl salicyclate, is the chief constituent of the oil formed from gaultherin (glycoside) on hydrolysis by the enzyme gaultherase, in the presence of water.

In addition to methyl salicylate, it also contain an ester that hydrolyse into ethyl alcohol and acid. The ethanolic alcohol have characteristic odour that distinguish wintergreen oil from the synthetic methyl salicylate.

Cosmetic Uses

It has been used as a **flavour** for many years. It is used as local irritant, antiseptic and as antirheumatic, in the concentration of 10–25% in **lotion** and solution.

WITCH HAZEL (*Hamamelis virginiana* Linn.)

Witch Hazel is the dried leaves of *Hamamelis virginiana* (Hamamelidaceae), common in the woods of Eastern American continent (Virginia).

The branches of the plants are ramified and bear leaves on short petioles which are asymetrical at the base, and have crenate margins. The tetramerous flowers blossom after the leaves fall.

This imparts the ornamental characters to this species. The drug is dull green or reddish and slightly astringent in taste.

Chemical Constituents

The leaves contain about 0.06% volatile oil (characterised by the presence of acetaldehyde, and ionones), flavonol glycosides (astragalin, myricitrin) and upto 10.5% tannins (gallic acid, polygalloylglucose, hamamelitannin and analogues) leaves also contain polyphenolic constituents, procyanidins and procyanidin-prodelphinidin co-polymers are the chief constituents. The bark of the plant mainly contains hamamelitannin, upto 65% in hydroalcoholic extract.

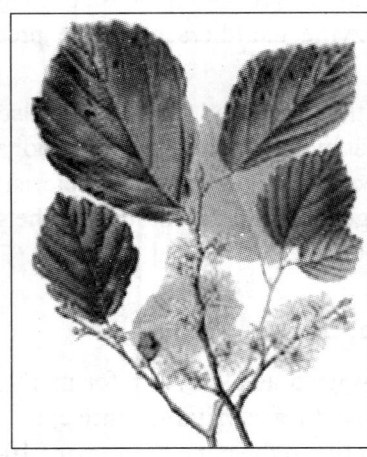

WITCH HAZEL (Hamamelis virginiana Linn)
(for colour, see Plate 8, Fig. 9)

Cosmetic Uses

The drug is used in **cosmetology** as Hamamelis water or distilled Witch Hazel extract in **astringent preparation**. Hamamelis leaf based phytomedicine are traditionally used locally to relieve eye irritation or discomfort due to strain, sea water, swimming pool water and smoky atmospheres.

COMMERCIAL HERBAL COSMETIC FORMULATIONS

Cosmetics

Wordly meaning of the cosmetic is any preparation relating to treatment intended to restore or improve a person's appearance or serving to improve the appearance of the body, especially the face.

Classification

Herbal cosmetics can be classified on the basis of:

(i) Dosage form

(ii) Part or organ of the body to be applied for

(i) Dosage forms

1. *Emulsions :* Cold cream, vanishing cream, liquid cream
2. *Powders :* Face powder, talcum powder, tooth powder
3. *Cakes :* Rouge compacts, make-up cake
4. *Oils :* Hair oils
5. *Mucilages :* Hand lotion
6. *Jellies :* Hand jelly, wave set jelly and brilliantine jelly
7. *Suspensions :* Cosmetic stockings
8. *Paste :* Tooth paste, deodorant paste
9. *Soaps :* Shampoo soap, shaving soap and toilet soap
10. *Solutions :* After shave lotions, hair set solutions and lotions

(ii) Part or organ of the body to be applied for

Herbal cosmetics for skin

• Powders
• Creams

- Lotions
- Deodorants
- Bath and cleansing products
- Make-up preparations
- Suntan preparation

Herbal cosmetics for hairs

- Shampoos - soap and soapless
- Tonics
- Hair dressing and brilliantines
- Hair waving preparations
- Beard softeners
- Shaving media
- Depilatories for removing unwanted hairs

Herbal cosmetics for nails

- Nail polishes and polish removers
- Manicure preparations

Herbal cosmetics for teeth and mouth

- Tooth paste
- Dentifrices
- Mouth washes

Borderline and kindered preparations

- Eye preparations
- Foot powders and applications
- Insect repellants
- Miscellaneous products

Emulsions or Cosmetics Creams

Cold cream : O/w emulsion produce cooling effect on application to the skin because of water evaportion.

Formula:

COLD CREAM

No. 1

	by weight
White beeswax	8.00
Liquid paraffin	10.00
Ceresin	4.00

Almond oil	40.00
Borax	1.50
Water	35.50
Perfume	0.45
	100.00 gm

No. 2

Beeswax	15.00
Almond oil	55.00
Rose water	28.50
Borax	1.50
	100.00 gm

No. 3

Spermaceti	5.50
White beeswax	15.00
Lanolin	3.50
Peanut oil	51.70
Distilled water	24.00
Borax	0.50
Perfume (Herbal base)	0.50
	100.00 gm

No. 4

White beeswax	10.00
Vegetable lard	15.00
Sesame oil	20.00
Almond oil	20.00
Borax	1.00
Rose water	35.00
	100.00 gm

No. 5

Beeswax	25.00
Neem oil	35.50
Water	38.00
Borax	1.50
	100.00 gm

No. 6

Beeswax	15.00
Sandalwood oil	35.00
Water	50.00
Borax	1.00
	100.00 gm

No. 7

Beeswax	18.00
Turmeric oil	42.00
Water	37.00
Borax	3.00
	100.00 gm

CHAMOMILE CREAM

Chamomile flowers	60.00 gm
Purified water	500.00 ml
Lemon juice	7.50 ml
Sodium benzoate	1.50 gm

LUBRICATING CREAM

Heavy white petrolatum	30.00
Honey	20.00
Cod liver oil	45.00
Borax	1.50
Water Q.S. to make	100.00

Face Pack or Mask

The face pack or mask stimulate the blood circulation, rejuvenate the muscles and help to maintain the elasticity of the skin and remove the dirt. from skin pores.

Formula:

FACE PACK (1)

Honey	15.00 gm
Apricot extract	15.00 ml
Olive Oil	3.00 ml
Lemon juice	3.00 ml

Mix all the components and apply the paste on the face.

FACE PACK (2)

Cucumber juice	26.00 ml
Peppermint extract	2.50 ml
Mint juice	2.50 ml

FACE PACK (3)

Brewer's yeast	120.00 gm
Witch hazel extract	7.50 ml
Peppermint extract	7.50 ml
Lemon juice	4.00 ml

This pack is for better blood circulation.

Lotions

Lotions are used for washing the skin, to remove the oily secretions, and thus help to open the skin pores consequently freshen the skin and increase the blood circulation.

Formula:

WITCH HAZEL SKIN TONING LOTIONS

Sunflower oil	45.00 ml
Wheat germ oil	7.50 ml
Witch hazel extract	25.00 ml
Sodium benzoate	5.00 gm.
Lanolin Q.S. to make	100.00 gm.

No. 1

	By weight
Boric acid	1.50
Menthol	0.05
Glycerin	2.50
Lemon juice	8.00
Witch hazel	88.00
Perfume	0.50
Oxyquinoline sulfate	0.50

Skin protective and hand cream

Herbal base formula for a skin protective, against the corrosive chemicals and the harmful UV rays. It is quite cheap and quite elegant cosmetically.

Formula:

Turmeric paste	3.50 gm

White bees wax	1.00 gm
White petrolatum	3.50 gm
Neem oil	2.50 gm
Triethanolamine (emulsifier)	4.00 gm
Magnesium stearate	2.00 gm
Boiling water sufficient to make.......	25.00 gms

Liquid Cream

The advantages of the liquid cream as against solid creams are that they may be applied easily and uniformly over large surface of the skin and they are more easily absorbed and they spread out in very thin layers.

Formula:

Amino glycol	1-5/4 gm
Glycerin	20.00 gm
Neem oil	45.00 gm
Sesame oil	20.00 gm
Cetyl alcohol	4.00 gm
Stearic acid	3-5/4 gm
Rose water	115.00 gm

ASTRINGENT CREAMS

Zinc oxide	10.00 gm
Bismuth subnitrate	2.50 gm
Balsam of Peru	5.00 gm
Mehndi	4.00 gm
Tulsi	4.00 gm
Perfume	1.50 ml
White Soft paraffrin Q.S. to make....	100.00 gm

MEDICATED HERBAL CREAMS

Olive oil	15.00 gm
Oil of cade	15.00 gm
Cetyl alcohol	10.00 ml
Cocoa butter	10.00 gm
Lanolin	15.00 gm
Ammonium sulfo-ichthyolate	5.00 gm
Oil of wintergreen	1.00 ml

Petrolatum Q.S. to make	100.00 gm

LEMON HAND LOTION

	by weight
Pectin	2.50 gm
Lemon juice	10.50 ml
Citric acid	2.50 gm
Benzoic acid	0.150 gm
Glycerin	6.00 gm
Alcohol	15.00 ml
Perfume	0.50 ml
Water Q.S. to make	100.00 gm

Skin freshner (astringent) Lotion

It is generally used to freshen the skin and to remove the residual traces of creams.

Formula:

No. 1

Boric acid	1.50 gm
Witch hazel	15.50 gm
Rose water	15.00 ml
Alcohol	10.00 ml
Orange flower water Q.S. to make....	100.00

No. 2

Sandal-wood oil	2.50 lt.
Glycerin	0.01 lt.
Perfume	0.02 lt.
Boric acid	3.00 gm
Sodium aluminium sulfate	100.00 ml
Distilled water distilled Q.S. to make...	1.00 lt.

BLEACHING LOTION

Henna paste 3%	9.50 gm
Turmeric	0.50 gm
Tincture of benzoin	1.00 ml
Perfume	0.30 ml
Rose water Q.S. to make..................	100.00 ml

SUNSCREEN LOTION

Quinine oleate	2.50 gm
Olive oil	450 gm
Oil of cassia	0.50 gm
Perfume oil	0.50 gm
Reafined peanut oil Q.S. to make..... 100.00 gm	

BURN OINTMENT

Tannic acid	4.50 gm
Oil of cade	6.00 gm
Cod liver oil	15.00 gm
Vegetable lard	40.00 gm
Phenol	0.20 gm
Water Q.S. to make ....100.00 gm	

LIME SHAMPOO

Amla	110.00 gms
Shikakai	180.00 gms
Char	110.00 gms
Charilla	100.00 gms
Khus	100.00 gms
Reetha	200.00 gms
Glycerine	165.00 ml
Lime juice	75.00 ml
Sodium benzoate	2.00 gm
Water Q.S. to make............................... 2.50 litres	

LAVENDER SHAMPOO

Amla	105.00 gm.
Shikakai	180.00 gm.
Henna	105.00 gm.
Khus	105.00 gm.
Char	100.00 gm.
Charilla	100.00 gm.
Reetha	200.00 gm.
Sodium Benzoate	2.50 gm.
Lavender oil	160.00 gm.
Water purified Q.S. to make ....2.50 litre	

NEEM SHAMPOO

Gram flour	1.00 kg.
Sandalwood powder	245.00 gm.
Neem leaves powder	165.00 gm.
Shikakai powder	1.00 kg.
Purified water Q.S. to make...................2.50 litres	

METHI-SHIKAKAI SHAMPOO

Methi	250.00 gm.
Shikakai	1.00 kg.
Orange peels	handful
Purified water Q.S. to make...................2.00 litres	

HERBAL MOUTH WASH

Boric acid	24.50 gm.
Thymol	1.00 gm.
Oil of Eucalyptus	1.50 ml
Menthol	1.50 gm.
Oil gaultheria	1.50 ml
Oil thyme white	0.30 ml
Benzoic acid	1.00 gm.
Ethyl alcohol	250.00 ml
Talc	5.00 gm.
Distilled water Q.S. to make............. 100.00 ml	

HERBAL HAIR RINSE

Lemon juice	15.00 ml
Tamarind	10.00 gm.
Alcohol	40.00 ml
Perfume	0.50 ml
Water Q.S. to make ....100.00 ml	

HERBAL HAIR TONIC FORMULATION

Castor oil, sulfonated	10.00 gm.
Oil of bergamot	1.10 ml
Oil of cinnamon	0.10 ml
Oil of clove	0.10 ml

Oil of lavender	0.75 ml
Tincture of capsicum	0.75 ml
Alcohol 90% Q.S. to make	100.00 ml

QUININE HAIR TONIC

Quinine sulfate	2.00 gm.
Tincture of krameria	2.50 ml
Tincture of cantharides	1.50 ml
Spirit of lavender	7.50 ml
Glycerin	9.00 gm.
Alcohol 90% Q.S. to make	100.00 ml

HAIR ZEST

Brandy	70.00 ml
Eucalyptus bark	1.50 gm.
Eucalyptus leaves	2.00 gm.
Cinchona bark	2.00 gm.
Burdock root	1.50 gm.
Acid free tincture of iron	0.50 ml
Distilled water Q.S. to make	100.00 ml

HERBAL TOOTH PASTE

Triphala/jaiphal	45.00 gm.
Collodial clay	2.50 gm.
Gum tragacanth mucilage (2%)	2.50 gm.
Glucose	4.00 gm.
Honey	17.50 gm.
Water	30.00 ml
Flavor	0.50 ml
Methyl parahydroxybenzoate	0.20 gm.
Milk of magnesia	24.00 gm.
Black pepper (Kalimirch)	30.00 gm.
White powder soap	2.00 gm.
Glycerine of tragacanth	10.00 gm.
Honey	10.00 gm.
Lavang oil	1.00 ml
Saccharine (soluble)	0.10 gm.
Methyl p-hydroxy benzoate	0.10 gm.
Flavour	0.80 ml
Distilled water Q.S. to make..............	100.00 gm.

HERBAL MOUTH WASH

	by volume
Eucalyptol	1.50
Menthol	1.50
Clove oil	0.50
Wintergreen oil	0.10
Heliotropine	0.01
Chlorophyll alcohol soluble	0.20
Alcohol	45.00
Purified Water Q.S. to make.............	100.00 ml

SUNTAN OIL

Peanut oil, refined	45.00 gm.
Sesame oil	5.00 gm.
Oil of thuja	1.00 ml
Perfume	1.00 ml
Coconut oil Q.S. to make..................	100.00 gm.

SUNBURN OINTMENT

	by weight
Oxyquinoline benzoate	0.15
Camphor-phenol	3.50
Linseed oil	21.50
Olive oil	20.00
Cholesterin absorption base Q.S.100.0 gm.	

BURN CREAM

	by weight
Glyceryl monostearate	15.00
Cetyl alcohol	5.00
Lanolin	2.50
Lecithin	1.50
Linseed oil	15.00
Glycerin	10.00
Para-chloro-meta-cresol	0.05
Distilled Water Q.S. to make	100.00 gm.

HERBAL SOAP

Acorus calamus	3.00 mg
Andropogan muricatus	2.50 mg

Balsamodendron mukul	2.50 mg		Curcuma longa linn	20.00 gm
Berberis aristata	2.50 mg		Azadirachta indica oil	2.00 ml
Cedrus deodara	2.50 mg		Santalum album linn	1.00 ml
Celastrus paniculatus	2.50 mg		Ocimum sanctum oil	2.00 ml
Coriandrum sativum	1.50 mg		Citrus sinensis rind	2.00 gm
Cuminum cyminum	1.50 mg		Rosemary oil	5.00 ml
Embelia ribes	2.00 mg		Aloe vera gel	2.00 ml
Glycyrrhiza glabra	2.00 mg		Crocus sativa	1.00 gm
Hemidesmus indicus	10.00 mg		Cream base Q.S. to make................... 100.00 gm	
Holarrehena antidysentrica	2.00 mg			
Melia Azadirachta	4.00 mg			
Nigella sativa	3.00 mg			
Plumbago rosea	225.00 mg			
Psoralea corylifolia	2.00 mg			
Smilax regelii	2.00 mg			
Zingiber officinalis	105.00 mg			

The above soap is based on coconut oil.

ULTRA FAIR CREAM

Curcuma oil	2.00 ml
Azaderachta indica aqueous extract	1.50 gm
Santalum album	0.50 gm
Orange peel powdered	2.00 gm
Rose petals	2.00 gm
Aloe vera gel	2.00 gm
Walnut powder	1.00 gm
Jasmine	0.50 gm
Non greasy cream base	100.00 gm

FAIRNESS CREAM

Rose water	25.00 mg
Orange oil	25.00 mg
Aloe vera gel	50.00 mg
Walnut leaves extract	20.00 mg
Cream base Q.S. to make .... 1.00 gm	

STOP HAIR LOSS

Hibiscus rosa sinensis	15.00 mg
Lawsonia alba	7.50 mg
Eclipta alba	7.50 mg
Emblica officianlis	25.00 mg
Aloe barbadensis	750.00 mg
Water miscible gel base Q.S. to make. 1.00 gm	

SCAR REMOVER SKIN CREAM

Each 100 gm contain

Wheat germ oil	3.50 ml

ANNEXURE-I
MANUFACTURERS OF HERBAL FORMULATIONS

1. Ansar Drugs Laboratories
   Salabatpura, Moti Begumwade
   SURAT - 359 002

2. Acis Laboratories
   118/177, Kaushalpuri
   KANPUR - 208 012

3. Aimil Pharmaceuticals (India) Pvt. Ltd.,
   2699, Main Patel Road,
   Patel Nagar (W) NEW DELHI - 110 008

4. Alrasin Marketing Pvt. Ltd.
   Plot No. 2, A-32, Road No. 3, MIDC,
   P. Box No. 9416, Opp ESIS Hospital
   Andheri (E)
   BOMBAY -- 400 093

5. Allen Laboratories Pvt. Ltd.
   224/H, Maniktala Main Road,
   CALCUTTA - 700 054

6. Bharati Rasyanagar
   26, Nakuleswar Bhattacharjee lane
   CALCUTTA - 700 026

7. Dabur India Ltd.,
   22, Site IV, Sahibabad,
   GHAZIABAD - 201 005

8. Dattatraya Krishan Sandu Bros
   (Chembur) Pvt. Ltd.
   Sanduwadi, D.K. Sandu marg
   Chembur,
   BOMBAY - 400 071

9. Herbals (APS) Private Ltd.,
   B.M. Das Road,
   PATNA - 800 004

10. Herbo - Med (P) Ltd.,
    68, Hemchandra naskar Road,
    CALCUTTA - 700 010

11. The Himalaya Drug Co.,
    Shivsagar `E'
    Dr. Annie Besant Road,
    BOMBAY - 400 018

12. Indian Herba Research & Supply Co.,
    Post Box No. 5, Sharda Nagar,
    SAHARANPUR - 400 018

13. J & J Dechane Laboratories Pvt. Ltd.,
    4-1-324, Residency Road,
    HYDERABAD - 500 001

14. Madona Pharmaceutical Research Pvt. Ltd.,
    208/7, Rishi Bankim Chandra Road,
    CALCULTTA - 700 028

15. Kruzer Herbals
    B-20/2, Okhla Phase II,
    NEW DELHI - 110 020

16. Shilpachem
    47-D, Industrial Estate,
    Fort, INDORE - 452 006

17. Hamdard (Wakf) Laboratories
    Hamdard Marg, DELHI - 110 006

18. Zandu Pharmaceutical Works Ltd.,
    Gokhale Road (South)
    Dadar, BOMBAY - 400 025

19. Shri Baidyanath Ayurved Bhavan (P) Ltd.,
    Baidyanath Baven Road,
    PATNA - 1

20. Ayurved Sewashram Ltd.
    Station Road,
    UDAIPUR

21. Charak Pharmaceuticals
    501/A, Poonam Chambers,
    Dr. Annie Besant Road,
    Worli, BOMBAY - 400 015

References

Ahmedullah, M., Nayar, M.P. (1986). Endemic Plants of the Indian Flora, Peninsular India, Volume 1, Botanical Survey of India, Calcutta.

Akerele, O. Heywood, V. Synge, H. (eds.) (1991). Conservation of Medicinal Plants. Cambridge University Press, Cambridge, U.K.

Alan, Hamilton. International trade in medicinal plants. Conservation issues and potential roles for botanic gardens.

Atal, C.K. Kapur, B.M. (1989) Cultivation and Utilization of Medicinal Plants. R.R.L., Jammu.

Balandrin, M. Klocke, J. Wurtele, E. Bollinger, W. (1985). Natural Plant Chemicals: Source of Industrial and Medicinal Material Science, 228.

Ballick, M.J. (1990). In: Bioactive compounds from plants. CIBA Foundation Symposium, John Wiley and Sons. Chichester.

Barz, W. Reinhard, E. Zerk, M.H. Plant Tissue Culture and its Biotechnological Application. Springer, Berlin.

Bendz, G. 80 Santesson, J. (eds) (1974). Chemistry in botanical classification. Academic Press, London.

Botanic Garden Conservation Secretariat (1989). The Botanic Garden Conservation and Strategy. BGCI, Richmond, U.K.

Bruneton, Jean (1999). Pharmacognosy (Ed. TEC&DOC) Lavoisier, Paris.

Cardellina, H. (2002). Challenges and opportunities confronting the Botanical Dietary Supplement Industry (Review) J. Nat. Prod. 65. 1073-1084.

Chadha, K.L. Gupta, R. Advances in Horticulture Vol. II Medicinal and Aromatic Plants. Malhotra Publishing House, New Delhi.

Chandrika, M. (2000). Indian plants can play major role in world herbal market. The Economic Times, 9 May 2000, India.

Chatterjee, S. (1995). Global hotspots of biodiversity. Current Science 68: 1178-118.

Chowdhury, A.R. (2003). Indigenous production of essential oils. CIMAP Lucknow (India) pp 71-76. "Proceeding of first National Interactive Meet on Medicinal and Aromatic Plants".

Christine, K. O'Neil, Charles, W. Fetrow (2002). Plants as Drugs. In: Encyclopedia of Pharmaceutical Technology. Marcel Dekker, London.

Datta, S.C. Sanganeria, (1984). Export Possibilities of medicinal and Aromatic Plants and their Derivatives. NSA BMATP (Bot.Lab.Pharm.Anat.), (Calcutta University) pp 462-485.

Endress, R. (1994). Plant cell Biotechnology. Springer-Verlag, New York.

Export Potential of selected Medicinal Plants; prepared by Basic Chemicals, Pharmaceuticals and Cosmetic Export Promotion Council, Mumbai and other Reports.

Farmsworth, N.R. Soajarto, D. (1985). Potential consequence of plant extinction in the United States on the current and future availability of prescription drugs. Economic Botany 39.

Faulkner, D.J. Fenical, W.H. (1989). Marine Natural Products Chemistry (NATO Conference Series 4) Plenum Press, N.Y.

Fransworth, N.R. Soejarto, D.D. (1991). Global importance of medicinal plants: In: Conservation of medicinal plants (Ed. Akerele O. Heywood V and Synge H) Cambridge University Press. Cambridge, New York. p. 25-52.

Gamborg, O.L. Wetter, L.R. Plant Tissue Culture Methods. National Research Council of Canada, Saskatchewan.

Gibbs, R. (1974) Chemotaxonomy of flowering plants, of volumes. Montreal: McGill U.P.

Government of India (1991) Report on Export of Technology for Medicinal Plant and their derivatives. N. Delhi.

Government of India 2000. Report of the Task Force on Conservation and sustainable use of Medicinal Plants, New Delhi.

Govindachari, T.R. (1992). In: Introduction to selected medicinal plants of India, Ed. SPARC and Technical Committee, P. XIX, CHEMEXCIL, Bombay.

Govt. of India 2000 Report on Medicinal plants: Information from http://indianmedicine.nic.in/html/plants/medmain.htm.

Govt. of India 2002, Government of India, Ministry of Commerce Notification No. 2 available at http://www.Indianspice.com/html/s0420sts.htm.

Greger, J.L. (2001). Dietary supplement use: Consumer characteristic and interests. Presented at the Conference "Bioavailability of Nutrients and other Bioactive Components from Dietary supplements" held January 5-6, 2000 in Bethesdia Maryland Published as a supplement to the Journal of Nutrition.

http://dgftcom.nic.in/exim/2000/not/not98/not/298.htm.

http://indianmedicine.nic.in/html/plants/medmain.htm.

http://ww.indianspices.com/htm/s0420sts.htm.

http://www./indianspices.com.

http://www.borneofocus.com/vaic/statistics/article6.htm.

http://www.cbsg.org/reports/exec_sum/indian_med.plants_north_camp.pdf

http://www.fao.org/docrep/w7261E/w.7261e00.htm.

http://www.fao.org/docrep/w7261eo8.htm.

http://www.fao.org/docrep/x5326eoe.htm.

http://www.infac.org.in/offer/tlbo/rep/So61.htm.

Hamitton, A.C. Bensted, R. (eds.) (1989). Forest Conservation in East Usambara Mountains, Tanzania, IUCN, Gland, Switzerland.

Handa, S.S. (1992). Medicinal plants based drug industry and emerging plant drugs. Currt Res. Med Arom 14: 233-262.

Handa, S.S. (1996). Medicinal plants and Priorities in Indian medicines Diverse studies and implications. Suppl. to Cultivation and utilization of medicinal plants. RRL, Jammu (J&K), India.

Handa, S.S. (1992). Drug industry for Indian system of medicine. Pharma Times 24: 24-26.

Harleka, R. (2000). Prospects of India to evolve as a major resource for the world's supply of essential oils and aroma chemicals. Journal of Medicinal and Aromatic Plant Sciences 22, 233-235.

Harvilicz, H. (2000). New Activity for botanicals in personal care. Chemical Market Reporter. 257(4), 1-16.

Hegnauer, R. (1986). Phytochemistry and Plant taxonomy - An Essay on the chemotaxonomy of Higher Plants (Review article) Phytochemistry 25(7); 1519-1535.

Jain, S.K. (1990). Our vanishing plants. Science Reporter 27; 10-24.

Kalkar, G.D. (2003). Value addition in essential oils. CIMAP Lucknow 12-16.

Manju Sharma, (2002). Biodiversity Conservation and Socio-economic development: role and relevance of biotechnology. In: Role of plant tissue culture in biodiversity conservation and economic development. (eds S.K. Nandi, L.M.S. Palni and A. Kumar) Gyanodaya Prakashan, Nainital, India; pp 1-9.

Narayana, D.B.A. Brindavanam, N.B. Doriyal, R.M. Katiyar, K.C. (2000). Indian spices: an overview with special references to nutraceuticals. Journal of Medicinal and Aromatic Plant Sciences 22, 236-46.

Natesh, S. (2001). The Changing Scenario of herbal drugs: Role of Botanists. Phytomorphology Golden Jubilee issue. Trends in Plant Science.

Nath, S.C. Sarma, T.C. (1997). Promising Aromatic Plants of Industrial value from North east India Suppl. to Cultivation and Utilization of Medicinal plants. RRL, Jammu (J&K), India.

Nayar, M.P. Sastry A.R.K. (eds) (1987). Red Data Book of Indian Plantry, Volume 1, Botanical Survey of India, Calcutta.

Panda, H. (2003). Medicinal Plants Cultivation and their uses. Asian Pacific Business Press, N. Delhi.

Parikh, K.M. (2000). Expectation from R&D Institution regarding India's share in the world market of herbal products. Journal of Medicinal and Aromatic Plant Sciences 22, 231-32.

Principle, P.P. (1989). The Economic Significance of plants and their constituents as Drugs. Economic and Medicinal Plant Research, 3.

Principle, P. (1989). The economic value of biological Diversity Among Medicinal Plants. ECD Environment monograph, organization for economic cooperation and development, Paris.

Principle, P.P. (1991). Valuing the biodiversity of medicinal plants In: Conservation of Medicinal plants (Ed. Akerale O. Heywood V and Synge II.) Cambridge University Press, Cambridge, New York. pp 79-124.

Raskin llya (2002). Plants and human health in the twenty-first century (Review). Trends in Biotechnology 20 (12): 522-532.

Rishi A.K., Bhan M.K. Dhar, P.L. (1996). Dioscorea deltoidea Hook. Distribution and Agrotechnology. Suppl. to Cultivation and Utilization of Medicinal Plants. R.R.L. Jammu (J&K) India.

Robbres, E. Speedle, K. Tyler, E. (1996) Pharmacognosy and Pharmacobio-technology. Williams & Wilkins, USA.

Role of medicinal plants on national economy obtained from http://www.google.com. woc:tejas.Sarc.iisc. ernet.in/currsci.

Ross, A. Medicinal Plants of the World. Vol. 2, Humana Press, Totowa, New Jersey.

Satyavati, G.V. (1990). Use of plant drugs in Indian traditional system of medicine and their relevance to primary health care. In: Economic and Medicinal Plant Research (Ed. Wagner H and Fransworth NR) Academic Press, London, Volume 4.

Scheuer, P.J. (1978). Marine Natural Products. Academic Press, London.

Schultes, R.E. (1972). The future of plants as source of new biodynamic compounds. In: Plants in the Development of Modern Medicine (ed. T. Swain) Harvard Univ. Press, Cambridge, M.A.

Singh, J. Singh, A K. Pravesh, R. (2003). Production and trade potential of some important medicinal plants: An overview, CIMAP, Lucknow (India) 50-58.

Srinivasan, P. (1995) National health policy for traditional medicine in India. World Health Forum 16.

Staba, E.J. (1980). Plant Tissue Culture as a source of Biomedicinals. CRC Press, Florida.

Street, H.E. Tissue Culture and Plant Science (2nd edn.). Academic Press, London.

Sukh Dev, (1999). Ancient modern Concordance in Ayurvedic Plants. Some example Environmental Health Perspective 107(10): 783-789.

Swain, T (1963). Chemical Plant Taxonomy. Academic Press, London.

Swain, T (ed) (1966). Comparative phytochemistry, Academic Press, London.

The Ayurvedic Formerly of India (1978). Ministry of Health and Family Welfare, Government of India, New Delhi.

The Wealth of India (1987-94), Raw Materials (All Volumes) CSIR, New Delhi.

Trease and Evans. Pharmacognosy. (2002) (edn 15th) W.B. Saunders. London.

Tyler, E. Brady, R. Robbers, E. (1981). Pharmacognosy (8th Ed) K.M. Varghese. Bombay.

Vashisht Karan and Kumar Vishvajit (2003) Medicinal Plants and their utilization. ICS-UNIDO.

Vahsisht Karan and Kumar Vishavjit (2002). Trade and Production of Herbal Medicines and Natural Health Products ICS-UNIDO.

Wagner, H. Horhammer, (1970). Pharmacognosy and Phytochemistry. Springer-Verlag, New York.

Wallis, T.E. Textbook of Pharmacognosy (Fifth Edition) C.B.S. Publishers, New Delhi.

Whistler, R.L. Industrial Gums, Polysaccharides and their Derivatives. Academic Press, N.Y.

Wilkinson, A. (1993). The potential of Herbal Products for Nutraceutical and Pharmaceuticals Development. Presented at the international Business Communications (IBC) Fifth Annual Conference, "Function foods 1998" London available at http://www.google.com.nic.

WWF. International, Panda House, Weyside Park, Godalming, U.K.

Index